2011
YEAR BOOK OF
NEONATAL AND
PERINATAL MEDICINE®

The 2011 Year Book Series

Year Book of Anesthesiology and Pain Management™: Drs Chestnut, Abram, Black, Gravlee, Lien, Mathru, and Roizen

Year Book of Cardiology®: Drs Gersh, Cheitlin, Elliott, Gold, Graham, and Thourani

Year Book of Critical Care Medicine®: Drs Dellinger, Parrillo, Balk, Dorman, Dries, and Zanotti-Cavazzoni

Year Book of Dermatology and Dermatologic Surgery™: Dr Del Rosso

Year Book of Diagnostic Radiology®: Drs Osborn, Abbara, Elster, Manaster, Oestreich, Offiah, Rosado de Christenson, Stephens, and Walker

Year Book of Emergency Medicine®: Drs Hamilton, Bruno, Handly, Mullin, Quintana, and Ramoska

Year Book of Endocrinology®: Drs Schott, Apovian, Clarke, Eugster, Ludlam, Meikle, Schinner, Schteingart, and Toth

Year Book of Gastroenterology™: Drs Talley, DeVault, Harnois, Murray, Pearson, Philcox, Picco, and Smith

Year Book of Hand and Upper Limb Surgery®: Drs Yao and Steinmann

Year Book of Medicine®: Drs Barker, Garrick, Gersh, Khardori, LeRoith, Panush, Talley, and Thigpen

Year Book of Neonatal and Perinatal Medicine®: Drs Fanaroff, Benitz, Donn, Neu, Papile, Polin, and Van Marter

Year Book of Neurology and Neurosurgery®: Drs Klimo and Rabinstein

Year Book of Obstetrics, Gynecology, and Women's Health®: Drs Dungan and Shulman

Year Book of Oncology®: Drs Arceci, Bauer, Chiorean, Gordon, Lawton, Murphy, Thigpen, and Tsao

Year Book of Ophthalmology®: Drs Rapuano, Cohen, Flanders, Fudemberg, Hammersmith, Milman, Myers, Nagra, Nelson, Penne, Pyfer, Sergott, Shields, Talekar, and Vander

Year Book of Orthopedics®: Drs Morrey, Beauchamp, Huddleston, Swiontkowski, and Trigg

Year Book of Otolaryngology-Head and Neck Surgery®: Drs Sindwani, Balough, Franco, Gapany, and Mitchell

Year Book of Pathology and Laboratory Medicine®: Drs Raab, Parwani, Bejarano, and Bissell

Year Book of Pediatrics®: Dr Stockman

Year Book of Plastic and Aesthetic Surgery™: Drs Miller, Gosain, Gurtner, Gutowski, Ruberg, Salisbury, and Smith

Year Book of Psychiatry and Applied Mental Health®: Drs Talbott, Ballenger, Buckley, Frances, Krupnick, and Mack

Year Book of Pulmonary Disease®: Drs Barker, Jones, Maurer, Raza, Tanoue, and Willsie

Year Book of Sports Medicine®: Drs Shephard, Cantu, Feldman, Jankowski, Khan, Lebrun, Nieman, Pierrynowski, and Rowland

Year Book of Surgery®: Drs Copeland, Behrns, Daly, Eberlein, Fahey, Huber, Klodell, Mozingo, and Pruett

Year Book of Urology®: Drs Andriole and Coplen

Year Book of Vascular Surgery®: Drs Moneta, Gillespie, Starnes, and Watkins

2011

The Year Book of NEONATAL AND PERINATAL MEDICINE®

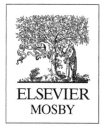

ELSEVIER
MOSBY

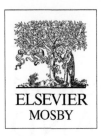

ELSEVIER
MOSBY

Vice President, Continuity: Kimberly Murphy
Editor: Kerry Holland
Production Supervisor, Electronic Year Books: Donna M. Skelton
Electronic Article Manager: Emily Ogle
Illustrations and Permissions Coordinator: Dawn Vohsen

2011 EDITION
Copyright 2011, Mosby, Inc. All rights reserved.

Composition by TNQ Books and Journals Pvt Ltd, India

Editorial Office:
Elsevier
Suite 1800
1600 John F. Kennedy Blvd.
Philadelphia, PA 19106-3399

International Standard Serial Number: 8756-5005
International Standard Book Number: 978-0-323-08417-8

Printed and bound by CPI Group (UK) Ltd, Croydon, CR0 4YY

Transferred to Digital Print 2011

Editorial Board

Contributing Editors

Francis Akita, MB, ChB
Assistant Professor of Clinical Pediatrics, Columbia University Medical Center; Division of Neonatology, Morgan Stanley Children's Hospital, New York, New York

Jill E. Baley, MD
Professor of Pediatrics, Case Western Reserve University School of Medicine; Medical Director, Neonatal Transitional Unit, Rainbow Babies & Children's Hospital, Cleveland, Ohio

John Donald E. Barks, MD
Professor of Pediatrics, Director, Neonatal-Perinatal Medicine, C.S. Mott Children's Hospital, University of Michigan Health System, Ann Arbor, Michigan

David A. Bateman, MD
Associate Professor of Clinical Pediatrics, Columbia University College of Physicians and Surgeons, Columbia University Medical Center, New York, New York

Michael S. Caplan, MD
Clinical Professor of Pediatrics, University of Chicago, Pritzker School of Medicine; Chairman, Department of Pediatrics, NorthShore University HealthSystem, Chicago, Illinois

Rachel L. Chapman, MD
Clinical Associate Professor of Pediatrics, University of Michigan School of Medicine, C.S. Mott Children's Hospital, Ann Arbor, Michigan

Jonathan M. Fanaroff, MD, JD
Associate Professor of Pediatrics, Case Western Reserve University School of Medicine; Director, Rainbow Center for Pediatric Ethics; Co-Director, Neonatal Intensive Care Unit, Rainbow Babies & Children's Hospital, Cleveland, Ohio

Jonathan Hellman, MBBCh, FRCPC, MHSc
Professor of Paediatrics, University of Toronto; Clinical Director, Neonatal Intensive Care Unit, The Hospital for Sick Children, Toronto, Canada

Marc Hershenson, MD
Huetwell Professor of Pediatrics and Communicable Diseases, Professor of Molecular and Integrative Physiology, University of Michigan School of Medicine, Ann Arbor, Michigan

Elia M. Pestana Knight, MD
Assistant Professor of Pediatrics and Neurology, Case Western Reserve University School of Medicine, Rainbow Epilepsy Center, Rainbow Babies & Children's Hospital, Cleveland, Ohio

Naomi Laventhal, MD
Department of Pediatrics and Communicable Diseases, Division of Neonatal-Perinatal Medicine, University of Michigan, Ann Arbor, Michigan

Jane S. Lee, MD, MPH

Assistant Clinical Professor of Pediatrics, Columbia University College of Physicians & Surgeons; Neonatologist; Director, Neonatal Follow-Up Program, New York Presbyterian Morgan Stanley Children's Hospital, Columbia University Medical Center, New York, New York

M. Jeffrey Maisels, MD, DSc

Professor and Chair, Department of Pediatrics, Oakland University William Beaumont School of Medicine, Beaumont Children's Hospital, Royal Oak, Michigan

Richard J. Martin, MD

Professor, Pediatrics, Reproductive Biology, Physiology and Biophysics, Case Western Reserve University School of Medicine; Drusinsky/Fanaroff Professor, Interim Chief, Pediatric Cardiology, Rainbow Babies & Children's Hospital, Cleveland, Ohio

Anand K. Rajani, MD

Attending Neonatologist, Assistant Clinical Professor of Pediatrics, UCSF Fresno Medical Education Program, Fresno, California

Rakesh Sahni, MBBS

Professor of Clinical Pediatrics, Columbia University College of Physicians & Surgeons, New York, New York

Istvan Seri, MD, PhD

Professor of Pediatrics, Keck School of Medicine of the University of Southern California; Director, Center for Fetal and Neonatal Medicine; Head, USC Division of Neonatal Medicine, Children's Hospital Los Angeles and LAC-USC Medical Center, Los Angeles, California

Renee A. Shellhaas, MD, MS

Clinical Assistant Professor, Department of Pediatrics and Communicable Diseases, Division of Pediatric Neurology, Department of Pediatrics, University of Michigan, Ann Arbor, Michigan

Eileen K. Stork, MD

Professor of Pediatrics, Case Western Reserve University School of Medicine; Director, Neonatal ECMO Program; Director, Neonatal Consult Services, Rainbow Babies & Children's Hospital, Cleveland, Ohio

Helen M. Towers, LRCP & SI, MBBCh

Division of Neonatology, Columbia University Medical Center; Associate Medical Director, Morgan Stanley Children's Hospital, New York, New York

Table of Contents

Journals Represented

Journals represented in this YEAR BOOK are listed below.

Acta Obstetricia et Gynecologica Scandinavica
Acta Paediatrica
Advances in Neonatal Care
Air Medical Journal
American Journal of Clinical Nutrition
American Journal of Epidemiology
American Journal of Obstetrics and Gynecology
American Journal of Perinatology
Annals of Neurology
Annals of Surgery
Archives of Dermatology
Archives of Disease in Childhood
Archives of Disease in Childhood & Fetal Neonatal Edition
Archives of Pediatrics & Adolescent Medicine
Australia & New Zealand Journal of Obstetrics & Gynaecology
British Medical Journal
Circulation
Clinical Pediatrics
European Respiratory Journal
Infant Behavior & Development
International Journal of Cardiology
International Journal of Developmental Neuroscience
International Journal of Gynaecology & Obstetrics
Journal of Child Neurology
Journal of Clinical Microbiology
Journal of Clinical Neurophysiology
Journal of Medical Ethics
Journal of Pediatric Gastroenterology and Nutrition
Journal of Pediatric Surgery
Journal of Pediatrics
Journal of Perinatology
Journal of the American Medical Association
Lancet
Nature Reviews Microbiology
New England Journal of Medicine
Obstetrics & Gynecology
Pain
Pediatric Critical Care Medicine
Pediatric Neurology
Pediatric Research
Pediatrics
Placenta
Proceedings of the National Academy of Sciences of the United States of America
Psychologie Medicale
Public Library of Science One
Respiratory Medicine

Schizophrenia Bulletin
Transfusion
Ultrasound in Obstetrics & Gynecology

STANDARD ABBREVIATIONS

The following terms are abbreviated in this edition: acquired immunodeficiency syndrome (AIDS), cardiopulmonary resuscitation (CPR), central nervous system (CNS), cerebrospinal fluid (CSF), computed tomography (CT), deoxyribonucleic acid (DNA), electrocardiography (ECG), health maintenance organization (HMO), human immunodeficiency virus (HIV), intensive care unit (ICU), intramuscular (IM), intravenous (IV), magnetic resonance (MR) imaging (MRI), ribonucleic acid (RNA), and ultrasound (US).

NOTE

The YEAR BOOK OF NEONATAL AND PERINATAL MEDICINE® is a literature survey service providing abstracts of articles published in the professional literature. Every effort is made to assure the accuracy of the information presented in these pages. Neither the editors nor the publisher of the YEAR BOOK OF NEONATAL AND PERINATAL MEDICINE® can be responsible for errors in the original materials. The editors' comments are their own opinions. Mention of specific products within this publication does not constitute endorsement.

To facilitate the use of the YEAR BOOK OF NEONATAL AND PERINATAL MEDICINE® as a reference tool, all illustrations and tables included in this publication are now identified as they appear in the original article. This change is meant to help the reader recognize that any illustration or table appearing in the YEAR BOOK OF NEONATAL AND PERINATAL MEDICINE® may be only one of many in the original article. For this reason, figure and table numbers will often appear to be out of sequence within the YEAR BOOK OF NEONATAL AND PERINATAL MEDICINE®.

Introduction

It is with a great sense of pride that we present the 2011 YEAR BOOK OF NEONATAL AND PERINATAL MEDICINE and celebrate the 25th such publication. Despite advances in technology and an expanded editorial board, it has not become any easier to put together this YEAR BOOK. This relates in part to the proliferation of medical journals but also the paucity of definitive trials. It has become commonplace to conclude most investigations with "large multicenter trials are necessary to answer this important question." Too often the conclusion from the Cochrane reviews or other meta-analyses are "There is insufficient evidence to establish the safety or effectiveness of the treatment," and "the quality of the trials was such that with the inclusion of randomized and quasi-randomized trials meta-analysis and subgroup analysis were not possible." We plead with investigators to do their homework and plan the trials and interventions so that they are sufficiently powered to meaningfully answer the question. We recognize that large trials are costly and take a long time, but the outcomes become relevant and hopefully generalizable.

The past year has again provided much provocative reading. Here are a few highlights from this issue: The Eunice Kennedy Shriver NICHD Neonatal Research Network SUPPORT trial concluded that setting lower oxygen saturations in very low birth weight infants reduced the incidence of retinopathy of prematurity, but at an unacceptable price: an increase in mortality. The Management of Myelomeningocele Study demonstrated the benefits to the fetus of in utero correction of a neural tube defects, but with significantly increased maternal morbidity and preterm delivery. The balance between risk and benefits emerges in all the trials. Hypothermia has an established role in the treatment of moderate and severe hypoxic ischemic encephalopathy, but there are still too many babies who die or have severe neurohandicap, so additional therapies are needed. The report on inter-alpha protein inhibitor as a marker of sepsis and necrotizing enterocolitis is intriguing because it also has the possibility to be a therapy. We included the summary of the consensus conference on inhaled nitric oxide as a lead article. The conclusion "Taken as a whole, the available evidence does not support use of inhaled nitric oxide (iNO) in early routine, early rescue, or later rescue regimens in the care of infants less than 34 weeks gestation who require respiratory support" is not in the least bit ambiguous and obviously very disappointing.

The YEAR BOOK provides insight into the major events in the field of Neonatal Medicine over the past year. As editors we hope that it is stimulating and interesting and not simply a reservoir of information. In contrast to text books, the gestation is shorter and the information timely and up to date. The editors are extremely grateful to our colleagues who willingly share their expertise. We welcome Linda Van Marter and Richard Polin to the editorial staff and thank John Hellman for his ongoing thoughtful contributions. We welcome Kerry Holland as our new editor and thank her and the Elsevier YEAR BOOK team for their continued assistance, professionalism, and support.

Avroy A. Fanaroff, MD, FRCPE, FRCP&CH

William E. Benitz, MD

Steven M. Donn, MD

Josef Neu, MD

Lu-Ann Papile, MD

Richard A. Polin, MD

Linda J. Van Marter, MD, MPH

National Institutes of Health Consensus Development Conference Statement

NIH Consensus Development Conference: Inhaled Nitric Oxide Therapy for Premature Infants October 27–29, 2010

National Institutes of Health (NIH) consensus and state-of-the-science statements are prepared by independent panels of health professionals and public representatives on the basis of (1) the results of a systematic literature review prepared under contract with the Agency for Healthcare Research and Quality (AHRQ), (2) presentations by investigators working in areas relevant to the conference questions during a 2-day public session, (3) questions and statements from conference attendees during open discussion periods that are part of the public session, and (4) closed deliberations by the panel during the remainder of the second day and morning of the third. This statement is an independent report of the panel and is not a policy statement of the NIH or the Federal Government.

The statement reflects the panel's assessment of medical knowledge available at the time the statement was written. Thus, it provides a "snapshot in time" of the state of knowledge on the conference topic. When reading the statement, keep in mind that new knowledge is inevitably accumulating through medical research.

Abstract

Objective

To provide healthcare providers, patients, and the general public with a responsible assessment of currently available data on the use of inhaled nitric oxide in early routine, early rescue, or later rescue regimens in the care of premature infants <34 weeks gestation who require respiratory support.

Participants

A non-Department of Health and Human Services, nonadvocate 16-member panel representing the fields of neonatology, pediatric pulmonology, pediatric neurology, perinatal epidemiology, ethics, neurodevelopmental follow-up, nursing, and family-centered care. In addition, 18 experts from pertinent fields presented data to the panel and conference audience.

Evidence

Presentations by experts and a systematic review of the literature prepared by the Johns Hopkins University Evidence-based Practice Center, through the Agency for Healthcare Research and Quality (ARHQ). Scientific evidence was given precedence over anecdotal experience.

Conference Process

The panel drafted its statement based on scientific evidence presented in open forum and on published scientific literature. The draft statement was presented on the final day of the conference and circulated to the audience for comment. The panel released a revised statement later that day at http://consensus.nih.gov. This statement is an independent report of the panel and is not a policy statement of the National Institutes of Health (NIH) or the Federal Government.

Conclusions

(1) Taken as a whole, the available evidence does not support use of inhaled nitric oxide in early routine, early rescue, or later rescue regimens in the care of premature infants <34 weeks gestation who require respiratory support. (2) There are rare clinical situations, including pulmonary hypertension or hypoplasia, that have been inadequately studied in which inhaled nitric oxide may have benefit in infants <34 weeks gestation. In such situations, clinicians should communicate with families regarding the current evidence on its risks and benefits as well as remaining uncertainties. (3) Basic research and animal studies have contributed to important understandings of inhaled nitric oxide benefits on lung development and function in infants at high risk of bronchopulmonary dysplasia. These promising results have only partly been realized in clinical trials of inhaled nitric oxide treatment in premature infants. Future research should seek to understand this gap. (4) Predefined subgroup and post hoc analyses of previous trials showing potential benefit of inhaled nitric oxide have generated hypotheses for future research for clinical trials. Prior strategies shown to be ineffective are discouraged unless new evidence emerges. The positive results of one multicenter trial, which was characterized by later timing, higher dose, and longer duration of treatment, require confirmation. Future trials should attempt to quantify the individual effects of each of these treatment-related variables (timing, dose, and duration), ideally by randomizing them separately. (5) Based on assessment of currently available data, hospitals, clinicians, and the pharmaceutical industry should avoid marketing inhaled nitric oxide for premature infants <34 weeks gestation.

Introduction

Premature birth is a major public health problem in the United States and internationally. Despite clinical, educational, and scientific efforts, the frequency of preterm birth has risen in the United States from 10.6 percent in 1990 to 12.7 percent in 2007. Worldwide, approximately 13 million infants are born prematurely every year. Infants born at or before 32 weeks gestation (2 percent of all births in the United States in 2007) are at extremely high risk for death in the neonatal period or for pulmonary, visual, and neurodevelopmental morbidities with lifelong consequences, including bronchopulmonary dysplasia (BPD, a form of chronic lung disease seen in premature infants), retinopathy of prematurity (ROP, the leading cause of blindness in children in the developed world), and brain injury.

Reduced lung function associated with prematurity may persist throughout childhood and adolescence. Neurodevelopmental problems—including cerebral palsy, blindness, hearing loss, and learning disabilities—create life-long challenges for many of these children and their families. Risks for adverse outcomes increase with decreasing gestational age. The economic costs to care for these infants are also substantial (estimated at $26 billion in 2005 in the United States). In addition, the emotional and indirect economic costs for families are substantial. Unfortunately, however, the multifactorial biological, behavioral, and environmental causes and the heterogeneity of preterm birth make it extremely unlikely that all premature births can be prevented.

Over the past 20 years, continuing advances in high-risk obstetrical management and neonatal intensive care have resulted in increased survival of extremely premature infants. For example, based on recent Cochrane reviews, administration of antenatal steroids to women with impending premature birth reduces the risk of in-hospital neonatal death by 23 percent, neonatal respiratory distress syndrome by 34 percent, and cerebroventricular hemorrhage by 46 percent. Exogenous surfactant administered to premature infants to either treat or prevent respiratory distress syndrome improves respiratory function and reduces risk of in-hospital death by 32 to 40 percent. After demonstration of efficacy and safety in multiple randomized controlled trials (RCTs), both of these interventions have been adopted into clinical practice.

Many clinical practices integrated into the care of these infants have been inadequately studied for safety and efficacy, with potentially serious consequences; yet, the smallest and sickest infants are the most vulnerable to adverse effects of the treatments they receive. The broad boundaries of accepted clinical practices in neonatal intensive care units lead to practice variations among centers. Large variations among centers in outcomes of premature infants, including BPD and adverse neurodevelopmental outcomes, persist after adjusting for risk factors such as gestational age, sex, and disease severity. The extent to which these differences in outcomes are due to differences in care practices or in patient characteristics is poorly understood. Clearly, the need for strategies to improve outcomes for this high-risk population is great, and this need has prompted testing of new therapies with the potential to decrease pulmonary and other complications of prematurity. Inhaled nitric oxide (iNO) emerged as one such therapy.

Nitric oxide is a gas that is ubiquitously produced in the human body. It serves as a signaling molecule with numerous regulatory effects on multiple human organ systems, including blood vessels, the lung, the heart, the nervous system, the immune system, and stem cells, and on the development of cancer. First discovered as a factor that relaxes resistance in blood vessels in 1980, nitric oxide was recognized by *Science* as the "Molecule of the Year" in 1992. The scientists who discovered its important role in diverse disease processes, including atherosclerosis, diabetes, impotence, and hypertension, were recognized with the Nobel Prize for Medicine or Physiology in 1998. More than 85,000 independent scientific articles about nitric oxide have been published since 1980. Over the past decade, the efficacy of nitric oxide in reducing blood vessel resistance and its easy administration via endotracheal tube to infants with respiratory distress led to trials in term and near-term newborns suffering from persistent pulmonary hypertension, a condition that results from failure of normal fetal lung blood vessel relaxation immediately following birth. Prior to iNO trials, many infants severely affected with pulmonary hypertension were treated using extracorporeal membrane oxygenation (ECMO), an invasive heart-lung bypass system, as a short-term strategy (up to 14 days) to improve survival by "buying time" for lung blood vessel resistance to decrease spontaneously. ECMO therapy is expensive, not widely available, and associated with considerable morbidity (e.g., bleeding). Large, placebo-controlled trials showed that nitric oxide decreases death or the need for ECMO in term and near-term infants with persistent pulmonary hypertension and led the Food and Drug Administration (FDA) to approve iNO as a therapy for that disease.

Findings from a substantial body of experimental work in developing animals and other model systems suggest that nitric oxide may enhance lung growth and reduce lung inflammation independently of its effects on blood vessel resistance. Although this work demonstrates biologic plausibility and the results of RCTs in term and near-term infants were positive, combined evidence from the 14 RCTs of iNO treatment in premature infants ≤34 weeks gestation have shown equivocal effects on pulmonary outcomes, survival, and neurodevelopmental outcomes. Despite these equivocal results, the off-label use of iNO has increased substantially. Controversy about its use in premature infants has been fueled by the refusal of some third-party payers to cover the substantial costs for iNO administration (up to $3,000 a day).

To provide healthcare professionals, families, and the general public with a responsible assessment of currently available data regarding the benefits and risks of iNO in premature infants, the *Eunice Kennedy Shriver* National Institute of Child Health and Human Development, the National Heart, Lung, and Blood Institute, and the Office of Medical Applications of Research of the National Institutes of Health convened a Consensus Development Panel that included experts in the fields of neonatology, pediatric pulmonology, pediatric neurology, perinatal epidemiology, ethics, neurodevelopmental follow-up, nursing, and family-centered care to review available data, to hear scientific summaries from investigators involved in this field, and to solicit input from the general public. A Planning Committee developed six questions to be addressed by the Consensus Development Panel.

As part of a comprehensive data review, an independent group, the Johns Hopkins University Evidence-based Practice Center (JHU EPC), generated a systematic review of all available human studies concerning use of iNO in premature infants. This review (available at http://www.ahrq.gov/clinic/tp/inoinftp.htm), along with an as yet unpublished, updated Cochrane review and an unpublished individual patient data meta-analysis (the Meta-Analysis of Preterm Patients on Inhaled Nitric Oxide [MAPPiNO]

IPD meta-analysis), provided the Panel with summaries of the available evidence from these trials. One of the published trials, and therefore the JHU EPC systematic review, included infants of 34 weeks gestation. The Panel's review of the published evidence is therefore based on infants ≤34 weeks gestation. Its recommendations for clinical use of iNO, however, are limited to infants <34 weeks to avoid contradiction and confusion with the FDA's labeled indications for iNO use.

Combining results of studies is complicated by differences in dose, timing, and duration of iNO administration, inclusion criteria (e.g., gestational age, chronologic age, severity of lung disease) of infants studied, and diversity of neurodevelopmental and pulmonary outcome measures. Where applicable, the Panel chose to follow the Cochrane review approach of subdividing the 14 trials into 3 clinically relevant groups based on characteristics of the participating infants and specific treatment strategies: early routine (initiation at <3 days, routine use in intubated infants), early rescue (initiation at <3 days based on oxygenation status), and later rescue (initiation at >3 days based on BPD risk).

Many of the trials and meta-analyses examined results in clinical or demographic subgroups. When treatment effects differ across subgroups, however, as they did in some of the iNO studies, it is unwise to make firm inferences about subgroup differences when those differences are observed post hoc. Post hoc analysis of treatment effects in specific subgroups (e.g., dose of iNO, gestational age, early versus late initiation of treatment), whether within or across trials, is prone to false-positive results. The Consensus Development Panel therefore considered the subgroup results of these analyses as hypothesis-generating, rather than hypothesis-testing, and used them as a basis for recommending future research directions.

The six questions considered by the Consensus Development Panel are listed below and addressed in the following sections.

1. Does inhaled nitric oxide therapy increase survival and/or reduce the occurrence or severity of bronchopulmonary dysplasia among premature infants who receive respiratory support?
2. Are there short-term risks of inhaled nitric oxide therapy among premature infants who receive respiratory support?
3. Are there effects of inhaled nitric oxide therapy on long-term pulmonary and/or neurodevelopmental outcomes among premature infants who receive respiratory support?
4. Does the effect of inhaled nitric oxide therapy on bronchopulmonary dysplasia and/or death or neurodevelopmental impairment vary across subpopulations of premature infants?
5. Does the effect of inhaled nitric oxide therapy on bronchopulmonary dysplasia and/or death or neurodevelopmental impairment vary by timing of initiation, mode of delivery, dose and duration, or concurrent therapies?
6. What are the future research directions needed to better understand the risks, benefits, and alternatives to nitric oxide therapy for premature infants who receive respiratory support?

Terminology surrounding disease processes in premature infants has been used in inconsistent ways. For clarity throughout this document, the Panel has chosen to define the following terms:

- *Premature infant:* The International Classification of Diseases (ICD) has eliminated the term "prematurity," because its prior definition was based on birth weight. This term is commonly used and understood as a synonym for preterm birth, defined by ICD as a gestational age at birth <37 completed weeks. Because the questions posed to the Panel used *premature infant*, this term is used throughout this consensus statement as a synonym for preterm infant. In this document, "near term" is used as it reflects the specific language in the FDA-approved label for inhaled nitric oxide. The Panel recognizes that "late preterm" is currently used to describe infants at 34 and up to 36 weeks and 6 days gestation.
- *Bronchopulmonary dysplasia (BPD):* First described in 1967, BPD is a heterogeneous lung disease observed in premature infants and diagnosed within the first months of life. The clinical picture and definition of BPD have evolved substantially since its first description, complicating comparisons of studies that use BPD as an outcome. In analyzing the studies of iNO discussed in this report, the Panel decided to follow the definitions of BPD used by there searchers who designed the different clinical trials.
- *Cerebroventricular hemorrhage (CVH):* This term is used as an inclusive term to refer to the spectrum of hemorrhagic brain injury most typically occurring in the first week of life in very premature infants. The location of hemorrhage may be periventricular, intraventricular, or intraparenchymal. Most studies report both the presence of any brain hemorrhage and severe hemorrhage. Severe hemorrhage most often refers to a large intraventricular hemorrhage or hemorrhage into white matter that surrounds the ventricles.
- *White matter injury (WMI):* WMI is a spectrum of brain pathology that includes (1) the classic lesion of periventricular leukomalacia (PVL), which comprises focal cystic damage to white matter tracts (made of nerve axons that connect different brain regions covered by the insulating substance, myelin), and (2) diffuse, noncystic lesions that result in disturbances in myelination.

1. Does inhaled nitric oxide therapy increase survival and/or reduce the occurrence or severity of bronchopulmonary dysplasia among premature infants who receive respiratory support?

A body of evidence is strongest when results are consistent across trials despite heterogeneity in study design and populations. Therefore, the Panel chose to address this question by including all of the trials that enrolled premature infants ≤34 weeks gestation irrespective of the timing, dosing regimen, duration of inhaled nitric oxide (iNO) therapy, or subcategorization of the subjects.

None of the individual trials included in the systematic reviews showed a statistically significant effect of iNO on survival in this population. Meta-analysis by the Johns Hopkins University Evidence-based Practice Center (JHU EPC) of 11 randomized controlled trials (RCTs) revealed that treatment with iNO did not increase survival. The individual patient data (IPD) approach used in the MAPPiNO study of pooled data from 11 RCTs demonstrated no statistically significant effect of iNO on death at any time, death by 36 weeks postmenstrual age (PMA), or death before discharge. Given that the mortality of premature infants is highest during the first week after birth, age at the time of study enrollment is likely to be a particularly important factor in analyzing the effect of iNO on survival. However, inclusion or exclusion of the one trial with enrollment exclusively after 1 week did not affect the results of the meta-analysis. Thus overall, in premature infants ≤34 weeks gestation requiring respiratory support, current evidence shows that treatment with iNO in the neonatal period does not increase survival.

Bronchopulmonary dysplasia (BPD) is defined in the Introduction. The evolution of BPD over decades has been reflected in numerous and various definitions, usually based on the persistence of respiratory symptoms, pulmonary radiographic appearance, and the persistent need for treatments at a specified age (e.g., requiring supplemental oxygen at 28 days of age, requiring supplemental oxygen at 36 weeks PMA).

Interpretation of results from RCTs was complicated by different studies calculating BPD rates using survivors versus the total group as the denominator, and by the competing risks of death and BPD. In other words, an infant who dies in the first weeks of life is not at risk for developing BPD, which is usually based on criteria at 28 days. Since most of the trials and the JHU EPC systematic review included analyses of BPD alone, however, the Panel also examined that evidence. None of the individual trials included in the systematic reviews showed statistically significant differences in BPD at 36 weeks PMA in those who received iNO compared with controls. The JHU EPC meta-analysis (8 RCTs) of BPD among surviving infants at 36 weeks PMA found no statistically significant differences in rates of BPD between iNO and control groups. The approach utilized in the MAPPiNO IPD meta-analysis did not report on BPD as a sole outcome variable. Thus, among premature infants who required respiratory support and were surviving at 36 weeks PMA, current evidence does not support the hypothesis that treatment with iNO in the neonatal period reduces the occurrence of BPD.

The composite outcome of "death or BPD at 36 weeks PMA" was reported, although not always as a primary outcome, in 11 iNO RCTs. Two individual trials found statistically significant reductions in the composite outcome of death or BPD in the iNO treated group. The JHU EPC meta-analysis of 11 RCTs showed a small, statistically significant reduction in the composite variable death or BPD at 36 weeks PMA. Exclusion of the one trial with enrollment after 1 week of age did not change the results of the meta-analysis. The MAPPiNO IPD meta-analysis of pooled data from 10 trials showed a similarly small effect size for BPD or death as the JHU EPC analysis, but did not achieve statistical significance. The small effect on this composite outcome should be interpreted cautiously.

The JHU EPC systematic review of the effect of iNO on the severity of BPD in the RCTs was compromised by the wide variation in BPD definitions and other study parameters. The JHU analysis concluded that insufficient data are available to perform a meta-analysis for any measure of severity due to the lack of uniformity in definitions and study measures used. There is insufficient evidence to support the hypothesis that treatment with iNO in the neonatal period reduces the severity of BPD. Two individual trials reported a statistically significant favorable effect of iNO on pulmonary outcomes reflecting severity of BPD; rates of hospitalization and respiratory support at 40 and 44 weeks PMA; and a statistically significant reduction in the average duration of supplemental oxygen. Although these trials raise intriguing questions, the effects of iNO on the severity of BPD have not been adequately studied in subpopulations, a subject addressed in the Panel's response to Question 4.

The available evidence therefore is insufficient to recommend the routine use of iNO in clinical care of premature infants <34 weeks gestation requiring respiratory support.

2. Are there short-term risks of inhaled nitric oxide therapy among premature infants who receive respiratory support?

Premature infants are at risk for short-term complications, including patent ductus arteriosus (PDA), late-onset (>7 days) sepsis, necrotizing enterocolitis (NEC), retinopathy of prematurity (ROP), pulmonary complications (e.g., air leak, pulmonary hemorrhage), and brain injury (e.g., intraventricular hemorrhage [IVH], intraparenchymal hemorrhage [IPH], and periventricular leukomalacia [PVL]). Although these are morbidities seen in premature infants which might be exacerbated by iNO, there may be other important indicators to evaluate shortterm risks. However, iNO may lead to accumulation of methemoglobin, formed by the reaction of nitric oxide with hemoglobin.

The JHU EPC analyses showed no evidence for an increased risk of PDA, late-onset sepsis, NEC, ROP, pulmonary complications, or toxic levels of methemoglobin. The MAPPiNO IPD meta-analysis also showed no statistically significant difference in the incidence of air leak, pulmonary hemorrhage, or severe ROP.

The JHU EPC systematic evidence review showed no overall difference between iNO-treated and control infants with respect to IVH, IPH, or PVL.

The updated Cochrane meta-analysis showed no statistically significant effects on brain injury, either severe IVH or the combined outcomes of severe IVH or PVL with early routine administration of iNO. Early rescue administration of iNO was associated with a nonsignficant trend toward increased severe IVH.

The MAPPiNO IPD meta-analysis showed a nonsignificant trend toward increased severe neurological events (e.g., IVH, IPH, cystic PVL) with iNO treatment.

In summary, there is no evidence that treatment with iNO either increases or decreases the risk of several short-term complications of prematurity, including PDA, late-onset sepsis, severe ROP, and pulmonary complications (e.g., air leaks, pulmonary hemorrhage). The risks for these complications are greatest for the infants born earliest (at 22 to 27 weeks gestation), and the iNO trials have not reported on these risks stratified by either birth weight or gestational age with the exception of studies described in the Panel's response to Question 4. Future research should attempt to fill this gap.

In these trials, administration of iNO at doses up to 20 ppm did not produce levels of methemoglobin that would be considered toxic in term infants or adults.

Considering all trials together, there is no convincing evidence to support the hypothesis that iNO administration increases or decreases the risk of PVL or IVH in premature infants ≤34 weeks gestation. These studies varied in design, and only three had baseline head sonograms before treatment with iNO. When head ultrasound studies were obtained, the timing of these studies and the categorization of brain injury were not uniform.

3. Are there effects of inhaled nitric oxide therapy on long-term pulmonary and/or neurodevelopmental outcomes among premature infants who receive respiratory support?

LONG-TERM PULMONARY OUTCOMES

The Johns Hopkins University Evidence-based Practice Center (JHU EPC) reported two randomized controlled trials (RCTs) examining long-term pulmonary outcomes. One large study demonstrated a statistically significant decrease in use of lung-related medications and fewer parental reports of respiratory symptoms at 12 months in children receiving inhaled nitric oxide (iNO) compared with controls; a smaller study found no statistically significant difference in reported use of lung medications or reports of symptoms at 12 months. Neither study found a statistically significant difference in rates of hospitalization for lung problems or wheezing at 12 months. The lack of a difference in hospitalization or wheezing casts doubt on the clinical importance of a difference in medication use between those who received iNO and the controls.

When the results of the two 12-month pulmonary follow-up studies were combined in a metaanalysis by the JHU EPC, the statistically significant decrease in the reported use of pulmonary medications in children who received iNO remained, because the smaller study did not have an influence on the overall results.

No studies of long-term pulmonary outcome have included available measurements of pulmonary function, gas exchange, or radiologic appearance. An important deficit of these studies was a failure to account for common confounders following discharge from the neonatal intensive care unit known to have substantial effects on the use of pulmonary medications.

The Panel concludes, as did the JHU EPC, that there is evidence in one trial of an advantage in long-term pulmonary outcome for the use of iNO, but that this evidence is not strong enough to justify the widespread use of iNO to prevent long-term pulmonary disease.

LONG-TERM NEURODEVELOPMENTAL OUTCOMES

None of the trials examining long-term neurodevelopmental outcomes in children have convincingly demonstrated a long-term neurodevelopmental effect of iNO. Individually, none of the trials found a statistically significant difference in the incidence of motor delay between those who had received iNO and controls. Few individual trials and none of the meta-analyses revealed a statistically significant association between neonatal iNO treatment and any neurodevelopmental outcome up to 5 years of age. For cerebral palsy, the two trials that did show associations conflicted in the direction of association. There is insufficient evidence to determine whether there is an effect of iNO on motor impairment or if it differs by the birth weight of the treated infants. There also were no significant differences between the iNO and control groups in the proportion of children with visual or hearing impairment.

Studies of long-term neurodevelopment in preterm infants ≤34 weeks gestation treated with iNO have been hampered by variation in measures used to assess neurodevelopmental status and the ages at which outcomes are measured, and by the lack of physiologic, radiologic, functional, or quality-of-life measures used as outcomes. Most studies of long-term effects typically have used overly broad measures of development in the absence of physiologic or anatomic examinations; many also have used the measure at too young an age. While 18 to 24 months is appropriate for detecting cerebral palsy, testing at school age is more appropriate for diagnosing intellectual disability. Newer methods of assessment, including correlated neuroimaging and standardized behavioral testing, should be included in any future assessments of the long-term neurodevelopmental consequences of iNO.

Long-term studies of pulmonary and neurodevelopmental health following premature birth are logistically challenging and expensive. Funding agencies should support the expense of longterm follow-up, and investigators should provide comprehensive plans for retention of subjects over the life of the trial.

4. Does the effect of inhaled nitric oxide therapy on bronchopulmonary dysplasia and/or death or neurodevelopmental impairment vary across subpopulations of premature infants?

In response to this question, the Panel elected to review common clinical variables that may interact with inhaled nitric oxide (iNO) treatment apart from timing or duration of treatment, which is covered in the Panel response to Question 5. Analysis of subpopulations is limited by the fact that few trials have identified subgroups, subgrouping results in small sample sizes in each subcategory, and trials are often not powered to detect subgroup differences. In addition, when trials did define subgroups, definitions varied across trials and were usually post hoc.

Based on the Johns Hopkins University Evidence-based Practice Center (JHU EPC) systematic review, there is insufficient evidence to evaluate whether factors such as sex, gestational age, ethnic group/race, and socioeconomic status were associated with increased benefit or risk from iNO therapy. There is no information regarding effects of growth restriction, antenatal steroid use, multiple gestation, chorioamnionitis, or other antenatal factors.

The JHU EPC systematic review reveals insufficient evidence of decreased incidence of death or bronchopulmonary dysplasia (BPD) particular to any subgroup of premature infants treated with iNO. Five studies (representing three independent clinical trials) reported outcomes by birth weight. Two of the three trials demonstrated a significant reduction in the composite outcome of death or BPD when iNO was administered to premature infants ≥1,000 grams, but not in those <1,000 grams.

This review raises a concern for safety of iNO in premature infants <1,000 grams. Three studies of infants of this birth weight treated within 48 hours of delivery reported an increased risk of death, severe intraventricular hemorrhage (IVH) and periventricular leukomalacia (PVL), neurodevelopmental impairment, BPD, and/or oxygen dependence at 1 year of age. However, in another large study that initiated iNO at 7 days of life, no such safety concerns were noted in this birth-weight category.

Based on the JHU EPC systematic review of published studies, there is insufficient evidence of improvement in neurodevelopmental outcomes in any subgroup of premature infants treated with iNO.

Published trials have shown insufficient evidence of benefit to premature infants with pulmonary hypoplasia or hypertension, likely due to small numbers of such patients and severity of illness. Additional studies in this population will be difficult to accomplish. Therefore, clinical use in this population should be left to clinical discretion.

Based on published data, the Panel recommends special caution in studies of early rescue use of iNO in premature infants <34 weeks gestation weighing <1,000 grams.

5. Does the effect of inhaled nitric oxide therapy on bronchopulmonary dysplasia and/or death or neurodevelopmental impairment vary by timing of initiation, mode of delivery, dose and duration, or concurrent therapies?

As previously stated in the Introduction, in the trials published to date, three distinct subgroups have been identified by a Cochrane meta-analysis, by timing of initiation, clinical phase, or severity of illness: (1) early (<3 days) routine initiation in preterm infants receiving respiratory support ("early routine"), (2) early (<3 days) initiation in ventilated infants by oxygenation criteria ("early rescue"), and (3) later (>3 days) initiation in infants at high risk of developing bronchopulmonary dysplasia (BPD), as defined by persistent need for respiratory support ("later rescue"). There is a clinical and biological rationale for this subdivision of trials. This meta-analysis within the first two subgroups reveals no significant reduction in death, BPD, or the composite outcome of death or BPD in the iNO study groups. However, the later rescue group is predominantly represented by one, large multicenter trial. In this trial, the treatment protocol, designed to test a novel hypothesis, was unique not only in the timing of initiation, but also in dosing and duration. This trial revealed an overall reduction in the composite outcome of death or BPD and a post hoc finding of greater efficacy when treatment was initiated during the second postnatal week, as compared with the third postnatal week. The method of treatment allocation and statistical analysis of multiples enrolled in the trial made it difficult to integrate this trial's findings in a conventional meta-analysis. Nevertheless, different statistical approaches to the analysis of multiples did not substantially change the estimate of the effect of iNO.

The effect of mode of ventilation (conventional versus high frequency) on efficacy and safety of iNO was evaluated in two trials, in one by prospective randomization and in the other by post hoc analysis. No studies have directly compared delivery by continuous positive airway pressure (CPAP) or nasal cannula versus endotracheal positive pressure ventilation. There is insufficient evidence to determine whether mode of ventilation impacts outcome from iNO treatment.

None of the trials published to date randomized subjects by dose or treatment duration of iNO. Despite this limitation, these trials can be subdivided into three broad dosage groups: 5 parts per million (ppm), 10 ppm, and 20 ppm. In a dose-stratified meta-analysis by the Johns Hopkins University Evidence-based Practice Center (JHU EPC), which combined all three treatment initiation subgroups, iNO therapy in the group that received a maximum dose of 10 ppm was associated with a statistically significant reduction in the risk of BPD, but not death, or the composite outcome of death or BPD. These results do not form a basis for deciding that one dosing regimen was superior, because they were based on post hoc comparisons and there was too much variability among the study designs within each dose group. A more focused examination of dosing and treatment duration within clinically meaningful subgroups is needed.

Little is known about the effect of concurrent therapies on the efficacy and safety of iNO. Only one trial directly addressed the effect of iNO with a concurrent therapy, glucocorticoids. Further research is needed to determine the effect of concurrent therapies—such as antenatal and postnatal glucocorticoids, surfactant, vitamin A, indomethacin, and caffeine—on the efficacy and safety of iNO.

There is no evidence to suggest that variations in these treatment regimen factors (e.g., dose, timing, mode of administration) are harmful in terms of BPD, death, or neurodevelopmental outcome. The design of future trials comparing treatment regimens should include a longer duration of follow-up to ensure long-term safety.

There is insufficient evidence to conclude that the efficacy of iNO therapy with respect to BPD and/or death, or neurodevelopmental impairment, varies by timing of initiation, mode of delivery, dose and duration of therapy, or concurrent therapies. A major limitation is that only one trial reporting these outcomes has randomized infants by treatment subgroups. Regimens vary considerably among the published studies, such that only broad categorizations of timing or dosing are appropriate for meta-analysis. Although the evidence suggests that some treatment regimens may provide greater benefit, further randomized controlled trials (RCTs) designed to address these specific hypotheses must be undertaken. Among the treatment regimen factors examined in RCTs, timing of initiation, dosing, and treatment duration currently show the most promise for further research.

6. What are the future research directions needed to better understand the risks, benefits, and alternatives to nitric oxide therapy for premature infants who receive respiratory support?

1. Understanding risks, benefits, and alternatives to inhaled nitric oxide (iNO) therapy for premature infants requires investigation of iNO's mechanisms of action through additional basic research in developmentally relevant experimental models. In particular, future animal and model system studies should focus on understanding the respective roles of dosing, delivery, and timing of therapy and of accompanying ventilation strategies, oxygen management, and concurrent therapies that optimize the benefits of iNO and reduce the risk of adverse short- or long-term effects. A clearer understanding of the pharmacology and toxicology of iNO in premature infants is needed to identify better markers of its toxicity and short-term risks. In addition, studies that focus on increasing tissue-specific production of endogenous nitric oxide should be considered.
2. Future trials for evaluation of safety and efficacy of iNO for premature infants should be informed by prior trials as well as by future studies in premature animals or other model systems. These trials and preclinical studies should examine both short- and long-term pulmonary and neurodevelopmental outcomes and investigate effect-modifying factors (e.g., pharmacokinetic, genetic, racial/ethnic, and disease risk factors).
3. Future randomized trials should be designed to assess variations in the timing, dose, and duration of treatment, to include a placebo control, to ensure a sample size sufficient to detect a significant interaction between gestational age category and treatment arm, and to consider an appropriate developmental window for efficacy and safety. The positive results of one multicenter trial, which was characterized by later timing, higher dose, and longer duration of treatment, require confirmation. Future trials should attempt to quantify the individual effects of each of these treatment12 related variables (timing, dose, and duration), ideally by randomizing them separately.
4. Future trials should assess the long-term effects of iNO treatment. Important safety and efficacy questions require that study subjects be followed to a minimum of school age with standardized assessments of behavior, cognitive ability, neuroanatomy, and neurophysiology.

5. Design of future efficacy and safety trials of iNO for premature infants should include interdisciplinary teams of experts in high-risk obstetrics, neonatology, pediatric pulmonology, pediatric neurology, neurodevelopmental follow-up, neonatal pharmacology, lung development, brain development, nitric oxide physiology, biostatistics, and clinical trial design, as well as ethicists, nurses, respiratory therapists, and families.
6. Given the large differences in outcomes of death and bronchopulmonary dysplasia (BPD) among neonatal intensive care units, new strategies should be considered which improve outcomes by reducing neonatal intensive care unit-specific variations in care.
7. In addition to the Panel's iNO research recommendations, future research should pursue promising strategies other than iNO.
8. Delay between treatment use and assessment of important outcomes creates a barrier to rapid progress in testing potentially effective treatments. Biomarker, neuroimaging, pulmonary function testing, pulmonary imaging, and other techniques with potentially better predictive accuracy should be developed and tested.

Conclusions

1. Taken as a whole, the available evidence does not support use of inhaled nitric oxide (iNO) in early routine, early rescue, or later rescue regimens in the care of premature infants <34 weeks gestation who require respiratory support.
2. There are rare clinical situations, including pulmonary hypertension or hypoplasia, that have been inadequately studied in which iNO may have benefit in infants <34 weeks gestation. In such situations, clinicians should communicate with families regarding the current evidence on its risks and benefits as well as remaining uncertainties.
3. Basic research and animal studies have contributed to important understandings of iNO benefits on lung development and function in infants at high risk of BPD. These promising results have only partly been realized in clinical trials of iNO treatment in premature infants. Future research should seek to understand this gap.
4. Predefined subgroup and post hoc analyses of previous trials showing potential benefit of iNO have generated hypotheses for future research for clinical trials. Prior strategies shown to be ineffective are discouraged unless new evidence emerges. The positive results of one multicenter trial, which was characterized by later timing, higher dose, and longer duration of treatment, require confirmation. Future trials should attempt to quantify the individual effects of each of these treatment-related variables (timing, dose, and duration), ideally by randomizing them separately.
5. Based on assessment of currently available data, hospitals, clinicians, and the pharmaceutical industry should avoid marketing iNO for premature infants <34 weeks gestation.

Consensus Development Panel

Panel Chairperson: F. Sessions Cole, M.D.
Panel and Conference Chairperson
Park J. White, M.D.
Professor of Pediatrics, Assistant Vice Chancellor for Children's Health, Vice Chairperson, Department of Pediatrics, Director, Division of Newborn Medicine, Washington University School of Medicine, Chief Medical Officer, St. Louis Children's Hospital, St. Louis, Missouri
Claudia Alleyne, M.D.
Medical Director, Neonatal Intensive Care Unit, Kaiser Permanente Anaheim Medical Center, Anaheim, California
John D.E. Barks, M.D.
Professor, Department of Pediatrics and Communicable Diseases, University of Michigan Medical School, Director, Division of Neonatal-Perinatal Medicine, C.S. Mott Children's Hospital, University of Michigan Health System, Ann Arbor, Michigan
Robert J. Boyle, M.D., FAAP
Professor of Pediatrics, Associate Faculty, Center for Biomedical Ethics, Department of Pediatrics, Division of Neonatology, University of Virginia Medical Center, Charlottesville, Virginia
John L. Carroll, M.D., FAAP
Professor, Department of Pediatrics, College of Medicine, University of Arkansas for Medical Sciences, Section Chief, Pediatric Pulmonary Division, Arkansas Children's Hospital, Little Rock, Arkansas
Deborah Dokken, M.P.A.
Family Health Care Advocate, Consultant in Family-Centered Care, Chevy Chase, Maryland
William H. Edwards, M.D.
Professor and Vice Chair of Pediatrics, Neonatology Section Chief, Medical Director CHaD Nurseries, Children's Hospital at Dartmouth Co-Director, Vermont Oxford Network, Lebanon, New Hampshire
Michael Georgieff, M.D.
Martin Lenz Harrison
Professor of Pediatrics and Child Psychology, Director, Division of Neonatology, Director, Center for Neurobehavioral Development, University of Minnesota School of Medicine, Twin Cities, Minneapolis, Minnesota
Katherine Gregory, Ph.D., R.N.
Assistant Professor of Nursing, William F. Connell School of Nursing, Boston College, Nurse Scientist, Brigham and Women's Hospital, Chestnut Hill, Massachusetts
Michael V. Johnston, M.D.
Chief Medical Officer and Executive, Vice President, Blum/Moser Professor for Pediatric, Neurology, Kennedy Krieger Institute, Professor

of Neurology, Pediatrics and Physical Medicine and Rehabilitation, Johns Hopkins University School of Medicine, Baltimore, Maryland

Michael Kramer, M.D.
Scientific Director, Institute of Human Development, Child and Youth Health, Canadian Institutes of Health Research

James McGill
Professor, Departments of Pediatrics and of Epidemiology, Biostatistics and Occupational Health, McGill University Faculty of Medicine, Montreal Children's Hospital, Montréal, Québec, CANADA

Christine Mitchell, M.S., M.T.S., R.N.
Associate Director, Clinical Ethics, Division of Medical Ethics, Harvard Medical School, Director, Office of Ethics, Children's Hospital Boston, Boston, Massachusetts

Josef Neu, M.D.
Professor of Pediatrics, Director, Neonatology Fellowship Training Program, Division of Neonatology, Department of Pediatrics, College of Medicine, University of Florida, Gainesville, Gainesville, Florida

DeWayne M. Pursley, M.D., M.P.H.
Chair, Section on Perinatal Pediatrics, American Academy of Pediatrics, Assistant Professor of Pediatrics, Harvard Medical School, Chief, Department of Neonatology, Beth Israel Deaconess Medical Center, Boston, Massachusetts

Walter Robinson, M.D., M.P.H.
Senior Research Scientist, Center for Applied Ethics, Education Development Center, Inc., Associate Professor of Pediatrics, Department of Pediatrics, Division of Pediatric Allergy, Immunology, and Pulmonary Medicine, Center for Biomedical Ethics and Society, Vanderbilt University School of Medicine, Nashville, Tennessee

David H. Rowitch, M.D., Ph.D.
Professor of Pediatrics and Neurological Surgery Investigator, Howard Hughes Medical Institute, Chief of Neonatology, University of California, San Francisco, San Francisco, California

Speakers

Steven H. Abman, M.D.
Professor, Department of Pediatrics, Director, Pediatric Heart Lung Center, Director, Ventilator Care Program, Co-Director, Pediatric Pulmonary Hypertension Program, University of Colorado School of Medicine, Children's Hospital, Aurora, Colorado

Marilee C. Allen, M.D.
Professor of Pediatrics, Johns Hopkins School of Medicine, Division of Neonatology, Johns Hopkins Children's Center, Neurodevelopmental Disabilities, Co-Director of Neonatal Intensive Care Unit, Development Clinic, Kennedy Krieger Institute, Baltimore, Maryland

Roberta A. Ballard, M.D.
Professor of Pediatrics, Division of Neonatology, Department of Pediatrics, University of California, San Francisco, Emeritus Professor of Pediatrics, University of Pennsylvania, San Francisco, California

Keith J. Barrington, M.D., M.B.Ch.B.
Professor of Pediatrics, University of Montreal, Chief of Neonatology, University Hospital Center, Sainte-Justine, Montréal, Québec, CANADA

Elizabeth A. Cristofalo, M.D., M.P.H.
Assistant Professor of Pediatrics, Neonatal-Perinatal Medicine, Johns Hopkins Children's Center, Johns Hopkins Hospital, Baltimore, Maryland

Maureen M. Gilmore, M.D.
Assistant Professor, Neonatal-Perinatal Medicine, Johns Hopkins Children's Center, Johns Hopkins Hospital, Division of Neonatology, Johns Hopkins Bayview Medical Center, Baltimore, Maryland

Alan E. Guttmacher, M.D.
Director, Eunice Kennedy Shriver National Institute of Child Health and Human Development, National Institutes of Health, Bethesda, Maryland

Susan R. Hintz, M.D., M.S. Epi
Associate Professor of Pediatrics, Division of Neonatal Medicine and Developmental Medicine, Stanford University School of Medicine, Director, Center for Comprehensive Fetal Health, Lucile Packard Children's Hospital, Palo Alto, California

Kathleen A. Kennedy, M.D., M.P.H.
Richard W. Mithoff Professor of Pediatrics, Director, Division of Neonatal-Perinatal Medicine, Director, M.S. in Clinical Research Degree Program, University of Texas-Houston Medical School, Houston, Texas

John P. Kinsella, M.D.
Professor of Pediatrics, Section of Neonatology, Medical Director, Newborn/Young Child Transport Service, Director of Clinical Research, Pediatric Heart Lung Center, Children's Hospital, University of Colorado, Denver, Aurora, Colorado

Jean-Christophe Mercier, M.D., M.Sci.
Professor of Pediatrics, University of Paris 7 Denis Diderot, Chief, Department of Pediatric Emergency Care, Hôpital Robert-Debré, Paris, FRANCE

Barbara K. Schmidt, M.D., M.Sc.
Kristine Sandberg Knisely Chair in Neonatology, Department of Pediatrics, University of Pennsylvania School of Medicine, Children's Hospital of Philadelphia, Philadelphia, Pennsylvania

Michael D. Schreiber, M.D.
Professor and Executive Vice Chairperson, Department of Pediatrics, University of Chicago, Chicago, Illinois

Philip W. Shaul, M.D.
Professor of Pediatrics, Director, Division of Pulmonary and Vascular, Biology, Lowe Foundation Professor of Pediatric, Critical Care Research, Department of Pediatrics, University of Texas Southwestern Medical Center at Dallas, Dallas, Texas

Roger F. Soll, M.D.
President, Vermont Oxford Network, Wallace Professor of Neonatology, Department of Pediatrics, University of Vermont College of Medicine, Burlington, Vermont

Robin H. Steinhorn, M.D.
Raymond and Hazel Speck Berry, Professor of Pediatrics, Vice Chairperson, Pediatrics, Chief, Division of Neonatology, Children's Memorial Hospital, Feinberg School of Medicine of Northwestern University, Chicago, Illinois

Robert S. Tepper, M.D., Ph.D.
Mary Agnes Kennedy and Kathryn Kennedy, Weinberger Professor, Pediatric Pulmonology and Critical, Care Section, Department of Pediatrics Herman B. Wells Center for Pediatric Research, Indiana University School of Medicine, James Whitcomb Riley Hospital for Children, Indianapolis, Indiana

Krisa P. Van Meurs, M.D.
Professor of Pediatrics, Neonatology, Associate Chief, Clinical Programs, Division of Neonatal and Development Medicine, Associate Chairperson, Clinical Research, Department of Pediatrics, Stanford University School of Medicine, Lucile Packard Children's Hospital, Palo Alto, California

Michele C. Walsh, M.D., M.S.
Professor of Pediatrics, Case Western Reserve University, Medical Director, Neonatal Intensive Care Unit, Co-Chief, Division of Neonatology, Rainbow Babies & Children's Hospital, University Hospitals Case Medical Center, Cleveland, Ohio

Planning Committee:

Planning Chairperson: Rosemary D. Higgins, M.D.
Program Scientist for the Neonatal Research Network, Pregnancy and Perinatology Branch, Center for Developmental and Perinatal Medicine, Eunice Kennedy Shriver National Institute of Child Health and Human Development, National Institutes of Health, Bethesda, Maryland

Lisa Ahramjian, M.S.
Communications Specialist, Office of Medical Applications of Research, Office of the Director, National Institutes of Health, Bethesda, Maryland

Carol J. Blaisdell, M.D.
Medical Officer, Lung Developmental Biology and Pediatric Pulmonary Diseases, Division of Lung Diseases National Heart, Lung and Blood Institute, National Institutes of Health, Bethesda, Maryland

Stephanie Chang, M.D., M.P.H.
Medical Officer, Evidence-Based Practice Centers Program, Center for Outcomes and Evidence, Agency for Healthcare Research and Quality, Rockville, Maryland

F. Sessions Cole, M.D.
Panel and Conference Chairperson

Park J. White, M.D.
Professor of Pediatrics, Assistant Vice Chancellor for Children's Health, Vice Chairman, Department of Pediatrics, Director, Division of Newborn Medicine, Washington University School of Medicine, Chief Medical Officer, St. Louis Children's Hospital, Division of Newborn Medicine, St. Louis, Missouri

Jennifer Miller Croswell, M.D.
Acting Director, Office of Medical Applications of Research, Office of the Director, National Institutes of Health, Bethesda, Maryland

Anthony G. Durmowicz, M.D.
Medical Officer, Division of Pulmonary and Allergy Products, Center for Drug Evaluation and Research, U.S. Food and Drug Administration, Silver Spring, Maryland

Alan H. Jobe, M.D., Ph.D.
Professor of Pediatrics, Division of Pulmonary, Biology/Neonatology, Cincinnati Children's Hospital Medical Center, Cincinnati, Ohio

Barnett S. Kramer, M.D., M.P.H.
Associate Director for Disease Prevention, Office of Disease Prevention, Office of the Director, National Institutes of Health, Bethesda, Maryland

Kelli K. Marciel, M.A.
Communications Director, Office of Medical Applications of Research, Office of the Director, National Institutes of Health, Bethesda, Maryland

Lawrence M. Nogee, M.D.
Professor, Department of Pediatrics, Johns Hopkins University School of Medicine, Baltimore, Maryland

Tonse N.K. Raju, M.D., D.C.H.
Medical Officer, Pregnancy and Perinatology Branch, Eunice Kennedy Shriver National Institute of Child Health and Human Development, National Institutes of Health, Bethesda, Maryland

Barbara K. Schmidt, M.D., M.Sc.
Director of Clinical Research, Division of Neonatology, Department of Pediatrics, Children's Hospital of Philadelphia, Philadelphia, Pennsylvania

Philip W. Shaul, M.D.
Professor of Pediatrics, Department of Pediatrics, University of Texas Southwestern Medical Center, Dallas, Texas

Barbara Stonestreet, M.D.
Professor, Department of Pediatrics, The Warren Alpert Medical School, Brown University Women and Infants' Hospital of Rhode Island, Providence, Rhode Island

Robin H. Steinhorn, M.D.
Chief, Division of Neonatology, Children's Memorial Hospital, Chicago, Illinois

Linda J. Van Marter, M.D., M.P.H.
Associate Professor of Pediatrics, Newborn Medicine, Harvard Medical School, Children's Hospital Boston, Boston, Massachusetts

Conference Sponsors

Eunice Kennedy Shriver National Institute of Child Health and Human Development
Alan Guttmacher, M.D., Director

Office of Medical Applications of Research
Jennifer M. Croswell, M.D., M.P.H., Acting Director

Conference Cosponsors

National Heart, Lung and Blood Institute
Susan B. Shurin, M.D., Acting Director

Conference Partners

Agency for Healthcare Research and Quality
Carolyn Clancy, M.D., Director

Centers for Disease Control and Prevention
Thomas R. Frieden, M.D., M.P.H., Director

1 Behavior and Pain

Early Opioid Infusion and Neonatal Outcomes in Preterm Neonates ≤28 Weeks' Gestation

Shah PS, the Canadian Neonatal Network (Univ of Toronto, Ontario, Canada; et al)

Am J Perinatol 28:361-366, 2011

We sought to assess risk-adjusted neonatal outcomes of extremely preterm infants who received opioid infusion during early postnatal period. A retrospective analysis of preterm infants ≤28 weeks' gestational age (GA) admitted to neonatal intensive care units in the Canadian Neonatal Network was conducted comparing infants on the basis of receipt of opioid infusion during day 1 and day 3 after birth. Rates of mortality, severe neurological injury, severe retinopathy of prematurity, and chronic lung disease were compared. A total 362 infants received opioid infusion on day 1 and day 3, whereas 4419 infants did not receive opioid infusion. Baseline comparison revealed higher number of males, infants of GA <26 weeks, low Apgar score, and higher Score for Neonatal Acute Physiology scores among those who received opioid infusion. Neonates who received opioid infusion had higher risk for mortality (adjusted odds ratio [AOR] 1.57, 95% confidence interval [CI] 1.13, 2.18), severe neurological injury (AOR 1.63, 95% CI 1.30, 2.04), severe retinopathy of prematurity (AOR 1. 39, 95% CI 1.08, 1.79), and bronchopulmonary dysplasia (AOR 1.36, 95% CI 1.03, 1.79). Early exposure to opioid infusion in the first 3 days was associated with higher risk of adverse outcomes in extremely preterm infants.

▶ Management of pain in extremely preterm infants remains a conundrum. By definition, the subjective experience of pain cannot be ascertained in preverbal subjects. Surrogate measures of pain in the extremely preterm infant are significantly limited by this lack of a reference standard for pain assessment. Nonetheless, the seminal work of Anand et al[1] and others has appropriately led to abandonment of the belief that these patients do not experience or are not harmed by pain. Recent work, including the NEOPAIN trial,[2] has raised concerns that opiates may be both ineffective and harmful to ventilated preterm infants. The results reported from the 27 centers in the Canadian Neonatal Network in this article add to those concerns. Although retrospective in nature, this well-done regression analysis demonstrates a significant relationship between early exposure to opiates and mortality, severe neurological injury, severe retinopathy of prematurity, and bronchopulmonary dysplasia among preterm infants at gestational age of 28 weeks or less, after adjustment for gestational age, sex, growth restriction, illness severity by the Score for Neonatal Acute Physiology, Apgar score, and antenatal steroid use. Infants with lethal congenital anomalies, who were born at less than 23 weeks of gestational age, and those who were moribund on admission were excluded. There are 2 ways to explain these observations: either opiates are bad for tiny babies or the care providers across this large consortium somehow recognize at-risk extremely preterm infants and compassionately provide opiate analgesia for them preferentially. How the latter might be achieved based on clinical signs not included in the regression model is a mystery. Routine opiate use should probably be avoided in this vulnerable population. If used, opiates should be used sparingly (for invasive procedures, for example), and caution is warranted. There is an urgent need to develop other methods for alleviating pain and stress in critically ill extremely preterm neonates.

W. E. Benitz, MD

References

1. Anand KJ, Sippell WG, Aynsley-Green A. Randomised trial of fentanyl anaesthesia in preterm babies undergoing surgery: effects on the stress response. *Lancet.* 1987; 1:243-248.
2. Bhandari V, Bergqvist LL, Kronsberg SS, Barton BA, Anand KJ; NEOPAIN Trial Investigators Group. Morphine administration and short-term pulmonary outcomes among ventilated preterm infants. *Pediatrics.* 2005;116:352-359.

Oral sucrose as an analgesic drug for procedural pain in newborn infants: a randomised controlled trial
Slater R, Cornelissen L, Fabrizi L, et al (Univ of Oxford, UK; Univ College London, UK; et al)
Lancet 376:1225-1232, 2010

Background.—Many infants admitted to hospital undergo repeated invasive procedures. Oral sucrose is frequently given to relieve procedural pain in neonates on the basis of its effect on behavioural and physiological pain scores. We assessed whether sucrose administration reduces pain-specific brain and spinal cord activity after an acute noxious procedure in newborn infants.

Methods.—In this double-blind, randomised controlled trial, 59 newborn infants at University College Hospital (London, UK) were randomly assigned to receive 0·5 mL 24% sucrose solution or 0·5 mL sterile water 2 min before undergoing a clinically required heel lance. Randomisation was by a computer-generated randomisation code, and researchers, clinicians, participants, and parents were masked to the identity of the solutions. The primary outcome was painspecific brain activity evoked by one time-locked heel lance, recorded with electroencephalography and identified by principal component analysis. Secondary measures were baseline behavioural and physiological measures, observational pain scores (PIPP), and spinal nociceptive reflex withdrawal activity. Data were analysed per protocol. This study is registered, number ISRCTN78390996.

Findings.—29 infants were assigned to receive sucrose and 30 to sterilised water; 20 and 24 infants, respectively, were included in the analysis of the primary outcome measure. Nociceptive brain activity after the noxious heel lance did not differ significantly between infants who received sucrose and those who received sterile water (sucrose: mean $0 \cdot 10$, 95% CI $0 \cdot 04 - 0 \cdot 16$; sterile water: mean $0 \cdot 08$, $0 \cdot 04 - 0 \cdot 12$; p=$0 \cdot 46$). No significant difference was recorded between the sucrose and sterile water groups in the magnitude or latency of the spinal nociceptive reflex withdrawal recorded from the biceps femoris of the stimulated leg. The PIPP score was significantly lower in infants given sucrose than in those given sterile water (mean $5 \cdot 8$, 95% CI $3 \cdot 7 - 7 \cdot 8$ *vs* $8 \cdot 5$, $7 \cdot 3 - 9 \cdot 8$; p=$0 \cdot 02$) and significantly more infants had no change in facial expression after sucrose administration (seven of 20 [35%] *vs* none of 24; p<$0 \cdot 0001$).

Interpretation.—Our data suggest that oral sucrose does not significantly affect activity in neonatal brain or spinal cord nociceptive circuits, and therefore might not be an effective analgesic drug. The ability of sucrose to reduce clinical observational scores after noxious events in newborn infants should not be interpreted as pain relief (Fig 3, Table 2).

▶ This is an intriguing article that addresses the important issue of pain management and recognition in newborn babies. We have come a long way

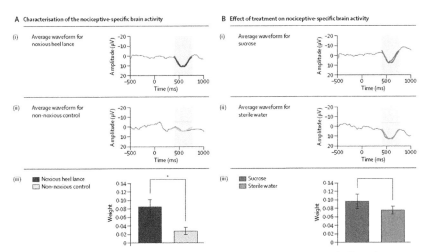

FIGURE 3.—Characterisation of the nociceptive-specific brain activity (A) and effect of sucrose or sterile water on the nociceptive-specific brain activity (B). (A) Average waveform of the group data after (i) noxious heel lance and (ii) non-noxious control stimulus (alignment window 400—750 ms). (iii) Mean (SE) weight of the second principal component after the noxious heel lance and non-noxious control stimulus (*p=$0 \cdot 006$). (B) Average waveform of the group data after the noxious heel lance, separated into two groups: (i) infants administered sucrose and (ii) infants administered sterile water (alignment window 400—750 ms). (iii) Mean (SE) weight of the nociceptive-specific component in the sucrose and sterile water groups (p=$0 \cdot 46$). (Reprinted from The Lancet, Slater R, Cornelissen L, Fabrizi L, et al. Oral sucrose as an analgesic drug for procedural pain in newborn infants: a randomised controlled trial. *Lancet.* 2010;376:1225-1232. Copyright 2010, with permission from Elsevier.)

TABLE 2.—Primary and Secondary Outcomes

	Sucrose (N=20)	Sterile Water (N=24)	p Value
Primary outcome			
Nociceptive-specific brain activity (mean weight)	0·10 (0·04—0·16)	0·08 (0·04—0·12)	0·46
Secondary outcomes			
Mean baseline heart rate (bpm)	132·6 (124·3—140·9)	131·8 (122·2—141·5)	0·90
Mean baseline oxygen saturation (%)	99·4% (98·8—100·1)	97·4% (95·0—99·8)	0·13
Baseline behavioural score (from PIPP)	1·3 (0·8—1·7)	1·3 (0·8—1·8)	0·91
PIPP score	5·8 (3·7—7·8)	8·5 (7·3—9·8)	0·02
Latency to change in facial expression (s)	3·8 (1·3—6·4)	3·5 (1·0—6·1)	0·86
Facial non-responders	7/20 (35%)	0/24 (0%)	<0·0001
Mean nociceptive reflex withdrawal activity (μV)	36·11 (24·20—48·02)	30·82 (18·51—43·13)	0·49
Mean latency to nociceptive reflex withdrawal activity (ms)	363·3 (256·4—470·1)	413·5 (262·0—564·9)	0·56

Data are mean (95% CI) or n/N (%). bpm=beats per min. PIPP=premature infant pain profile.

since the primitive notions that neonates neither felt nor remembered pain and were subjected to major surgical procedures without the benefit of anesthesia or analgesia. Pain management is an integral part of modern neonatal intensive care. However, there are still many unanswered questions. Stevens et al[1] completed a Cochrane review that included 44 studies enrolling 3496 infants. Results from only a few studies could be combined in meta-analyses. Sucrose significantly reduced the duration of total crying time but did not reduce the duration of the first cry. No significant differences were found for the percentage change in heart rate from baseline at 1 and 3 minutes after the heel lance or for mean heart rate at 3 minutes after the heel lance.

Oxygen saturation was significantly lower in infants given sucrose during the retinopathy of prematurity (ROP) examination compared with controls.

Infants given sucrose after the heel lance had significantly lower premature infant pain profile (PIPP) scores at 30 and 60 seconds. For ROP examinations, sucrose did not significantly reduce PIPP scores. There were no differences in adverse effects between sucrose and control groups. Slater's double-blind, randomized, controlled trial used new electrophysiological methods to assess the effectiveness of analgesic drugs in newborn infants. The primary outcome measure was pain-specific brain activity evoked by 1 time-locked heel lance, recorded with electroencephalogram, and identified by principal component analysis (Fig 3, Table 2). Secondary measures were baseline behavioral and physiological measures, observational pain scores (PIPP), and spinal nociceptive reflex withdrawal activity. The primary hypothesis was that administration of sucrose 2 minutes before a heel lance would reduce the evoked nociceptive-specific brain activity. Slater commented that the conclusions drawn from this study are limited by the small sample size (n = 44), which could mean that this study was not powered to observe subtle effects that sucrose might have on central nervous system processing. Significant group differences in infant nociceptive brain activity have, however, been recorded in sample sizes of only 15 infants.[2] Although true pain perception cannot be measured in nonverbal populations, neural activity in nociceptive pathways is a more direct measure than behavioral and physiological assessment. The finding that sucrose does not change neural activity strongly suggests that pain perception is not affected by this intervention. However, Lasky and van Drongelen,[3] in an accompanying editorial, are of the opinion that this conclusion is premature. They critically analyzed the study and concluded that despite the limitations outlined by Slater et al, this study adds an important and innovative measurement to evaluating pain management in newborn babies. Such research has just begun but promises better understanding of pain and more effective pain management. However, until we better understand pain pathways and the short-term and long-term sequelae of painful procedures, it seems premature to conclude that sucrose might not be an effective analgesic for newborn babies. We concur and are of the opinion that this single-center trial should be repeated in a larger sample of infants and this new method used to test the effect of other known pharmacological analgesic agents, such as morphine.

A. A. Fanaroff, MD, FRCPE, FRCP&CH

References

1. Stevens B, Yamada J, Ohlsson A. Sucrose for analgesia in newborn infants undergoing painful procedures. *Cochrane Database Syst Rev.* 2010;(1). CD001069.
2. Slater R, Fabrizi L, Worley A, Meek J, Boyd S, Fitzgerald M. Premature infants display increased noxious-evoked neuronal activity in the brain compared to healthy age-matched term-born infants. *Neuroimage.* 2010;52:583-589.
3. Lasky RE, van Drongelen W. Is sucrose an effective analgesic for newborn babies? *Lancet.* 2010;376:1201-1203.

Pain in neonates is different
Johnston CC, Fernandes AM, Campbell-Yeo M (McGill Univ School of Nursing, Montreal, Canada; Coimbra School of Nursing, Portugal; IWK Health Centre, Halifax, Canada)
Pain 152:S65-S73, 2011

Pain processing and management in neonates, especially preterm neonates, differs from older populations. In this review, a brief background on pain processing in neonatal life, pain exposure in Neonatal Intensive Care Units (NICU), the consequences of untreated pain, and the difficulties in treating procedural pain pharmacologically will be presented. A more detailed review of non-pharmacological interventions for procedural pain in neonates will include sensory stimulation approaches, oral sweet solutions, and maternal interventions. Some possible mechanisms for the effectiveness of non-pharmacological interventions are offered. Finally, avenues of research into similar interventions as adjuvant therapies or drug-sparing effects in older populations are suggested (Table 1).

▶ We have come a long way since the "old days," when a common misconception was that neonates, especially preterms, do not experience pain and it was

TABLE 1.—Non-Pharmacological Interventions

Intervention	Population of Neonates	Painful Procedure	Effects	Overall Effectiveness to Reduce Pain Responses
Containment/facilitated tucking (Ward-Larson, 2004; Axelin, 2006, 2009) Swaddling (Fearon, 1997; Campos, 1989; Prasopkitikun, 2003 [SR]; Huang, 2004 [SR]) Prone position (Grunau, 2004)	Term preterm very preterm	Endotracheal/pharyngeal suctioning IM injections heel stick	↓ Physiological and behavioral pain responses ↓ Arousal and sustained reduction in HR and crying with swaddling	Containment and swaddling are effective Prone position alone is not effective
Rocking (Campos, 1989; Mathai, 2006) Simulated rocking (Johnston, 1997)	Full term preterm	Heel stick	↓ Total cry duration ↓ Pain scores with rocking combined with NNS, compared to sucrose	Rocking is effective during and after heel stick but not simulated rocking
NNS* (Field, 1984; Carbajal, 1999, 2002; Corbo, 2000; Mathai, 2006; Stevens, 1999; Tsao, 2009 [SR])	Term preterm	Venepuncture heel stick	↓ Heart rate ↑ Oxygenation	Effective, potentiates the effect of sweet taste
Sweet taste (Gaspardo, 2005) (SR*); Tsao, 2009 (SR*); (Stevens, 2010 (SR*))	Full term preterm very preterm	Heel stick venepuncture	↓ Cry and grimacing ↓ Pain scores compared to placebo ↓ In pain scores when associated to NNS.	Effective for single and repeated heel lance Insufficient evidence for other procedures
Maternal holding and touch (Huang, 2004 (SR*); Phillips, 2005)	Full term very preterm	Heel stick pharyngeal suctioning	↓ Crying when held by mothers	Effective
Auditory recognition: maternal heart rate (Kurihara, 1996) music therapy (Bo, 2000; Butt, 2000; Hardling, 2009) (SR*) recorded maternal voice (Johnston, 2007)	Full term preterm	Heel stick	↓ HR, ↑ oxygenation and quicker recovery Strongest effect combined with NNS	Maternal heart beat or music are effective but not recorded maternal voice
Olfactory recognition: own mother's milk or familiar odor (Goubet, 2003, 2007; Rattaz, 2005; Nishitani, 2009)	Full term preterm	Heel stick venepuncture	↓ Crying and grimacing during venepuncture	Effective during venepuncture but not heel lance
Sensorial saturation (Bellieni, 2001, 2002, 2007)	Full term preterm	Heel stick	↓ Cry	Effective Potentiates the effect of sweet taste

Intervention (references)	Population	Procedure	Findings	Conclusion
Breastfeeding and expressed breast milk (Shah, 2008 (SR); Efe, 2007; Osinaike, 2007; Codipietro, 2008)	Full term preterm	Venepuncture heel stick	↓ Crying time and smaller increase in HR with breastfeeding compared to swaddling ↓ Pain scores with breastfeeding compared to placebo Mixed results when comparing breastfeeding to sweet solutions	Breastfeeding is effective; conflicting results regarding expressed breast milk
Skin-to-skin care (Gray, 2000; Johnston, 2003; Ludington-Hoe, 2005; Castral, 2008; Ferber, 2008; Freire, 2008; Johnston, 2008; Kashaninia, 2008; Kostandy, 2008; Akcan, 2009; Chermont, 2009; Razek, 2009)	Full term preterm very preterm	Heel stick venepuncture intramuscular injection	↓ Crying, less variation in HR ↓ Pain scores Better results when combined with breastfeeding or sweet taste	Effective

Editor's Note: Please refer to original journal article for full references.
Abbreviations: NNS, non-nutritive sucking; SR, systematic review; HR, heart rate.

not unusual for surgical procedures, such as ductal ligations, to be performed without analgesia. We are certainly much more concerned about pain in this population than previously, and a good body of knowledge has developed surrounding how babies respond to pain and measures that can be taken to ameliorate pain caused by procedures. This article provides an interesting and helpful review, even providing a summary of research that evaluates responses to pain in individuals who are neonatal intensive care unit (NICU) graduates who underwent many versus few painful procedures. Needless to say, there are long-term effects, including greater cortisol production, increased stress levels, and other indications that previous pain in the NICU has long-lasting effects. A very useful table (Table 1) is provided that summarizes the effects of various interventions for painful procedures, their effects, and their overall effectiveness to reduce pain responses. Furthermore, some of the modalities mentioned in this article to reduce pain (skin-to-skin care, sweet taste, containment) have not been studied to the same extent in older individuals.

J. Neu, MD

Randomized controlled trial of early skin-to-skin contact: effects on the mother and the newborn
Gabriel MAM, Martín IL, Escobar AL, et al (Hosp Madrid-Torrelodones, Madrid, Spain)
Acta Paediatr Int J Paediatr 99:1630-1634, 2010

Objective.—To estimate the influence of skin-to-skin care on the thermal regulation of the infant and the rate of breastfeeding at different points of time. We also aim to establish whether skin-to-skin contact reduces maternal pain during episiotomy repair and decreases the time to expel the placenta.

Methods.—A randomized control study was performed with 137 patients in each branch of the study. Differences between the study groups were analysed with the unpaired t-test, Fisher test or chisquare test as appropriate.

Results.—Greater thermal stability in the skin-to-skin care group was found where an average temperature rise of 0.07°C was observed. Mothers in the skin-to-skin care group exclusively breastfed more frequently at discharge. Mean time to expel the placenta was lesser in the skin-to-skin care group.

Conclusion.—This study shows that skin-to-skin care implies better thermal regulation and a better proportion of exclusive breastfeeding at hospital discharge.

▶ My colleagues and mentors John Kennell and Marshall Klaus first demonstrated that mothers who were offered early contact with their premature infants showed differences in attachment behavior when compared with mothers whose first contact with their infants was 3 weeks after delivery. Furthermore, mothers who had 1 hour of close physical contact with their nude full-term infants within the first 2 hours after delivery and who had 15 extra hours of contact in the first 3 days behaved significantly differently during a physical examination of the infant at 1 month and 1 year, and in their speech to their infants at 2 years, from a control group of mothers who had only routine contact. They concluded that shortly after birth, there is a sensitive period that appears to have long-lasting effects on maternal attachment and may ultimately affect the development of the child.[1] This heralded the "bonding" era in which babies and mothers were offered immediate skin-to-skin contact (SSC), and intensive care nurseries were opened for visitors. Many randomized trials have now demonstrated the advantages of early SSC. Moore et al[2] have updated a Cochrane review that includes 30 randomized and quasi-randomized clinical trials, involving 1925 participants (mother-infant dyads) comparing early SSC with usual hospital care. Limitations included methodological quality, variations in intervention implementation, and outcome variability. The intervention may benefit breast-feeding outcomes (number and duration), early mother-infant attachment, infant crying, and cardiorespiratory stability (in late preterm infants) and has no apparent short- or long-term negative effects. Gouchon et al[3] demonstrated that Cesarean-delivered newborns who experienced SSC within 1 hour of delivery are not at risk for hypothermia and that not only were the mothers more satisfied with the experience, they were also more successful at establishing breast-feeding.

Despite all this evidence, Bystrova et al[4] noted "A tradition of separation of the mother and baby after birth still persists in many parts of the world, including some parts of Russia, and often is combined with swaddling of the baby." In a prospective randomized trial, SSC for 25 to 120 minutes after birth, early suckling, or both positively influenced mother-infant interaction 1 year later when compared with routines involving separation of mother and infant.

It is therefore not surprising to see the benefits of SSC reported by Marin Gabriel and colleagues from Spain. Not only was there greater thermal stability in the SSC group but the placenta was expelled earlier, and the mothers exclusively breast-fed more frequently. There were some concerns about the distribution of the groups, with treating physicians only being assigned to one limb of the study, and the room temperature was higher in the control room. Nevertheless, the SSC babies were warmer. The authors also for the first time examined the effects of SSC on pain relief during episiotomy repair but found no difference. SSC is simple to apply, has many benefits, and causes no harm. It should be universally applied.

A. A. Fanaroff, MD, FRCPE, FRCP&CH

References

1. Kennell JH, Trause MA, Klaus MH. Evidence for a sensitive period in the human mother. *Ciba Found Symp*. 1975;(33):87-101.
2. Moore ER, Anderson GC, Bergman N. Early skin-to-skin contact for mothers and their healthy newborn infants. *Cochrane Database Syst Rev*. 2007;(3). CD003519.
3. Gouchon S, Gregori D, Picotto A, Patrucco G, Nangeroni M, Di Giulio P. Skin-to-skin contact after cesarean delivery: an experimental study. *Nurs Res*. 2010; 59:78-84.
4. Bystrova K, Ivanova V, Edhborg M, et al. Early contact versus separation: effects on mother-infant interaction one year later. *Birth*. 2009;36:97-109.

Maternal attachment representations after very preterm birth and the effect of early intervention

Meijssen D, Wolf M-J, van Bakel H, et al (Tilburg Univ, Netherlands; Academic Med Ctr, Amsterdam, Netherlands; et al)
Infant Behav Dev 34:72-80, 2011

Objective.—For very preterm infants the mother–infant relationship may be compromised. Maternal attachment representations 18 (corrected) months after very preterm birth and the effect of the post-discharge Infant Behavioral Assessment and Intervention Program (IBAIP) were studied. The IBAIP is designed to assist parents to support and enhance their infant's regulatory competence and development. The intervention consisted of 6–8 home visits during the first 8 months after birth.

Method.—Seventy-eight mothers of very preterm infants (<32 weeks and/or <1500 g) were interviewed, who participated in a randomized controlled trial: 41 from the intervention group and 37 from the control group. Maternal attachment representations were assessed with the Working Model of the Child Interview (WMCI). The interviews resulted in a classification of the attachment representations into balanced or non-balanced.

Results.—30% of the mothers had non-balanced attachment representations. Qualitative content analysis of the answers showed that negative feelings when first seeing their baby and negative or ambivalent feelings in the first weeks at home with their baby are related to non-balanced attachment representations. The WMCI revealed no differences between the intervention and control group.

Conclusion.—Early support for mothers of very preterm born infants to develop a healthy mother–infant relationship is recommended especially for mothers who report negative first experiences.

▶ This study measured a mother's perception of attachment to her preterm infant and explored the impact of a home-based developmental intervention program on this perception. The developmental intervention program used an observational tool based on the conceptual framework that underlies the Newborn Individual Developmental Care and Assessment Program.[1] The purpose of the tool was to make parents aware of their baby's responses to information and assist them in supporting their infant's self-regulatory behavior. Maternal interviews were conducted when their infants were 18 months corrected age to assess the long-term effects of the intervention program. Overall, the distribution of balanced versus nonbalanced attachment was similar to that found in studies involving mothers who delivered term infants, with 70% having a balanced attachment representation. No differences were found in maternal attachment representations between mothers who received the intervention and the control mothers. The latter is surprising and suggests that involving mothers in an intervention program designed to improve infant mental and motor development does not necessarily enhance maternal feelings of attachment.

L. A. Papile, MD

Reference

1. Als H. A syndactive model of neonatal behavioral organization: framework for the assessment of neurobehavioral development in the premature infants and for support of infants and parents in the neonatal intensive care environment. *Phys Occup Ther Pediatr.* 1986;6:3-55.

Perceptions of Parents, Nurses, and Physicians on Neonatal Intensive Care Practices

Latour JM, Hazelzet JA, Duivenvoorden HJ, et al (Erasmus MC — Sophia Children's Hosp, Rotterdam, The Netherlands; Netherlands Inst for Health Science and Erasmus Univ Med Centre, Rotterdam)
J Pediatr 157:215-220, 2010

Objective.—To identify satisfaction with neonatal intensive care as viewed by parents and healthcare professionals and to explore similarities and differences between parents and healthcare professionals.

Study Design.—A 3-round Delphi method to identify neonatal care issues (round 1) and to determine the importance of these issues (rounds 2 and 3) was conducted among nurses (n = 84) and physicians (n = 14), followed by an exploratory survey among parents (n = 259). Main outcome measures were 92 neonatal care-related items.

Results.—Sixty-eight nurses and 13 physicians completed all 3 rounds. The first round yielded 419 neonatal care related statements, which were clustered into 92 items. The survey was completed by 148 (57%) parents. Parents rated 25 of 92 care items significantly higher than did the professionals (effect size of Cohen's d, 0.31 to1.14, $P \le .02$). Two items related to medication administration had the largest effect size. Professionals rated 7 items significantly higher than did parents (Cohen's d, −0.31 to −0.58, $P \le .04$). One of these was assigning a physician and a nurse to the parents. Three were related to multicultural care.

Conclusions.—This study revealed disparities between parents and neonatal intensive care unit staff on a number of care issues reflecting incongruity in recognizing parents' desires.

▶ Family centered care is considered a cornerstone of modern-day neonatal intensive care unit (NICU) care. Yet as this study highlights, there is frequently a gap between knowledge and practice. The survey was divided into 5 domains: information, treatment and care, organization, parental participation, and professional attitude. Most of the items that parents considered more important than professionals were in the information and care-giving domains. The items most rated as very important by parents were "parents are informed about the adverse effects of medication" (information domain) and "the correct medication is given at the right time" (treatment and care domain). Among the 7 items ranked more important by professionals, there were 2 that concerned multicultural care: "parents are offered religious/spiritual support" and "caregivers communication with non—Dutch-speaking parents is through an interpreter or the interpreter-phone." These statements were ranked significantly less important by both Dutch-speaking and non—Dutch-speaking parents. Although the survey results may be somewhat limited because they reflect the opinions of parents in 1 NICU, the results will hopefully stimulate a review by other NICU nurses and physicians of their practices in light of the opinions of parents.

L. A. Papile, MD

2 Cardiovascular System

Congenital Heart Defects in Europe: Prevalence and Perinatal Mortality, 2000 to 2005
Dolk H, European Surveillance of Congenital Anomalies (EUROCAT) Working Group (Univ of Ulster, UK; et al)
Circulation 123:841-849, 2011

Background.—This study determines the prevalence of Congenital Heart Defects (CHD), diagnosed prenatally or in infancy, and fetal and perinatal mortality associated with CHD in Europe.

Methods and Results.—Data were extracted from the European Surveillance of Congenital Anomalies central database for 29 population-based congenital anomaly registries in 16 European countries covering 3.3 million births during the period 2000 to 2005. CHD cases (n=26 598) comprised live births, fetal deaths from 20 weeks gestation, and terminations of pregnancy for fetal anomaly (TOPFA). The average total prevalence of CHD was 8.0 per 1000 births, and live birth prevalence was 7.2 per 1000 births, varying between countries. The total prevalence of nonchromosomal CHD was 7.0 per 1000 births, of which 3.6% were perinatal deaths, 20% prenatally diagnosed, and 5.6% TOPFA. Severe nonchromosomal CHD (ie, excluding ventricular septal defects, atrial septal defects, and pulmonary valve stenosis) occurred in 2.0 per 1000 births, of which 8.1% were perinatal deaths, 40% were prenatally diagnosed, and 14% were TOPFA (TOPFA range between countries 0% to 32%). Live-born CHD associated with Down syndrome occurred in 0.5 per 1000 births, with >4-fold variation between countries.

Conclusion.—Annually in the European Union, we estimate 36 000 children are live born with CHD and 3000 who are diagnosed with CHD die as a TOFPA, late fetal death, or early neonatal death. Investing in primary prevention and pathogenetic research is essential to reduce this burden, as well as continuing to improve cardiac services from in utero to adulthood.

▶ Congenital heart disease (CHD) is a common form of congenital malformation associated with significant morbidity and mortality. Antenatal diagnosis of life-threatening forms of CHD not only may help to improve survival and morbidity but also may prepare and inform the families so they can make rational rather than rushed decisions.

This article by Dolk presents a wonderful overview of the prevalence of CHD. It is particularly notable that at these many centers in Europe, terminations of pregnancies for fetal anomalies ranged from 0% to 32%, and there was a greater than 4-fold difference in the incidence of anomalies associated with trisomy 21. The mortality for nonchromosomal-associated CHD was less than 5%. This study presents the background for improved detection of CHD. Has the time come for universal screening using history and physical examination complemented by pulse oximetry of the upper and lower extremities?

Newborn screening is a complex process requiring skilled personnel and a comprehensive system to track and communicate results of testing with public health departments, health care providers, and families. Prior to 2010, newborn hearing screening was the only condition that did not rely on the double mass spectrometry dried blood analysis. Pulse oximetry is gaining momentum to be added to the techniques of screening. The experience from Sweden[1] and Germany[2] certainly supports such an approach, and it is my impression that the pediatric cardiologists will readily adopt such an approach. Certainly even the best cardiologists may miss critical CHD (cCHD), and this approach will reduce the chances of missing many lesions.

The modern generation pulse oximeters are stable and reliable, and the evidence to date is that the false positives will be considerably less than 1%. It is particularly encouraging that Riede et al[2] reported a negative predictive accuracy of 99.9% among 42 240 newborns from 34 institutions that were screened.

Traditionally the arterial pulse oximetry screening (foot and/or right hand) has been put forth as the most useful strategy. The left hand, however, has always been ignored, as it was unclear if the ductus arteriosus influences left-hand arterial perfusion. Rüegger et al[3] studied 251 term or near-term neonates to determine the value of readings from the left wrist. They reported that mean pulse oximetry saturation (POS) for the overall study population was 95.7% (90% confidence interval [CI], 90%-100%) on the right hand, 95.7% (90% CI, 90%-100%) on the left hand, and 94.9% (90% CI, 86%-100%) on the foot. Multivariate logistic regression did not identify any associated factors influencing the oximeters readings on the left hand.

They concluded that with the exception of some children with complex or duct-dependent congenital heart defects and some children with persistent pulmonary hypertension, POS on both hands can be considered equally preductal. This may or may not be surprising information for our readers.

With pulse oximetry as an adjunct to prenatal diagnosis, physical examination, and clinical observation, the percentage of newborns with late diagnosis of cCHD was 4.4%.[2] Riede et al[2] concluded that "pulse oximetry screening can substantially reduce the postnatal diagnostic gap in cCHD, and false-positive results leading to unnecessary examinations of healthy newborns are rare. Pulse Oximetry Saturation should be implemented in routine postnatal care."

Indeed this is likely to happen soon in the United States where a draft copy of the "Strategies for Implementing Screening for Critical Congenital Heart

Disease: Recommendations of the United States Health and Human Services Secretary's Advisory Committee on Heritable Disorders in Newborns and Children" is being reviewed and will in all probability be endorsed by the American Academy of Pediatrics.

A. A. Fanaroff, MD, FRCPE, FRCP&CH

References

1. de-Wahl AGW, Wennergren M, Sandberg K, et al. Impact of pulse oximetry screening on the detection of duct dependent congenital heart disease: a Swedish prospective screening study in 39,821 newborns. *BMJ.* 2009;338:a3037.
2. Riede FT, Wörner C, Dähnert I, Möckel A, Kostelka M, Schneider P. Effectiveness of neonatal pulse oximetry screening for detection of critical congenital heart disease in daily clinical routine—results from a prospective multicenter study. *Eur J Pediatr.* 2010;169:975-981.
3. Rüegger C, Bucher HU, Mieth RA. Pulse oximetry in the newborn: is the left hand pre- or post-ductal? *BMC Pediatr.* 2010;10:35.

Delivery mode shapes the acquisition and structure of the initial microbiota across multiple body habitats in newborns
Dominguez-Bello MG, Costello EK, Contreras M, et al (Univ of Puerto Rico, San Juan; Univ of Colorado, Boulder; Venezuelan Inst for Scientific Res, Caracas; et al)
Proc Natl Acad Sci U S A 107:11971-11975, 2010

Upon delivery, the neonate is exposed for the first time to a wide array of microbes from a variety of sources, including maternal bacteria. Although prior studies have suggested that delivery mode shapes the microbiota's establishment and, subsequently, its role in child health, most researchers have focused on specific bacterial taxa or on a single body habitat, the gut. Thus, the initiation stage of human microbiome development remains obscure. The goal of the present study was to obtain a community-wide perspective on the influence of delivery mode and body habitat on the neonate's first microbiota. We used multiplexed 16S rRNA gene pyrosequencing to characterize bacterial communities from mothers and their newborn babies, four born vaginally and six born via Cesarean section. Mothers' skin, oral mucosa, and vagina were sampled 1 h before delivery, and neonates' skin, oral mucosa, and nasopharyngeal aspirate were sampled <5 min, and meconium <24 h, after delivery. We found that in direct contrast to the highly differentiated communities of their mothers, neonates harbored bacterial communities that were undifferentiated across multiple body habitats, regardless of delivery mode. Our results also show that vaginally delivered infants acquired bacterial communities resembling their own mother's vaginal microbiota, dominated by *Lactobacillus, Prevotella,* or *Sneathia* spp., and C-section infants harbored bacterial communities similar to those found on the skin surface, dominated by *Staphylococcus, Corynebacterium,* and *Propionibacterium* spp. These findings establish an important baseline for studies tracking the human microbiome's successional development in different body habitats following different delivery modes, and their associated effects on infant health.

▶ Hypoxic-ischemic encephalopathy (HIE) and multiorgan failure are feared complications of perinatal asphyxia. The introduction of therapeutic hypothermia and more appropriate supportive measures has resulted in improvements in the outcome of asphyxiated neonates suffering from HIE and multiorgan failure. In the future, further improvements in outcomes are expected by the use of targeted brain-protective treatment modalities such as erythropoietin, xenon, melatonin, topiramate, magnesium sulfate, and stem cell therapy. In addition, improved diagnostic approaches to the frequently associated myocardial dysfunction, as well as a more appropriate, pathophysiology-directed treatment for it, may contribute to improvements in the outcome of neonates suffering from perinatal asphyxia. The article by Martin Kluckow entitled "Functional Echocardiography in Assessment of the Cardiovascular System in Asphyxiated Neonates"[1] addresses these aspects of perinatal asphyxia.

With improvements in our understanding of the physiology and pathophysiology of cardiovascular adaptation immediately after delivery and with the use of targeted neonatal echocardiography by trained neonatologists in the neonatal intensive care unit (NICU) over the past 10 to 15 years, timely recognition and more appropriately tailored management of cardiovascular compromise in asphyxiated neonates have emerged, mostly in larger academic centers, as part of the clinical practice. Dr Kluckow discusses these advances in the article, including the complex requirements for training and skill maintenance for neonatologists in using echocardiography in the NICU. It is of note, however, that we do not have high-level evidence that our improved understanding of transitional hemodynamics, the use of comprehensive hemodynamic monitoring, including targeted neonatal echocardiography, and the associated changes in management of shock in the asphyxiated neonate have resulted in improved outcomes. Since the pathophysiology and management of cardiovascular compromise, multiorgan failure, and HIE are extremely complex, it is possible that such evidence will never be produced. However, it is tempting to speculate that timely diagnosis and appropriately tailored cardiovascular management of these infants may indeed contribute to improvements in long-term outcomes of asphyxiated neonates.

I. Seri, MD, PhD

Reference

1. Kluckow M. Functional echocardiography in assessment of the cardiovascular system in asphyxiated neonates. *J Pediatr.* 2011;158:e13-e18.

Distribution of and Mortality From Serious Congenital Heart Disease in Very Low Birth Weight Infants

Archer JM, Yeager SB, Kenny MJ, et al (Univ of Florida, Gainesville; Univ of Vermont, Burlington; et al)
Pediatrics 127:293-299, 2011

Objective.—To characterize serious congenital heart disease in very low birth weight (VLBW) infants (born at <1500 g or a gestational age of 22–29 weeks) in a large, international database.

Patients and Methods.—We analyzed a database of 99 786 VLBW infants born or treated at 703 NICUs between calendar years 2006 and 2007. We defined serious congenital heart disease as 1 of 14 specific lesions or any other structural congenital heart disease that required surgical or medical treatment by initial hospital discharge or by the age of 1 year. We reviewed records for all infants with cardiac diagnoses and other genetic syndromes and associations to determine which had serious congenital heart disease. We excluded nonstructural disease as well as isolated and untreated atrial or ventricular septal defects. We determined the frequency of serious congenital heart disease, compared overall mortality rates of those with and without serious congenital heart disease, and determined the distribution of specific lesions and mortality for each diagnosis.

Results.—Of 99 786 VLBW infants studied, 893 had serious congenital heart disease (8.9 per 1000). The most common lesions were tetralogy of Fallot ($n = 166$ [18.6% of those with serious congenital heart disease]), aortic coarctation ($n = 103$ [11.5%]), complete atrioventricular canal ($n = 81$ [9.1%]), pulmonary atresia ($n = 73$ [8.2%]), and double-outlet right ventricle ($n = 68$ [7.6%]). The mortality rate of those with serious congenital heart disease was 44%, compared with 12.7% in those without serious congenital heart disease ($P < .0001$).

Conclusions.—Serious congenital heart disease is probably more frequent in VLBW infants treated in NICUs than in the general live-born population, and the distribution reflects lesions associated with extracardiac malformations. VLBW infants with serious congenital heart disease have higher a mortality rate than those without, independent of other risk factors.

▶ A birth defect is defined as an abnormality of structure, function, or body metabolism (inborn error of body chemistry) present at birth that results in physical or mental disability or is fatal. There are more than 4000 known birth defects. In the United States, birth defects are the leading cause of infant mortality, directly responsible for 1 of every 5 infant deaths.[1] Heart defects, which are present about 1 in every 125 births, are the most common birth defect—related cause of infant deaths.

Birth defects threaten the lives of infants of all racial and ethnic backgrounds and can be caused by exposure to environmental hazards or adverse health conditions during pregnancy, including drug and alcohol ingestion, infections, or genetic mutations. Public awareness strategies, such as programs using folic acid vitamin supplements to prevent neural tube defects and alcohol avoidance programs to prevent Fetal Alcohol Syndrome, are essential.

A decade ago, Rasmussen et al[2] investigated the relationship between prematurity and birth defects in a population-based cohort study using the Metropolitan Atlanta Congenital Defects Program. Among 264 392 infants with known gestational ages born between 1989 and 1995, 7738 were identified as having birth defects (2.93%). Premature infants (< 37 weeks' gestation) were more than 2 times as likely to have birth defects as term infants (37-41 weeks; risk ratio, 2.43; 95% confidence interval, 2.30-2.56). This relationship was evident for several categories of birth defects. The rate of birth defects varied by gestational age categories, with the highest risk in the 29- to 32-week gestational age category (risk ratio, 3.37).

Archer et al have used the very extensive Vermont-Oxford Network (VON) database to accumulate the largest cohort of preterm very low birth weight (VLBW) infants with serious congenital heart disease (sCHD). The VON database contained records for 104 339 VLBW infants born in 2006 and 2007 and treated at 703 VON centers in 24 countries. After excluding the 4553 infants who died in the delivery room, a staggering 99 786 records were available for analysis. Of these, 893 infants had sCHD, for an overall frequency of 8.9 per 1000. The most common lesions are noted in the abstract, and the mortality data are self-explanatory. As would be anticipated, the left-sided and single ventricle lesions were associated with the highest mortality (around 85%), whereas two-thirds of the infants with tetralogy of Fallot survived, and less than 10% with pulmonic stenosis died. Aortic stenosis amenable to balloon correction and coarctations also did well. The authors set out to determine the prevalence and outcome of sCHD in VLBW infants. The discovery that VLBW infants have a higher incidence of sCHD than term infants together with a much higher mortality rate than those without sCHD, independently of the presence of extracardiac malformation and other variables known to affect mortality, was in support of their primary hypothesis.

A. A. Fanaroff, MD, FRCPE, FRCP&CH

References

1. Mathews TJ, Miniño AM, Osterman MJ, Strobino DM, Guyer B. Annual summary of vital statistics: 2008. *Pediatrics*. 2011;127:146-157.
2. Rasmussen SA, Moore CA, Paulozzi LJ, Rhodenhiser EP. Risk for birth defects among premature infants: a population-based study. *J Pediatr*. 2001;138:668-673.

Functional cardiac MRI in preterm and term newborns
Groves AM, Chiesa G, Durighel G, et al (Hammersmith Hosp, London, UK; et al)
Arch Dis Child Fetal Neonatal Ed 96:F86-F91, 2011

Objective.—To use cardiac MRI techniques to assess ventricular function and systemic perfusion in preterm and term newborns, to compare techniques to echocardiographic methods, and to obtain initial reference data.

Design.—Observational magnetic resonance and echocardiographic imaging study.

Setting.—Neonatal Unit, Queen Charlotte's and Chelsea Hospital, London, UK.

Patients.—108 newborn infants with median birth weight 1627 (580–4140) g, gestation 32 (25–42) weeks.

Results.—Mean (SD) flow volumes assessed by phase contrast (PC) imaging in 28 stable infants were left ventricular output (LVO) 222 (46), right ventricular output (RVO) 219 (47), superior vena cava (SVC) 95 (27) and descending aorta (DAo) 126 (32) ml/kg/min, with flow being higher at lower gestational age. Limits of agreement for repeated PC assessment of flow were LVO ±50.2, RVO ±55.5, SVC ±20.9 and DAo ±26.2 ml/kg/min. Mean (SD) LVO in 75 stable infants from three-dimensional models were 245 (47) ml/ kg/min, with limits of agreement ±58.3 ml/kg/min. Limits of agreement for repeated echocardiographic assessment of LVO were ±108.9 ml/kg/min.

Conclusions.—Detailed magnetic resonance assessments of cardiac function and systemic perfusion are feasible in newborn infants, and provide more complete data with greater reproducibility than existing echocardiographic methods. Functional cardiac MRI could prove to be a useful research technique to study small numbers of newborn infants in specialist centres; providing insights into the pathophysiology of circulatory failure; acting as an outcome measure in clinical trials of inotropic intervention and so guiding clinical practice in the wider neonatal community.

▶ Noninvasive assessment of neonatal hemodynamics, particularly cardiac function and tissue perfusion, is an ongoing challenge in caring for ill newborns. Blood pressure is known to correlate only weakly with tissue perfusion. In this study, Groves and colleagues describe functional magnetic resonance imaging (MRI) techniques they applied to evaluate ventricular function and systemic perfusion among 108 newborn infants across a wide spectrum of gestational ages (25–42 weeks). Unsedated infants underwent cardiac MRI in a Phillips 3 Tesla scanner. Cardiac function was evaluated by phase-contrast and cine imaging of ventricles, superior vena cava, aortic and pulmonary outflow tracts, and descending aorta. Images were analyzed with automated and semiautomated proprietary software. The investigators showed feasibility and reproducibility of MRI in assessing cardiac output and systemic perfusion, obtaining high-quality images of cardiac filling, cardiac output, and systemic perfusion. Currently, this approach is likely to prove most useful for studies of neonatal cardiopulmonary physiology, hemodynamics, and vasopressors. Even now, however, it might prove useful in evaluating cardiac function and/or systemic perfusion in a small number of particularly vexing infants. As MRIs decrease in size and more often are built adjacent to or incorporated into neonatal intensive care units, such a technique might well be used routinely to augment other approaches, such as functional echocardiography, and prove useful in the clinical management of infants with a number of causes of cardiopulmonary dysfunction.

L. J. Van Marter, MD, MPH

Functional Echocardiography in Assessment of the Cardiovascular System in Asphyxiated Neonates
Kluckow M (Univ of Sydney, Australia)
J Pediatr 158:e13-e18, 2011

Perinatal asphyxia commonly results in multi-organ damage, and cardiovascular dysfunction is a frequent association. Myocardial damage, right ventricular dysfunction, abnormal circulatory transition, and impaired autoregulation may all contribute to postnatal neurological damage. Adequate monitoring and appropriate targeted treatment therefore are essential after an asphyxial insult. Standard methods of cardiovascular monitoring in the neonate have limitations. Point of care ultrasound scanning or functional echocardiography offers extra information to assist the clinician in identifying when there is significant cardiovascular impairment, classifying the underlying abnormal physiology and potentially targeting appropriate therapy, thereby optimizing the post-insult cerebral blood flow and oxygen delivery.

▶ Hypoxic-ischemic encephalopathy (HIE) and multiorgan failure are feared complications of perinatal asphyxia. The introduction of therapeutic hypothermia and more appropriate supportive measures has resulted in improvements in the outcome of asphyxiated neonates suffering from HIE and multiorgan failure. In the future, further improvements in outcomes are expected by the use of targeted brain-protective treatment modalities such as erythropoietin, xenon, melatonin, topiramate, magnesium sulfate, and stem cell therapy. In addition, improved diagnostic approaches to and a more appropriate, pathophysiology-directed treatment of the frequently associated myocardial dysfunction may contribute to improvements in the outcome of neonates suffering from perinatal asphyxia. The article by Martin Kluckow addresses these aspects of perinatal asphyxia.

With improvements in our understanding of the physiology and pathophysiology of cardiovascular adaptation immediately after delivery and with the use of targeted neonatal echocardiography by trained neonatologists in the neonatal intensive care unit (NICU) over the past 10 to 15 years, timely recognition and more appropriately tailored management of cardiovascular compromise in asphyxiated neonates have emerged, mostly in larger academic centers, as part of the clinical practice. Dr Kluckow discusses these advances, including the complex requirements for training and skill maintenance for neonatologists in using echocardiography in the NICU. It is of note, however, that we do not have high-level evidence that our improved understanding of transitional hemodynamics; the use of comprehensive hemodynamic monitoring, including targeted neonatal echocardiography; and the associated changes in management of shock in the asphyxiated neonate have resulted in improved outcomes. Since the pathophysiology and management of cardiovascular compromise, multiorgan failure, and HIE are extremely complex, it is possible that such evidence will never be produced. However, it is tempting to speculate that timely diagnosis and appropriately tailored cardiovascular management of these infants may indeed contribute to improvements in long-term outcomes of asphyxiated neonates.

I. Seri, MD, PhD

Functional Echocardiography in Assessment of the Cardiovascular System in Asphyxiated Neonates
Kluckow M (Univ of Sydney, Australia)
J Pediatr 158:e13-e18, 2011

Perinatal asphyxia commonly results in multi-organ damage, and cardiovascular dysfunction is a frequent association. Myocardial damage, right ventricular dysfunction, abnormal circulatory transition, and impaired autoregulation may all contribute to postnatal neurological damage. Adequate monitoring and appropriate targeted treatment therefore are essential after an asphyxial insult. Standard methods of cardiovascular monitoring in the neonate have limitations. Point of care ultrasound scanning or functional echocardiography offers extra information to assist the clinician in identifying when there is significant cardiovascular impairment, classifying the underlying abnormal physiology and potentially targeting appropriate therapy, thereby optimizing the post-insult cerebral blood flow and oxygen delivery.

▶ The neonatology group in Sydney, led by Drs Kluckow and Evans, has been instrumental in advancing the use of—and knowledge gained by—functional echocardiography. Their research has shown the importance of defining underlying pathophysiology in the determination of therapeutic strategies. We have learned that blood pressure measurement is a poor surrogate for blood flow and tissue oxygen delivery. Clearly, this is a huge problem in the neonatal intensive care in the United States.

During my travels in Eastern Europe, I was impressed by how many neonatal intensive care units possessed echocardiography devices and how many neonatologists were able to perform functional echocardiography. More importantly, they used the information gleaned from the study to decide whether the impairments to perfusion were related to preload, afterload, contractility, ductal steal, or other issues. In many places, there are only itinerant or no pediatric cardiologists.

The sad truth appears to be the turf war that thus far has precluded neonatologists from access to training and the use of functional echocardiography. Dr Kluckow presents a compelling argument as to why we need to revisit this issue. Our patients certainly deserve the best care, derived from physiologic information and good clinical evidence.

S. M. Donn, MD

Intrauterine Inflammation as a Risk Factor for Persistent Ductus Arteriosus Patency after Cyclooxygenase Inhibition in Extremely Low Birth Weight Infants

Kim ES, Kim E-K, Choi CW, et al (Seoul Natl Univ College of Medicine, Republic of Korea)
J Pediatr 157:745-750, 2010

Objectives.—To test the hypothesis that intrauterine inflammation increases prostaglandin production and may be a risk factor for persistent ductus arteriosus after therapy with indomethacin, a nonselective cyclooxygenase inhibitor.

Study Design.—Indomethacin therapy was started after confirming ductus arteriosus within 24 hours after birth in extremely low birth weight infants. After one cycle of therapy, infants with closed ductus were classified as responders, and those with patent ductus were classified as nonresponders. Multiple logistic regression analysis was used to determine important perinatal factors associated with persistent ductus arteriosus. Immunohistochemistry with cyclooxygenase antibodies and radioimmunoassay by 6-keto prostaglandin $F_{1\alpha}$ kit were used to determine the relationship between intrauterine inflammation and ductal patency.

Results.—Forty-one infants were responders, and 37 infants were nonresponders. Responders were frequently small for gestational age; nonresponders frequently had lower gestational age, respiratory distress syndrome, and intrauterine inflammation. By multiple logistic regression analysis, respiratory distress syndrome and intrauterine inflammation were more frequent in nonresponders. Cyclooxygenase-1 expression in the umbilical arteries and plasma 6-keto prostaglandin $F_{1\alpha}$ levels were higher in nonresponders.

Conclusions.—Respiratory distress syndrome and intrauterine inflammation were independent risk factors for persistent ductus arteriosus after indomethacin therapy in extremely low birth weight infants. Intrauterine inflammation may have a negative influence on ductus arteriosus closure via increased cyclooxygenase-1 activity.

▶ This report provides additional evidence of the entanglement of the fetal inflammatory response and persistent ductal patency. In this cohort of infants who received indomethacin therapy within the first 24 hours after birth, those with persistent ductal patency despite treatment had more evidence of intrauterine inflammation, which has also been associated with adverse events including chronic lung disease, necrotizing enterocolitis, intraventricular hemorrhage, and periventricular leukomalacia. Because early treatment to close the ductus fails to prevent those complications, it is likely that ductal patency is not a mediator of these injuries but rather a marker of the underlying systemic inflammatory response. We should hope that a deeper understanding of that pathophysiology, leading to strategies for modulation of the inflammatory cascade, will prove more effective in preventing those untoward outcomes than our efforts to do so through closure of the ductus have been.

W. E. Benitz, MD

Left Vocal Cord Paralysis After Extreme Preterm Birth, a New Clinical Scenario in Adults
Røksund OD, Clemm H, Heimdal JH, et al (Haukeland Univ Hosp, Bergen, Norway; et al)
Pediatrics 126:e1569-e1577, 2010

Objective.—The goal was to study the incidence and long-term consequences of left vocal cord paralysis (LVCP) after neonatal surgical treatment of patent ductus arteriosus (PDA) in a population-based cohort of adults who were born at gestational ages of ≤28 weeks or with birth weights of ≤1000 g in western Norway.

Methods.—Subjects with a history of neonatal PDA surgery were examined with transnasal flexible laryngoscopy, and those with LVCP were examined with continuous laryngoscopy during maximal treadmill exercise (continuous laryngoscopy exercise testing). All subjects underwent lung function testing, ergospirometry, and pulmonary high-resolution computed tomography. Symptoms were recorded with a questionnaire.

Results.—Forty-four (86%) of 51 eligible preterm infants participated in the study, 13 (26%) had a history of PDA surgery and 7 (54%) had LVCP, with the laryngeal appearances varying slightly. As a group, subjects with LVCP had significant airway obstruction, no decreases in aerobic capacity, and no obvious evidence of longstanding aspiration on high-resolution computed tomography scans. The continuous laryngoscopy exercise tests revealed increasing respiratory symptoms in parallel with increasing anteromedial collapse of the left aryepiglottic folds as the exercise load increased. Hoarseness and voice-related symptoms were the most typical complaints. Symptoms were attributed erroneously to other diseases for at least 2 subjects.

Conclusions.—LVCP is not uncommon in young adults exposed to PDA surgery as preterm infants. The condition may be overlooked easily, and symptoms may be confused with those of other diseases. Laryngoscopy should be offered on the basis of liberal indications after PDA ligation.

▶ Twenty-seven years passed between the first report of surgical ligation of a patent ductus arteriosus (PDA)[1] and description of associated injury to the left recurrent laryngeal nerve.[2] Another 22 years elapsed before this complication of ductal ligation was reported in preterm infants.[3] Early reports suggested that this complication is relatively benign, completely resolves clinically in several weeks, and could be minimized by closure using a surgical clip rather than suture ligature.[3] There is now ample evidence that these effects are neither transient nor inconsequential, but data on long-term outcomes in adults have been lacking. This population-based cohort study of infants born at gestational ages ≤28 weeks or birth weights ≤1000 g in Western Norway from 1982 to 1985 addresses that deficiency. Follow-up at adulthood (in 2008 and 2009) was obtained for 44 of 51 surviving infants (86%), including 13 of the 14 (93%) who had a history of surgical PDA closure, which was performed using a metal clip. Seven infants in the latter group (56% of those examined or at least 50% of those with PDA ligations) had persisting left vocal cord paralysis. Vocal cord paralysis was functionally consequential, as all subjects had prolongation of inspiration, wheezing, or stridor during heavy exercise, and all had weak or hoarse phonation and reported being uncomfortable singing or speaking loudly. Subjects with cord paralysis had significantly lower percent of predicted forced expiratory volume in the 25th to 75th second of expiration and percent of predicted forced expiratory volume in the first second of expiration/forced vital capacity values compared with those without cord paralysis. While the prevalence of this permanent injury in this series may not be representative of results from other regions, consideration of this hazard should become a part of the consent process for PDA ligation. Along with these data, the undefined nature of the benefit(s) of PDA ligation and accumulating evidence of other adverse consequences[4] should dampen enthusiasm for this intervention until well-designed clinical trials demonstrate long-term benefits and define the population of infants to whom those benefits may accrue.

W. E. Benitz, MD

References

1. Gross RE, Hubbard JP. Surgical ligation of a patent ductus arteriosus. Report of the first successful case. *JAMA*. 1939;112:729.
2. Hardy JD, Webb WR, Timmis H, Watson DG, Blake TM. Patent ductus arteriosus: operative treatment of 100 consecutive patients with isolated lesions without mortality. *Ann Surg*. 1966;164:877-882.
3. Davis JT, Baciewicz FA, Suriyapa S, Vauthy P, Polamreddy R, Barnett B. Vocal cord paralysis in premature infants undergoing ductal closure. *Ann Thorac Surg*. 1988;46:214-215.
4. Chorne N, Leonard C, Piecuch R, Clyman RI. Patent ductus arteriosus and its treatment as risk factors for neonatal and neurodevelopmental morbidity. *Pediatrics*. 2007;119:1165-1174.

Perinatal asphyxia and cardiac abnormalities
Dattilo G, Tulino V, Tulino D, et al (Univ of Messina, Italy; Univ Hosp of Messina, Italy; Hosp "G. Jazzolino," Vibo Valentia, Italy)
Int J Cardiol 147:e39-e40, 2011

The most common etiologies of myocardial infarction in the perinatal period are congenital heart disease, coronary artery lesions, thromboembolism and perinatal asphyxia. Cardiac abnormalities in perinatal asphyxia include tricuspid regurgitation and mitral regurgitation associated with transient myocardial ischemia of the newborn. Patent foramen ovale is a frequent remnant of the fetal circulation. Persistent hypoxia sometimes causes pulmonary arterial hypertension with consequent right to left shunt across patent ductus arteriosus and foramen ovale. We describe a case of tricuspid regurgitation, mitral regurgitation, and patent foramen ovale in a 15-day-old newborn male infant with a history of perinatal asphyxia. Also this case focuses attention on the perinatal asphyxia.

▶ Case reports and anecdotes do have a place in the medical literature. Accordingly, they should receive the same meticulous preparation by the authors and demand the same close scrutiny that reviewers would pay to research papers.

When I encountered this article by Dattilo et al, I was taken aback. These authors entitled a case report "Perinatal Asphyxia and Cardiac Abnormalities" with no (as in zero) evidence of perinatal asphyxia, which was apparently based on Apgar scores of 7 and 8 at 1 and 5 minutes, respectively. No information was provided about umbilical cord or neonatal arterial blood gases, other organ involvement, or even what the historical information was that led to this diagnosis. An echocardiography performed at 15 days of age showed some elements of mild pulmonary hypertension. Would anyone care to guess what the underlying problem was?

In addition, the terminology chosen also leaves much to be desired. We need to be more precise than to use the word perinatal to describe the timing of an event. It is too vague. Do we mean prenatal, intrapartum, or postnatal? Asphyxia should be defined either biochemically (acidosis, hypoxia, and hypercapnia) or functionally (failure of the organ of respiration).

Frankly, I am surprised that this article passed not only peer review but also editorial approval. The editor should be ashamed. Let's hope the lawyers don't get a hold of this one.

S. M. Donn, MD

Vasopressin for Refractory Hypotension in Extremely Low Birth Weight Infants
Bidegain M, Greenberg R, Simmons C, et al (Duke Univ Med Ctr, Durham, NC)
J Pediatr 157:502-504, 2010

Intravenous vasopressin at 0.01 to 0.04 units/kg/h increased median mean blood pressure from 26 mm Hg (range 18-44) to 41 mm Hg (range 17-90) by 12 hours of infusion ($P = .002$) and allowed weaning of catecholamines in a group of extremely low birth weight infants with refractory hypotension.

▶ Despite the ongoing lack of consensus on the criteria for diagnosis of hypotension in extremely low birth weight (ELBW) infants, the search for more effective treatments continues. This brief report describes the experience of using vasopressin by continuous infusion in 20 infants with birth weights

<1000 g who were unable to maintain mean systemic blood pressures above the 10th percentile for gestational and postnatal age, despite treatment with hydrocortisone, dopamine, and epinephrine. The data (Fig in the original article) suggest a therapeutic response, but these observations are difficult to interpret. No controls are compared, so it is possible that rising blood pressures were unrelated to the drug. It is not clear whether or how data attrition might have influenced the data, as 14 of the 33 courses were shorter than 12 hours in duration. Thirteen of the 20 subjects died. While demonstrating the technical feasibility of administration of vasopressin to ELBW infants, this report falls short of providing evidence that it is either safe or efficacious. The authors are correct in calling for "Further research evaluating the use of vasopressin in ELBW infants with refractory hypotension ... to determine the pharmacokinetics, timing of treatment, efficacy, and side effects of vasopressin."

W. E. Benitz, MD

Delayed cord clamping and blood flow in the superior vena cava in preterm infants: an observational study

Meyer MP, Mildenhall L (Middlemore Hosp, Auckland, New Zealand)
Arch Dis Child Fetal Neonatal Ed 2011 [Epub ahead of print]

Objective.—To determine if timing of cord clamping affects blood flow in the upper body, as measured by flow in the superior vena cava (SVC).
Design.—Observational study.
Setting.—Neonatal Unit, Middlemore Hospital, Auckland, New Zealand.
Patients.—30 preterm infants <30 weeks' gestational age.
Intervention.—Cord clamping was immediate in 17 infants and delayed by 30—45 s in 13.
Results.—Infants in the two groups did not differ significantly in terms of gestational age, gender or use of antenatal steroids. Median flow in the SVC in the first 24 h was significantly higher in the group with delayed clamping (median 91 ml/kg/min; IQR 81—101) compared with 52 ml/kg/min (IQR 42—100) in the immediate clamping group (p = 0.028). Fewer infants in the delayed group had low flow (1 compared with 9; p = 0.017). All three infants with intraventricular haemorrhage (IVH) (of any grade) had low flow.
Conclusions.—Blood flow in the SVC was higher in infants where delayed cord clamping was performed. The relationship of IVH, low flow and timing of cord clamping requires further study.

▶ In a recent meta-analysis of 10 randomized controlled studies of delayed cord clamping in preterm infants, the odds ratio for intraventricular hemorrhage (IVH) was reduced.[1] The mechanism of the reported benefit is unclear but may relate to increased circulating blood volume at birth. IVH has been associated with reduced blood flow to the upper part of the body, as measured by blood flow in the superior vena cava (SVC).[2] In this observational study, echocardiography was used to measure blood flow in the SVC. It had been previously shown that SVC blood flow is independent of blood pressure and cardiac output measurements, both of which are inconsistent gauges of systemic blood flow. Low SVC was defined as less than 55 mL/kg/min.[3] Nine of the 10 infants with low SVC were in the late cord clamping group as were all of the infants (n = 3) who were treated for hypotension. Low SVC blood flow was noted in the 3 infants with IVH, 1 of whom was in the late cord clamping group.

Although the results indicate that delayed cord clamping is associated with low SVC flow, the association between low SVC and IVH is less apparent. It will take additional studies examining the effects of early and late cord clamping on the dynamics of the transitional circulation and subsequent IVH.

L. A. Papile, MD

References

1. Rabe H, Reynolds G, Diaz-Rossello J. A systematic review and meta-analysis of a brief delay in clamping the umbilical cord of preterm infants. *Neonatology.* 2008;93:138-144.
2. Kluckow M, Evans N. Low superior vena cava flow and intraventricular haemorrhage in preterm infants. *Arch Dis Child Fetal Neonatal Ed.* 2000;82:F188-F194.
3. Groves AM, Kuschel CA, Knight DB, Skinner JR. Echocardiographic assessment of blood flow volume in the superior vena cava and descending aorta in the newborn infant. *Arch Dis Child Fetal Neonatal Ed.* 2008;93:F24-F28.

3 Central Nervous System and Special Senses

Carbon Dioxide and Glucose Affect Electrocortical Background in Extremely Preterm Infants
Wikström S, Lundin F, Ley D, et al (Uppsala Univ, Sweden; County Council of Värmland, Karlstad, Sweden; Lund Univ Hosp, Sweden)
Pediatrics 127:e1028-e1034, 2011

Objectives.—To investigate if $Paco_2$ and plasma glucose levels affect electrocortical activity.

Methods.—Ours was an observational study of 32 infants with a gestational age of 22 to 27 weeks. We performed simultaneous single-channel electroencephalogram (EEG) and repeated blood gas/plasma glucose analyses during the first 3 days ($n = 247$ blood samples with corresponding EEG). Interburst intervals (IBIs) and EEG power were averaged at the time of each blood sample.

Results.—There was a linear relationship between $Paco_2$ and IBI; increasing $Paco_2$ was associated with longer IBIs. One day after birth, a 1-kPa increase in $Paco_2$ was associated with a 16% increase in IBI in infants who survived the first week without severe brain injury. EEG power was highest at a $Paco_2$ value of 5.1 kPa and was attenuated both at higher and lower $Paco_2$ values. Corrected for carbon dioxide effects, plasma glucose was also associated with IBI. Lowest IBI appeared at a plasma glucose level of 4.0 mmol/L, and there was a U-shaped relationship between plasma glucose level and EEG with increasing discontinuity at glucose concentrations above and below 4.0 mmol/L.

Conclusions.—Both carbon dioxide and plasma glucose level influenced EEG activity in extremely preterm infants, and values considered to be within normal physiologic ranges were associated with the best EEG background. Increasing EEG discontinuity occurred at carbon dioxide levels frequently applied in lung-protection strategies; in addition, moderate hyperglycemia was associated with measurable EEG changes. The long-term effects of changes in carbon dioxide and glucose on brain function are not known.

▶ In this observational study, Wilkstrom et al documented the effect of PaCO2 and serum glucose on the electrocortical activity of extremely preterm infants by measuring their effect on 2 electroencephalographic parameters: the interburst interval (IBI) and the electroencephalogram (EEG) power; both are measurements of the EEG background.

The EEG provides an excellent tool to study the effects of systemic metabolic changes on the electrocortical function of extremely preterm infants. EEG does not significantly change during the awake/sleep cycle, and it is not affected by external stimulation. These EEGs are discontinuous. Periods of IBI alternate with burst intervals (periods of synchronized, high-voltage activity with mixed, mainly theta and delta, frequencies located primarily over the centrotemporal and occipital regions) and repeat at a fairly semiregular interval during awake and sleep stages. IBIs have clearly defined amplitude ($< 2 \mu V$) and duration (6-12 seconds, maximum 35 seconds) in preterm infants younger than 28 weeks. The consistent characteristics of the IBI make it a sensitive parameter for the study of metabolic changes in electrocortical function in this age group. The EEG spectral power analysis, although less used in clinical practice, offers a quantitative tool for the study of metabolic changes in electrocortical function in extremely preterm infants. It provides a good analysis of activities within the delta, theta, alpha, and beta frequency bands. There is clear documentation that the EEG background in neonates is affected by metabolic and toxic changes, including the administration of anesthetics, benzodiazepines, barbiturates, other antiepileptic drugs, opioids, and hypothermia. There is also good clinical documentation of the effects of hyperglycemia and hypoglycemia on neurodevelopment in children of mothers with diabetes. The clinical and neurophysiological effect of abnormal glucose and hypercapnia on the electrocortical activity of preterm infants has been less studied. The Wilkstrom et al study was well designed and considered the factors that could impact their EEG analysis very carefully. They excluded segments of the EEG recorded within 2 hours of administration of opioids and included segments of EEGs taken 5 to 10 minutes prior to blood sampling to minimize artifacts.

The study documented that, even when adjusted for postnatal age, an increase of PaCO2 resulted in prolonged IBI (linear association) and the EEG power was higher at normal PaCO2 values but attenuated at hypercapnic and hypocapnic levels (dome-shaped association). In contrast with the previous results, the serum glucose level had a nonlinear association with the IBI (U-shaped association) and no relationship with changes in the EEG power analysis. The lowest IBI was recorded with serum glucose levels of 4.0 mmol/L (74 mg/dL); IBIs were longer with lower and higher serum glucose levels. It is not surprising that the IBI lengthens in the setting of hyperglycemia and hypoglycemia or hypercapnia and hypocapnia because the IBI also lengthens in the presence of other toxic-metabolic or systemic changes that lead to various degrees of neonatal encephalopathy (ie, sedation or anesthesia). A less clear relationship was found between changes of the EEG power spectral analysis and changes in serum glucose in extremely premature infants. Results of this study may imply that the IBI is a better neurophysiological parameter than the EEG spectra analysis to measure the effect of the CO2 and glycemic changes in extremely premature infants. The lack of a relationship between changes in serum glycemia glucose and the spectra analysis could be because higher or lower levels of serum glucose than those encountered in the study ones are needed to produce a change in the typical delta-theta activity that dominates the burst portion of the EEG background in the extremely premature neonates. The effects of hyperglycemia and hypoglycemia on brain development and neurodevelopment has been previously documented, but the long-term effects on neurodevelopment of moderate hypercapnia, in premature infants who required ventilator support for prolonged periods of times, still need to be clarified.

E. M. Pestana Knight, MD

Cerebellar Hemorrhage on Magnetic Resonance Imaging in Preterm Newborns Associated with Abnormal Neurologic Outcome
Tam EWY, Rosenbluth G, Rogers EE, et al (Univ of California San Francisco)
J Pediatr 158:245-250, 2011

Objective.—To investigate the relationship between cerebellar hemorrhage in preterm infants seen on magnetic resonance imaging (MRI), but not on ultrasonography, and neurodevelopmental outcome.

Study Design.—Images from a cohort study of MRI in preterm newborns were reviewed for cerebellar hemorrhage. The children were assessed at a mean age of 4.8 years with neurologic examination and developmental testing using the Wechsler Preschool and Primary Scale of Intelligence, Third Edition.

Results.—Cerebellar hemorrhage was detected on both ultrasonography and MRI in 3 of the 131 preterm newborns evaluated, whereas smaller hemorrhages were seen only on MRI in 10 newborns (total incidence, 10%). Adjusting for gestational age at birth, intraventricular hemorrhage, and white matter injury, cerebellar hemorrhage detectable solely by MRI was associated with a 5-fold increased odds of abnormal neurologic examination compared with newborns without cerebellar hemorrhage (outcome data in 74%). No association with the Wechsler Preschool and Primary Scale of Intelligence, Third Edition score was found.

Conclusions.—Cerebellar hemorrhage is not uncommon in preterm newborns. Although associated with neurologic abnormalities, hemorrhage seen only on MRI is associated with much more optimistic outcomes than that visible on ultrasonography.

▶ Advances in imaging, including cranial ultrasound and MRI, have resulted in an increased recognition of cerebellar hemorrhage. Prior reports, including what must be considered an antique from our group,[1] concerned mainly infants with many perinatal risk factors, including traumatic delivery and coagulopathy. Cerebellar hemorrhage was only recognized at autopsy, and the rates of severe neurologic impairment were extraordinarily high. Although reports indicated that large cerebellar hemorrhage carries a high risk of mortality and severe neurodevelopmental deficits, the effects of smaller cerebellar hemorrhages seen on MRI but not on cranial ultrasound had not been reported prior to this prospectively collected cohort of 131 infants, with a 2% incidence of ultrasound-detected and 8% of solely MRI-detected cerebellar hemorrhage (1-3 mm).

The smaller cerebellar hemorrhages seen only on MRI were associated with an increased risk for abnormalities on neurologic examination but not with abnormalities of cognition at 3 to 6 years of age. Some infants demonstrated increased tone and hyperreflexia but were able to ambulate.

Although the effect of overall cerebellar injury on outcome could be detected, there were too few cases to compare unilateral versus bilateral cerebellar injury or to compare severity related with the side of the injury. However, Limperopoulos et al[2] provides some of the answers. She and her team measured volumes of cortical and subcortical gray matter and white matter in 38 preterm infants with MRI evidence of cerebellar injury. Unilateral cerebellar injury was associated with significantly smaller volumes of cortical gray and cerebral white matter in the contralateral cerebral hemisphere. Regions affected were dorsolateral prefrontal, premotor, sensorimotor, and midtemporal regions. With bilateral cerebellar injury, there were no significant interhemispheric differences. Hence, regional cerebral growth impairment results from the interruption of cerebrocerebral connectivity and loss of neuronal activation critical for development. In conclusion, cerebellar injury in the preterm infant is associated with impaired growth of the uninjured contralateral cerebral hemisphere with significant impairment evident as early as term equivalent.

Furthermore, in 18 term infants with cerebellar hemorrhage followed by Limperopoulos et al,[3] 39% had neurologic abnormalities. Gross-motor delays, expressive language deficits, and externalizing behavioral problems were the most common (44%). Cognitive deficits were present in one-third of cases. Larger cerebellar lesions were associated with significantly lower cognitive, gross motor, expressive language, and social-behavioral scores. They concluded that cerebellar injury in the term infant is associated with a broad spectrum of neurodevelopmental disabilities, particularly in infants with large cerebellar lesions.

A. A. Fanaroff, MD, FRCPE, FRCP&CH

References

1. Martin R, Roessmann U, Fanaroff A. Massive intracerebellar hemorrhage in low-birth-weight infants. *J Pediatr.* 1976;89:290-293.
2. Limperopoulos C, Chlingryan G, Guizard N, Robertson RL, Du Plessis AJ. Cerebellar injury in the premature infant is associated with impaired growth of specific cerebral regions. *Pediatr Res.* 2010;68:145-150.
3. Limperopoulos C, Robertson RL, Sullivan NR, Bassan H, du Plessis AJ. Cerebellar injury in term infants: clinical characteristics, magnetic resonance imaging findings, and outcome. *Pediatr Neurol.* 2009;41:1-8.

Cerebral Palsy Among Term and Postterm Births
Moster D, Wilcox AJ, Vollset SE, et al (Univ of Bergen, Norway; Natl Insts of Health, Durham, NC; et al)
JAMA 304:976-982, 2010

Context.—Although preterm delivery is a well-established risk factor for cerebral palsy (CP), preterm deliveries contribute only a minority of affected infants. There is little information on the relation of CP risk to gestational age in the term range, where most CP occurs.

Objective.—To determine whether timing of birth in the term and postterm period is associated with risk of CP.

Design, Setting, and Participants.—Population-based follow-up study using the Medical Birth Registry of Norway to identify 1 682 441 singleton children born in the years 1967-2001 with a gestational age of 37 through 44 weeks and no congenital anomalies. The cohort was followed up through 2005 by linkage to other national registries.

Main Outcome Measures.—Absolute and relative risk of CP for children surviving to at least 4 years of age.

Results.—Of the cohort of term and postterm children, 1938 were registered with CP in the National Insurance Scheme. Infants born at 40 weeks had the lowest risk of CP, with a prevalence of 0.99/1000 (95% confidence interval [CI], 0.90-1.08). Risk for CP was higher with earlier or later delivery, with a prevalence at 37 weeks of 1.91/1000 (95% CI, 1.58-2.25) and a relative risk (RR) of 1.9 (95% CI, 1.6-2.4), a prevalence at 38 weeks of 1.25/1000 (95% CI, 1.07-1.42) and an RR of 1.3 (95% CI, 1.1-1.6), a prevalence at 42 weeks of 1.36/1000 (95% CI, 1.19-1.53) and an RR of 1.4 (95% CI, 1.2-1.6), and a prevalence after 42 weeks of 1.44 (95% CI, 1.15-1.72) and an RR of 1.4 (95% CI, 1.1-1.8). These associations were even stronger in a subset with gestational age based on ultrasound measurements: at 37 weeks the prevalence was 1.17/1000 (95% CI, 0.30-2.04) and the relative risk was 3.7 (95% CI, 1.5-9.1). At 42 weeks the prevalence was 0.85/1000 (95% CI, 0.33-1.38) and the relative risk was 2.4 (95% CI, 1.1-5.3). Adjustment for infant sex, maternal age, and various socioeconomic measures had little effect.

Conclusion.—Compared with delivery at 40 weeks' gestation, delivery at 37 or 38 weeks or at 42 weeks or later was associated with an increased risk of CP.

▶ Cerebral palsy (CP) is an umbrella term encompassing a group of nonprogressive, noncontagious motor conditions that cause physical disability in human development, chiefly in the various areas of body movement. Most publications address the high rates and risk of CP with preterm delivery. Nonetheless, numerically, it is the term and near-term infants that account for most cases of CP despite significantly lower risk. This interesting article from a large cohort in Norway documents the prevalence of CP among term infants, clearly delineating a relationship between gestational age and CP. Furthermore, they document that the risk at term and beyond is not uniform. The risk of CP is lowest at 40 weeks, with the highest risks at 37 weeks and at 42 weeks or later. Other neurologic conditions have also been found to vary by gestational age at term. A U-shaped pattern for low IQ was recently reported among term and postterm births.[1] I was intrigued by the postulate that rather than the timing of delivery causing the association, it was the underlying brain injury that disrupted the timing of the delivery. The authors noted:

> "However, an equally plausible interpretation is that fetuses predisposed to CP have a disturbance in the timing of their delivery, which causes them to be more often delivered early or late. This apparently happens with other fetal conditions: there is a U-shaped pattern in the risk of congenital anomalies with gestational age after 37 weeks. Since congenital anomalies are not caused by the timing of delivery, the most plausible explanation is reverse causation; malformed infants experience disruptions in their time of delivery, with increased chance of delivery either earlier or later than 40 weeks."

This line of reasoning is very logical because brain injury and insults leading to CP frequently occur before labor and delivery. It will, however, not be easy to prove since "A definitive answer would require a randomized clinical trial of deliveries at various gestational ages—an impractical option, given the very low prevalence of CP."

A. A. Fanaroff, MD, FRCPE, FRCP&CH

Reference

1. Yang S, Platt RW, Kramer MS. Variation in child cognitive ability by week of gestation among healthy term births. *Am J Epidemiol.* 2010;17:399-406.

Cerebral Palsy, Developmental Delay, and Epilepsy After Neonatal Seizures
Garfinkle J, Shevell MI (Montreal Children's Hosp-McGill Univ Health Ctr, Quebec, Canada; McGill Univ, Montreal, Quebec, Canada)
Pediatr Neurol 44:88-96, 2011

This study sought to identify clinical prognostic factors for cerebral palsy, global developmental delay, and epilepsy in term infants with neonatal seizures. We completed a retrospective analysis of 120 term infants who experienced clinical neonatal seizures at a single academic pediatric neurology practice. Logistic regression analysis determined the significant independent prognostic ($P < 0.05$) indicators of cerebral palsy, global developmental delay, and epilepsy. Fifty-four (45%) infants were never diagnosed with a neurodevelopmental abnormality, whereas 37 (31%) manifested cerebral palsy, 51 (43%) manifested global developmental delay, and 38 (32%) manifested epilepsy. Global developmental delay was present in 92% of the children who manifested spastic quadraparetic cerebral palsy. Seizure type, seizure onset, electroencephalographic background findings, and 5-minute Apgar scores constituted independent predictors of cerebral palsy. None of the children who manifested less than two predictors developed the disorder. For global developmental delay, predictors included method of delivery, seizure onset, electroencephalographic background findings, and etiology. Only one infant (2%) who manifested less than two predictors exhibited global developmental delay. For epilepsy, predictors included seizure type and administration of a second antiepileptic drug. Only one infant (3%) who manifested neither predictor developed the disease.

▶ Drs Garfinkle and Shevell[1] present data on 120 term infants diagnosed clinically with neonatal seizures between 1991 and 2007 and provide data regarding their clinical outcomes and predictors thereof. The strengths of this article include its relatively large sample size and lengthy uniform follow-up (all children were followed clinically by the senior author). The critical weakness of this work is that the diagnosis of seizures was based on clinical criteria rather than electrographic criteria.

Neonatal seizures are notoriously difficult to diagnose based on clinical observation alone. A study by Murray et al[2] illustrates this problem. High-risk infants were monitored with video electroencephalogram, and the results were blinded to the clinical staff. Nurses and physicians were instructed to document clinical events concerning seizures in bedside logs. In all, 9% (48/526) of electrographic seizures were recognized and documented by clinical staff. Conversely, 73% (129/177) of the clinical events documented by the staff had no electrographic correlate: they were not seizures. Since most neonatal seizures are subclinical[3-5] and most abnormal movements are not seizures, studies that define neonatal seizures solely by their clinical manifestations are inherently flawed.

Regardless, this cohort of neonates was clearly at high risk for adverse neurodevelopmental outcomes, with 31% manifesting cerebral palsy, 43% with global developmental delay, and 32% with epilepsy after a median follow-up of 3.5 years for normal survivors and 6.0 years for those with abnormal outcomes. Nine percent of the infants died in the postneonatal period (median age at death was 21 months, range was 6-90 months), suggesting ongoing vulnerability even after the initial critical illness.

Those with cerebral palsy had high rates of comorbid epilepsy (58%) regardless of the cerebral palsy subtype. Among those with spastic quadriparetic cerebral palsy, 92% also manifested global developmental delay (vs 36% of those with hemiplegic cerebral palsy). Intrapartum asphyxia, diagnosed in 52% of the subjects, was closely associated with a later diagnosis of cerebral palsy and global developmental delay but not epilepsy. Overall, outcomes were relatively better for those with focal cerebral abnormalities (eg, stroke or hemorrhage) compared with those with diffuse injuries (eg, birth asphyxia).

The authors emphasize outcome predictors with high sensitivity but relatively low specificity. They found multiple individual variables to be associated with statistically significantly increased odds of cerebral palsy and global developmental delay, but fewer factors were associated with postneonatal epilepsy (in which acute neonatal seizures may resolve, but chronic epilepsy develops later in life).

These results, derived from a large cohort of high-risk infants, may help physicians to focus on particularly relevant factors in their at-risk patients' neonatal course. However, combinations of these predictors were quite sensitive but not terribly specific for the 3 defined adverse outcomes, which somewhat limits their clinical use. It is important to recognize that most of the predictors identified in this study were independent of the infants' clinical seizures (ie, the abnormal clinical events raised concern but may not have been the driving force behind the adverse neurodevelopmental outcomes). Finally, knowing which aspects of neurodevelopmental outcome are most significant to an individual family is important but often overlooked. Further study of families' perceptions of the value of outcome predictors could help to guide both clinicians and researchers in their care and assessments of this vulnerable population.

R. A. Shellhaas, MD, MS

References

1. Garfinkle J, Shevell MI. Cerebral palsy, developmental delay, and epilepsy after neonatal seizures. *Pediatr Neurol.* 2011;44:88-96.
2. Murray DM, Boylan GB, Ali I, Ryan CA, Murphy BP, Connolly S. Defining the gap between electrographic seizure burden, clinical expression and staff recognition of neonatal seizures. *Arch Dis Child Fetal Neonatal Ed.* 2008;93:F187-F191.
3. Clancy RR, Legido A, Lewis D. Occult neonatal seizures. *Epilepsia.* 1988;29:256-261.
4. Scher MS, Alvin J, Gaus L, Minnigh B, Painter MJ. Uncoupling of EEG-clinical neonatal seizures after antiepileptic drug use. *Pediatr Neurol.* 2003;28:277-280.
5. Scher MS, Aso K, Beggarly ME, Hamid MY, Steppe DA, Painter MJ. Electrographic seizures in preterm and full-term neonates: clinical correlates, associated brain lesions, and risk for neurologic sequelae. *Pediatrics.* 1993;91:128-134.

Cool treatment for birth asphyxia, but what's next?
Levene MI (Leeds General Infirmary, UK)
Arch Dis Child Fetal Neonatal Ed 95:F154-F157, 2010

Background.—Moderate hypothermia for 72 hours after severe birth asphyxia reduces both death and disability. The number of normal infants who survive birth asphyxia is significantly higher when hypothermia is used than with traditional treatment. It is likely that adding other neuroprotective agents could have an added benefit. Several neuroprotective agents were reviewed for their ability to improve outcome after asphyxia.

Drugs.—Erythropoietin is a naturally occurring glycoprotein that stimulates erythropoeisis in human newborns and helps avoid neonatal anemia. Postnatal recombinant human erythropoietin (EPO) reduces the need for blood transfusions in very low-birth weight infants. Among its neuroprotective properties are antiapoptotic action; inhibition of the intracerebral cellular inflammatory response; and amelioration of glutamate-induced injury, leading to higher intraneuronal calcium concentrations. Animal studies show that, compared to controls, neonatal rats or mice had better short-term outcomes after cerebral insult and less asymmetrical limb movement after middle cerebral artery occlusion. Studies in human infants reveal that EPO treatment for low-birth weight infants produce better neurodevelopmental outcome than placebo. With term infants having moderate or severe hypoxic ischemic encephalopathy, EPO treatment produces a significantly better primary outcome (death or disability rate) and possibly a neuroprotective effect that lasts over 6 hours after the asphyxial incident.

The naturally occurring hormone melatonin mediates circadian rhythms and is used in pediatric sleep disorders. Its powerful effects reduce neurotoxicity, but white matter is more susceptible to its influence than grey matter. Neuroprotective doses can be as low as 5 mg/kg.

Magnesium sulfate is used to treat hypomagnesemia in newborns. The standard dose is safe, but higher doses may lead to hypotension. It significantly reduces the rate of cerebral palsy in premature infants. Asphyxiated infants treated with magnesium sulfate have a better short-term outcome and lower rate of neurologic abnormalities than those receiving placebo. The effects are most beneficial when it is used shortly after the asphyxial event; adding it to hypothermia may improve the results.

The widely used antiepileptic drug topiramate modulates inhibitor gamma-aminobutyric acid (GABA)-n-mediated neuroreceptors and protects the immature brain after both focal and global asphyxial insult. In asphyxiated rat pups topiramate suppresses acute seizures, reduces neuronal fragmentation, and improves cognitive ability compared to no treatment. The higher (20 mg/kg) dose is more effective than the 10 mg/kg dose, markedly reducing the severity of neuronal injury compared to placebo or the lower dose. The combination of topiramate and hypothermia may be even more effective.

The rare noble gas xenon is commonly employed to measure cerebral blood flow in neonates. It is a potent inhibitor of the N-methyl-D-aspartate (NMDA) receptor channels, has presynaptic activity, and inhibits other glutamate receptor channels. Fifty percent xenon combined with hypothermia has an even more impressive effect in reducing brain damage and improving functional outcome in rats. Female animals respond better than male animals. The use of xenon in humans is limited by the cost and the need for an effective way of scavenging and a rebreathing technique plus ventilator.

Conclusions.—Hypothermia may delay damage from asphyxia and give neuroprotective drugs the chance to minimize adverse outcomes. Several agents are currently available that could be combined with hypothermia to manage infants who suffer asphyxiation. Trials are needed of the combined therapies.

▶ There is now sufficient evidence from multiple randomized controlled trials, as summarized in a recent meta-analysis, to recommend hypothermia as standard treatment for neonates of 36 weeks' gestation or greater with moderate or severe hypoxic-ischemic encephalopathy (HIE), when initiated within 6 hours of birth, in a well-resourced level 3 neonatal intensive care unit. Yet the benefit of hypothermia is modest, and still approximately 40% of hypothermia-treated infants have a poor outcome (disability or death). Thus, there is a need for further trials to improve upon the outcomes of the initial wave of hypothermia trials.

Two potential approaches to improving outcomes with therapeutic hypothermia are to modify cooling protocols (to cool longer and/or deeper, see postscript below) or to combine cooling with a pharmacologic adjunct. This review article focuses on the latter strategy. Given the evidence of safety and efficacy of cooling in a well-resourced setting, either approach to improving upon cooling will randomize infants to an established cooling regimen versus a new cooling regimen or will randomize to standard cooling versus drug + standard cooling.

This review article is suggested reading because it reviews the experimental and clinical evidence in support of several promising pharmacologic agents (erythropoietin, melatonin, magnesium sulfate, topiramate, and xenon) that are approved for human use (in at least some jurisdictions) and that could be tested as combined therapy with hypothermia in infants with HIE. Erythropoietin and magnesium sulfate have each shown promise in single published trials in normothermic infants with HIE. Erythropoietin is being evaluated in combination with hypothermia in a phase I trial (NCT00719407) in the United States, and xenon is being evaluated in combination with the Treatment of Perinatal Asphyxial Encephalopathy hypothermia regimen in a phase II randomized trial in the United Kingdom (NCT00934700).

Although most neonatologists or pediatricians will not directly participate in the clinical trials of drug + hypothermia combination therapy, it is crucial that they be aware of the scientific rationale behind these therapies, as reviewed in this article. The success of any future randomized trials to improve outcomes after hypothermia for HIE is dependent on the willingness of clinicians and families to refer eligible infants to nearby trial centers (where geographically feasible), rather than treating them locally.

Postscript: Although it is not directly related to the focus of this review, American readers should be aware of a clinical trial underway in the centers of the Eunice Kennedy Shriver National Institute of Child Health and Human Development (NICHD) Neonatal Research Network that compares the standard 72-hour NICHD whole body cooling regimen with regimens of longer duration, with lower target temperature, or both (NCT01192776).

J. D. E. Barks, MD

Early postnatal hypotension is not associated with indicators of white matter damage or cerebral palsy in extremely low gestational age newborns
Logan JW, for the ELGAN Study Investigators (Betty H Cameron Women's and Children's Hosp, Wilmington, NC; et al)
J Perinatol 31:524-534, 2011

Objective.—To evaluate, in extremely low gestational age newborns (ELGANs), relationships between indicators of early postnatal hypotension and cranial ultrasound indicators of cerebral white matter damage imaged in the nursery and cerebral palsy diagnoses at 24 months follow-up.

Study Design.—The 1041 infants in this prospective study were born at <28 weeks gestation, were assessed for three indicators of hypotension in the first 24 postnatal hours, had at least one set of protocol cranial ultrasound scans and were evaluated with a structured neurological exam at 24 months corrected age. Indicators of hypotension included: (1) lowest mean arterial pressure (MAP) in the lowest quartile for gestational age; (2) treatment with a vasopressor; and (3) blood pressure lability, defined as the upper quartile of the difference between each infant's lowest and highest MAP. Outcomes included indicators of cerebral white matter damage, that is, moderate/severe ventriculomegaly or an echolucent lesion on cranial ultrasound and cerebral palsy diagnoses at 24 months gestation. Logistic regression was used to evaluate relationships among hypotension indicators and outcomes, adjusting for potential confounders.

Result.—Twenty-one percent of surviving infants had a lowest blood pressure in the lowest quartile for gestational age, 24% were treated with vasopressors and 24% had labile blood pressure. Among infants with these hypotension indicators, 10% percent developed ventriculomegaly and 7% developed an echolucent lesion. At 24 months follow-up, 6% had developed quadriparesis, 4% diparesis and 2% hemiparesis. After adjusting for confounders, we found no association between indicators of hypotension, and indicators of cerebral white matter damage or a cerebral palsy diagnosis.

Conclusion.—The absence of an association between indicators of hypotension and cerebral white matter damage and or cerebral palsy suggests that early hypotension may not be important in the pathogenesis of brain injury in ELGANs.

▶ Clinicians undertake the treatment of early postnatal hypotension in the belief that doing so will prevent or at least mitigate brain injury. However, without tools to accurately measure regional oxygen delivery to brain tissue, it is not possible to determine a critical level of blood pressure that requires treatment and whether such treatment is efficacious. In this secondary analysis of the extremely low gestational age (ELGANs) study, the authors imply that early postnatal hypotension is not associated with brain injury.

ELGANs is a multicenter observational study that was designed to identify characteristics and exposures that increase the risk of structural and functional neurological disorders in infants who were delivered before 28 weeks of gestational age. The definitions of hypotension in the current report were based on retrospective analysis of prospectively collected data. Mean blood pressure less than gestational age, the most common definition of hypotension used by clinicians, was not included because approximately two-thirds of the cohort was hypotensive using this criterion. Similarly, volume expansion was not used, as 75% of the cohort received bolus infusions in the first 24 hours after birth.

One of the strengths of a multicenter observational study is that it reflects common clinical practice in each of the participating centers. This is also an inherent weakness, because clinical practice often varies between centers. The data presented suggest that hypotension as defined in the study was not associated with cranial ultrasound lesions considered indicators of white matter damage or cerebral palsy at 24 months of corrected age. However, as the authors acknowledge in the discussion, the data are confounded by several factors, such as the inclusion of blood pressure measurements obtained by oscillometry, variable frequency of blood pressure measurements, and the frequent use of volume expansion. In addition, 2 of the variables used to define hypotension (lowest mean arterial blood pressure in the lowest quartile for gestational age and blood pressure lability) are not clinically useful because they are unique to the data set. Until randomized clinical trials are used to evaluate the efficacy of treatments to raise blood pressure in extremely low birth weight infants, no consensus will be reached regarding the management of early postnatal hypotension.

L. A. Papile, MD

Efficacy of Intravitreal Bevacizumab for Stage 3+ Retinopathy of Prematurity

Mintz-Hittner HA, for the BEAT-ROP Cooperative Group (Univ of Texas Health Science Ctr at Houston—Med School)
N Engl J Med 364:603-615, 2011

Background.—Retinopathy of prematurity is a leading cause of childhood blindness worldwide. Peripheral retinal ablation with conventional (confluent) laser therapy is destructive, causes complications, and does not prevent all vision loss, especially in cases of retinopathy of prematurity affecting zone I of the eye. Case series in which patients were treated with vascular endothelial growth factor inhibitors suggest that these agents may be useful in treating retinopathy of prematurity.

Methods.—We conducted a prospective, controlled, randomized, stratified, multicenter trial to assess intravitreal bevacizumab monotherapy for zone I or zone II posterior stage 3+ (i.e., stage 3 with plus disease) retinopathy of prematurity. Infants were randomly assigned to receive intravitreal bevacizumab (0.625 mg in 0.025 ml of solution) or conventional laser therapy, bilaterally. The primary ocular outcome was recurrence of retinopathy of prematurity in one or both eyes requiring retreatment before 54 weeks' postmenstrual age.

Results.—We enrolled 150 infants (total sample of 300 eyes); 143 infants survived to 54 weeks' postmenstrual age, and the 7 infants who died were not included in the primaryoutcome analyses. Retinopathy of prematurity recurred in 4 infants in the bevacizumab group (6 of 140 eyes [4%]) and 19 infants in the laser-therapy group (32 of 146 eyes [22%], P = 0.002). A significant treatment effect was found for zone I retinopathy of prematurity (P = 0.003) but not for zone II disease (P = 0.27).

Conclusions.—Intravitreal bevacizumab monotherapy, as compared with conventional laser therapy, in infants with stage 3+ retinopathy of prematurity showed a significant benefit for zone I but not zone II disease. Development of peripheral retinal vessels continued after treatment with intravitreal bevacizumab, but conventional laser therapy led to permanent destruction of the peripheral retina. This trial was too small to assess safety. (Funded by Research to Prevent Blindness and others; ClinicalTrials.gov number, NCT00622726.)

▶ The frequency of retinopathy of prematurity (ROP) is inversely proportional to gestational age and, with increasing survival of the most immature infants, is commonplace in today's neonatal intensive care unit population. Recent statistics indicate that the overall rate is greater than 70% among infants born at less than 27 weeks of gestational age and that approximately 10% will develop stage 3 disease. Because ROP in zone 1 can progress rapidly to retinal detachment, ophthalmologists frequently recommend laser therapy when stage 3 is noted, whether or not plus disease is present. Laser therapy for zone 1 ROP is successful in approximately 50% of cases, but it inevitably causes permanent loss of peripheral visual fields and often induces clinically significant myopia.

ROP is thought to be a biphasic disease consisting of an initial phase of oxygen-induced vascular obliteration followed by a period of hypoxia-induced vessel proliferation; the latter phase is associated with elevated levels of vascular endothelial growth factor (VEGF). This study is the first randomized clinical trial in which bevacizumab, a humanized murine monoclonal antibody against all isoforms of human VEGF, was used as a primary treatment of ROP.

The results of the trial are enticing and most likely will result in the displacement of laser therapy as the preferred treatment of zone 1, stage 3 + ROP, especially since the editorial accompanying the report stated that bevacizumab should become the treatment of choice for zone 1 ROP. However, as noted by the authors, the sample size for the trial was insufficient to assess the safety of bevacizumab. As we have learned from previous studies, such as the use of dexamethasone for the prevention/amelioration of bronchopulmonary dysplasia, it is only after there is widespread use of promising therapies that the safety/efficacy can truly be assessed. Unfortunately, because the use of bevacizumab is off-label, there is no mechanism in place to track the potential adverse effects.

L. A. Papile, MD

Fish-Oil Fat Emulsion Supplementation May Reduce the Risk of Severe Retinopathy in VLBW Infants

Pawlik D, Lauterbach R, Turyk E (Jagiellonian Univ Med College, Kraków, Kopernika, Poland)
Pediatrics 127:223-228, 2011

Objective.—The retina contains rods and cones that have membranes highly enriched with docosahexaenoic acid (DHA). Infants born prematurely are at risk of DHA insufficiency, because they may not have benefited from a full third trimester of the mother's lipid stores. Moreover, within the first 2 to 3 weeks of life, the main sources of lipids for premature infants are fat emulsions, which do not contain DHA.

Patients and Methods.—This observational study was designed to compare the safety and efficacy outcomes of an intravenous fat emulsion that consists of fish-oil emulsion (contains DHA) with soybean and olive oil, administered from the first day of life to 40 infants who weighed <1250 g; results were obtained from a historical cohort of 44 preterm neonates who were given an emulsion of soybean and olive oil. The primary study outcomes were the occurrence of retinopathy and need for laser therapy and cholestasis. Infants in the 2 groups were comparable with regard to demographic and clinical characteristics and were subjected to the same conventional therapy.

Results.—There was a significantly lower risk of laser therapy for infants who received an emulsion of soybean, olive oil, and fish oil ($P = .023$). No significant differences were found in acuity and latency of visual evoked potentials between infants in the 2 groups. There was no infant with cholestasis among those who received fish-oil emulsion, and there were 5 subjects with cholestasis in the historical group ($P = .056$).

Conclusion.—Fish-oil–based fat emulsion administered from the first day of life may be effective in the prophylaxis of severe retinopathy.

▶ This article provides interesting preliminary information about the efficacy of providing intravenous docosahexaenoic acid (DHA) to preterm infants with birth weights less than 1250 g starting the first few days after birth. The investigators used a scheme where they increased the intravenous lipid intake in increments (which is based on tradition rather than science), with approximately one-third of the lipid being in the form of Omegaven, an intravenous preparation derived from fish oil that is rich in preformed DHA. A historical group that closely matched the experimental group was chosen as a control. The major outcome difference between the 2 groups was a lower incidence of retinopathy with laser therapy in the experimental DHA group versus the control group (7.5% vs 27%, $P = .023$). There was also a trend toward less cholestasis in the experimental group.

To my knowledge and that of the authors, this was the first study of an intravenous fish oil–based preparation to determine whether this would be effective in prevention of retinopathy and cholestasis. The results suggest a benefit along with safety, but the retrospective nature of the study begs for more extensive randomized trials. A concern for proceeding in the direction of intravenous supplementation in these infants is that they have a functioning gastrointestinal tract that should be able to tolerate long-chain lipids and may also benefit from the anti-inflammatory effect of the long-chain omega-3 on the intestine. Rather than designing prospective studies using intravenous omega-3 lipid, why can't this be supplied by the enteral route?

J. Neu, MD

Hypothermia after Perinatal Asphyxia: Selection for Treatment and Cooling Protocol

Thoresen M (Univ of Bristol, UK)
J Pediatr 158:e45-e49, 2011

Three large randomized controlled trials have demonstrated benefits from 3 days of cooling to 33-34°C after perinatal asphyxia. No serious adverse effects were documented. The trials excluded many infants for hypothermia (HT) therapy, including those of age >6 hours and those with prematurity of <36 weeks gestation, abnormal coagulation, persistent pulmonary hypertension, and congenital abnormalities. This article considers whether the foregoing trial exclusion criteria are feasible given current knowledge and evidence. HT affects the validity of some outcome predictors (eg, clinical examination, amplitude-integrated electroencephalography), but not of magnetic resonance imaging. HT is a time-critical emergency treatment after perinatal asphyxia that requires optimal collaboration among local hospitals, transport teams, and cooling centers.

▶ Dr Thoresen has been a pioneer in neonatal hypothermic neuroprotection. In this article, she reviewed 3 major randomized trials of cooling—the CoolCap, National Institute of Child Health and Human Development Neonatal Research Network Whole Body Cooling Trial, and the Total body hypothermia for neonatal encephalopathy trial (also whole-body cooling). Her focus was on exclusionary criteria; the article was an exceptional review of information derived from the 3 trials.

While neuroprotective hypothermia improved outcomes of infants treated under the rigorous observation of well-done clinical trials, are we likely to see the same results now that it has become the standard of care following severe intrapartum asphyxia? My hunch is that it won't. The seemingly incredibly low rate of complications and the number needed to treat of 9 make cooling an attractive treatment for clinicians to apply to even mildly encephalopathic newborns, perhaps even extend the therapy to less mature infants and to those older than the 6-hour limit imposed in the initial trials.

As Dr Thoresen cautions, and please pardon the pun, our understanding of hypothermia is just at the tip of the iceberg. We still have much to learn, and we will only accomplish this through more investigation.

S. M. Donn, MD

Clinical Seizures in Neonatal Hypoxic-Ischemic Encephalopathy Have No Independent Impact on Neurodevelopmental Outcome: Secondary Analyses of Data from the Neonatal Research Network Hypothermia Trial

Kwon JM, for the Eunice Kennedy Shriver National Institute of Child Health and Human Development Neonatal Research Network (Univ of Rochester, NY; et al)
J Child Neurol 26:322-328, 2011

It remains controversial as to whether neonatal seizures have additional direct effects on the developing brain separate from the severity of the underlying encephalopathy. Using data collected from infants diagnosed with hypoxic-ischemic encephalopathy, and who were enrolled in an National Institute of Child Health and Human Development trial of hypothermia, we analyzed associations between neonatal clinical seizures and outcomes at 18 months of age. Of the 208 infants enrolled, 102 received whole body hypothermia and 106 were controls. Clinical seizures were generally noted during the first 4 days of life and rarely afterward. When adjustment was made for study treatment and severity of encephalopathy, seizures were not associated with death, or moderate or severe disability, or lower Bayley Mental Development Index scores at 18 months of life. Among infants diagnosed with hypoxic-ischemic encephalopathy, the mortality and morbidity often attributed to neonatal seizures can be better explained by the underlying severity of encephalopathy.

▶ The results of the study need to be interpreted cautiously, because it is a secondary analysis of a large clinical trial. Limitations of the study include the accuracy of the data regarding the diagnosis of neonatal seizures and the power of the analysis to support the conclusion that neonatal seizures do not contribute to the poor outcome of infants with hypoxic-ischemic encephalopathy. The study is a secondary analysis of the National Institute of Child Health and Human Development (NICD) Neonatal Research Network clinical trial of therapeutic hypothermia and, as such, includes only infants categorized as having moderate to severe encephalopathy. The main trial did not include a standardized method for the diagnosis of clinical seizure, but rather relied on the judgment of site investigators. As the authors acknowledge in the discussion, there was wide variability in the rate of seizure diagnosis by center, suggesting that the criteria for diagnosing seizures differed among centers. In addition, the sample size was relatively small and was predicted to have 80% power to detect a 50% increase in adverse outcomes in the seizure group.

Clinical seizures were reported in 127 (61%) of the 208 infants enrolled in the trial. Of the 81 infants assigned to the no-seizure group, 25% (20/81) had missing data on the occurrence of clinical seizures. Significantly more infants with clinical seizures were classified as having severe hypoxic-ischemic encephalopathy (HIE) (44% vs 21%, $P \leq .001$). Although the allocation of infants with clinical seizures to the 2 treatment arms was not statistically different ($P = .09$), there was a higher proportion of infants with clinical seizures in the control group (57% vs 44%). On univariate analysis, a higher proportion of infants diagnosed as having clinical seizures were either dead or disabled ($P = .003$). When multivariate logistic regression modeling controlling for the effects of hypothermia treatment and severity of HIE was performed, the effects of seizures on neurodevelopmental outcome were no longer significant.

In the abstract, the authors state that the morbidity and mortality often attributed to neonatal seizures can be better explained by the underlying severity of HIE. Given the limitations of the data, this would seem to be an overstatement. It will require a more rigorous study with sufficient power and objective criteria for the ascertainment of seizures before the true impact of neonatal seizures in the setting of HIE can be determined.

L. A. Papile, MD

Long-Term Clinical Outcome of Neonatal EEG Findings
Almubarak S, Wong PKH (British Columbia Children's Hosp, Vancouver, Canada; Univ of British Columbia, Vancouver, Canada)
J Clin Neurophysiol 28:185-189, 2011

The aim of the study is to determine how specific EEG findings during neonatal period correlate with clinical outcome on follow-up. This is a retrospective study of 118 term newborns who had EEG in the first month of life and subsequent clinical assessment between 4 and 16 years. Clinical neurologic outcome was classified into "favorable" when patients had no or only mild limitation in assessment, "unfavorable" when patients had moderate to severe abnormalities in assessment, and "epilepsy" when patients had seizures. Of the 118 neonates, 36 (30.5%) had favorable and 82 (69.5%) had unfavorable outcome; 89 (75.4%) had epilepsy and 28 (23.7%) had not. Sixty-seven (57%) had abnormal EEG background of which 56 had both unfavorable outcome and epilepsy; 102 (86%) had sharp transient discharges of which 75 had unfavorable outcome; 20 (17%) had ictal epileptiform discharges of which 18 had unfavorable outcome; 98 (83%) had abnormal overall EEG impression of which 77 had unfavorable outcome and 80 had epilepsy. Abnormal EEG background (particularly suppression) during neonatal period may be predictive of Unfavorable outcome. Overall impression of EEG may be predictive of clinical outcome, even when individual parameters were not predictive. Other findings did not appear to be predictive.

▶ This study may be helpful to clinical neonatologists in their discussions with families regarding the prognosis of neonatal seizures in term infants.

The authors reviewed the electroencephalograph (EEG) database at British Columbia Children's Hospital for the period 1992 to 2009. Infants were included if they were 37 to 42 weeks of gestational age, had at least one EEG in the first month, and had at least 1 clinical follow-up assessment after 4 years of age. Clinical outcome was classified as unfavorable when there were moderate or severe limitations with regard to developmental milestones, school performance, and neurologic examination.

The most common findings on EEG were sharp transient discharges (86%) and an abnormal background (57%); ictal epileptiform discharges were noted in only 17%. Sharp transient discharges were associated with the lowest risk of an unfavorable outcome (74%), ictal epileptiform discharges were associated with the highest (90%), and abnormal background was intermediate (84%). The subsequent development of epilepsy was essentially the same regardless of EEG findings and ranged from 78% to 84%.

The etiology of seizures included hypoxic-ischemic encephalopathy (32%), metabolic (17%), and stroke (9%). No etiology was found in 17% of the cases. The frequency of both an unfavorable outcome and epilepsy was 82% for infants with hypoxic-ischemic encephalopathy. The prognosis was better for infants in whom the cause of seizures was unknown (unfavorable outcome 53%; epilepsy 74%). Neonatal stroke was associated with the best prognosis (unfavorable outcome 43%; epilepsy 74%).

L. A. Papile, MD

Oral D-penicillamine for the prevention of retinopathy of prematurity in very low birth weight infants: a randomized, placebo-controlled trial
Tandon M, Dutta S, Dogra MR, et al (Postgraduate Inst of Med Education and Res (PGIMER), Chandigarh, Punjab, India)
Acta Paediatr 99:1324-1328, 2010

Purpose.—To compare prophylactic enteral D-penicillamine (DPA) with placebo for prevention of 'retinopathy of prematurity (ROP) or death' among very low birth weight (VLBW) infants.

Methods.—This was a double-blind, single-centre, randomized, placebo-controlled trial with stratification (for birth weight <1250 and ≥1250 g) and blocking. Inborn neonates with birth weight 750−1500 g, gestation ≤32 weeks, age ≤5 days, who tolerated feeds were eligible. Neonates with gastro-intestinal malformations, life-threatening malformations and necrotizing enterocolitis were excluded. Enrolled subjects were randomly allocated to receive oral DPA suspension at 100 mg/kg/dose 8 h for 3 days, followed by 50 mg/kg/day for another 11 days or placebo. The primary outcome was 'any ROP or death'. Secondary outcomes included any ROP, treatable ROP, adverse effects and feed intolerance.

Results.—A total of 88 subjects were enrolled. Baseline characteristics were similar with the exception of multiple gestation. There were no significant differences in primary and secondary outcomes, even after adjusting for multiple gestation and on sub-group analysis. No adverse reaction was noted.

Conclusion.—Prophylactic enterally administered DPA suspension in a dose 100 mg/kg/dose 8 h for 3 days, followed by 50 mg/kg once per day for next 11 days, does not prevent 'any stage ROP or death' or

'ROP requiring treatment' in VLBW infants. DPA is well tolerated and does not have any major short-term adverse effects.

▶ It is interesting that after many years of evaluating the potential benefits of anti-oxidants such as vitamins E and A to prevent or treat retinopathy of prematurity, we have not been successful. Even the use of human milk, which appears to have so many other beneficial outcomes for preterm infants, has not shown definite benefit. This study, which also attempted to test another agent, D-penicillamine, a free radical scavenger that has been shown to protect biomembranes, also did not show benefit. So is it possible we are barking up the wrong tree with the use of antioxidants? Should we be considering other potentially useful therapies that act on vasculogenesis and angiogenesis, which seem to be more proximal components of the disease pathogenesis than oxidative stress and may be a rela-tively late component? Should we be evaluating specific nutrients, pharmacologic agents, or nutraceuticals that act on insulin-like growth factor and vascular endo-thelial growth factor and inflammatory pathways instead?

J. Neu, MD

Passive cooling for initiation of therapeutic hypothermia in neonatal encephalopathy
Kendall GS, on behalf of the Cooling on Retrieval Study Group (Univ College London, UK; et al)
Arch Dis Child Fetal Neonatal Ed 95:F408-F412, 2010

Objective.—To determine the feasibility of passive cooling to initiate therapeutic hypothermia before and during transport.

Methods.—Consensus guidelines were developed for passive cooling at the referring hospital and on transport by the London Neonatal Transfer Service. These were evaluated in a prospective study.

Results.—Between January and October 2009, 39 infants were referred for therapeutic hypothermia; passive cooling was initiated at the referring hospital in all the cases. Despite guidance, no rectal temperature measure-ments were taken before arrival of the transfer team. Cooling below target temperature (33°C−34°C) occurred in five babies before the arrival of the transfer team. In two of these infants, active cooling was performed, rectal temperature was not recorded and their temperature was lower than 32°C. Of the remaining 37 babies, 33 (89%) demonstrated a reduction in core temperature with passive cooling alone. The percentage of the babies within the temperature range at referral, arrival of the transfer team and arrival at the cooling centre were 0%, 15% and 67%, respectively. On arrival at the cooling centre, four babies had cooled to lower than 33°C by passive cool-ing alone (32.7°C, 32.6°C, 32.2°C and 32.1°C). Initiation of passive cool-ing before and during transfer resulted in the therapy starting 4.6 (1.8) h earlier than if initiated on arrival at the cooling centre.

Conclusions.—Passive cooling is a simple and effective technique if portable cooling equipment is unavailable. Rectal temperature monitoring is essential; active cooling methods without core temperature monitoring may lead to overcooling.

▶ Therapeutic hypothermia is currently the only effective therapy available for the treatment of neonatal encephalopathy. However, most babies who are eligible for treatment are born in community hospitals and there is often a delay in treatment until the baby can be transferred to a regional center. In animal models of neonatal encephalopathy, therapeutic hypothermia is most effective when treatment is initiated shortly after birth. As a consequence, the practice of passively cooling babies at the referring hospital and on transport is becoming more widespread.

In this observational study, the investigators evaluated the safety and efficacy of passive cooling after consensus guidelines were developed and disseminated. Since continuous rectal temperature was not available in any of the referring hospitals, the guidelines stipulated that skin temperature be monitored continuously and intermittent rectal temperature be monitored every 15 minutes. If it was not usual practice to take rectal temperatures, axillary temperatures could be used as a substitute. Notably, none of the babies had a rectal temperature recorded at the referral hospital, and only 15% of the babies were in the target temperature range when the transfer team measured rectal temperature upon arrival. Analysis of data regarding available rectal-skin and rectal-axillary temperatures revealed that skin temperature did not accurately reflect rectal temperature and axillary temperature correlated with rectal temperature with a mean difference of 0.1°C (95% limits of agreement -1.1°C to 1.3°C).

In order for passive cooling in referring hospitals to be applied successfully, it is essential that rectal temperatures be monitored. As in the United Kingdom, rectal temperatures of neonates are rarely taken in US hospitals and, in fact, are precluded for safety reasons. It behooves centers that offer therapeutic cooling to develop guidelines for their referral hospitals and to take an active role in educating personnel who care for newborns in their referral area about the need for rectal temperature monitoring when a baby is being passively cooled.

L. A. Papile, MD

Perinatal Events and Early Magnetic Resonance Imaging in Therapeutic Hypothermia
Bonifacio SI, Glass HC, Vanderpluym J, et al (Univ of California, San Francisco; Univ of Alberta, Edmonton, Canada)
J Pediatr 158:360-365, 2011

Objective.—To compare the association between perinatal events and the pattern and extent of brain injury on early magnetic resonance imaging in newborn infants with and without therapeutic hypothermia for hypoxic-ischemic encephalopathy.

Study Design.—We performed a cohort study of 35 treated and 25 non-treated neonates who underwent magnetic resonance imaging. The injury patterns were defined a priori as: normal, watershed, or basal ganglia/thalamuspredominant, as well as a dichotomous outcome of moderate-to-severe versus mild-no injury.

Results.—Neonates with hypothermia had less extensive watershed and basal ganglia/thalamus injuries and a greater proportion had normal imaging. Therapeutic hypothermia was associated with a decreased risk of both basal ganglia/thalamus injury (relative risk, 0.29; 95% CI, 0.10 to 0.81, *P* =.01) and moderate-severe injury. Neonates with sentinel events showed a decrease in basal ganglia/thalamus-predominant injury and an increase in normal imaging. All neonates with decreased fetal movements had injury, predominantly watershed, regardless of therapeutic hypothermia.

Conclusions.—These results validate reports of reduced brain injury after therapeutic hypothermia and suggest that perinatal factors are important indicators of response to treatment.

▶ In this observational study, the authors evaluated the impact of perinatal factors on brain injury among infants who did or did not undergo therapeutic hypothermia for presumed hypoxic-ischemic encephalopathy. Perinatal factors that were evaluated included maternal report of decreased fetal movement, fetal distress during labor (variable decelerations, late decelerations, fetal brady-cardia, fetal tachycardia, lack of heart rate variability), and perinatal sentinel events (placental abruption, uterine rupture, umbilical cord accident, neonatal anemia/hypovolemia). Therapeutic hypothermia was noted to be most effective when there was a sentinel event. Most treated infants who had an acute event (62%) had normal imaging compared with none of the nontreated infants. All of the infants with a history of decreased fetal movement had brain injury regard-less of treatment, although the extent of injury was less in treated infants. As the authors note, these observations support the hypothesis that hypothermia lessens secondary energy failure in the brain after an acute ischemic event and that it may not be as effective in situations where chronic ischemia or hypoxia contributes to the brain injury.

L. A. Papile, MD

Possible roles of bilirubin and breast milk in protection against retinopathy of prematurity
Kao JS, Dawson JD, Murray JC, et al (Univ of Iowa, Iowa City)
Acta Paediatr 100:347-351, 2011

Aim.—To explore the association of serum bilirubin level and breast milk feeding with retinopathy of prematurity (ROP) in preterm infants.

Methods.—We conducted a case—control study to examine the independent and combined effects of serum bilirubin and breast milk feeding on

ROP risk in infants <32 weeks gestation or with birth weight <1500 g. Cases (66 infants with ROP) were matched with controls (66 infants without ROP) based on factors known to affect ROP risk.

Results.—When analysed using the paired t-test, the peak bilirubin levels were lower in ROP cases than in controls (mean 7.2 vs. 7.9 mg/dL; p = 0.045). Using conditional logistic regression, we found a negative association between highest serum bilirubin level and risk of ROP (OR = 0.82 per 1-mg/dL change in bilirubin; p = 0.06). There was no significant association between breast milk feeding and risk of ROP.

Conclusion.—Bilirubin may help to protect preterm infants against ROP.

▶ Retinopathy of prematurity (ROP) is a major complication of preterm birth. The pathogenesis is complex and includes vasoobliteration and compensatory neovascularization steps.[1] Along with vasoobliteration, there is an increase in reactive oxygen species (ROS) concentrations that are cytotoxic to retinal microvasculature. The ability of the retina to generate excessive ROS is not counterbalanced by antioxidants, which are deficient in the immature subject relative to the adult since the low oxygen—exposed fetus has modest needs for antioxidants in utero.

Bilirubin, the end product of heme catabolism in mammals, is generally regarded as a potentially cytotoxic waste product that needs to be excreted. At micromolar concentrations in vitro, bilirubin efficiently scavenges peroxyl radicals. The antioxidant activity of bilirubin increases as the experimental concentration of oxygen is decreased from 20% (that of normal air) to 2% (physiologically relevant concentration). The data support the idea of a beneficial role for bilirubin as a physiological antioxidant.[2]

The concept that bilirubin may be a protective antioxidant is therefore not a new one, and as mentioned in this article, it has been previously studied, but the results have been equivocal. This study, unlike previous studies, examined the effects of 2 predictor variables (human milk feeding and bilirubin concentrations) on the development of ROP. This was done using a case-control analysis of the independent and combined effects of serum bilirubin and breast milk feeding on ROP risk in infants less than 32 weeks' gestation or with birth weight less than 1500 g. When analyzed using the paired t-test, the peak bilirubin levels were about 10% lower in ROP cases than in controls (mean 7.2 vs 7.9 mg/dL; $P = .045$). There was no significant association between breast milk feeding and risk of ROP. The authors conclude after several caveats about the pitfalls in the methodology of their analysis and urging future additional studies that bilirubin may help to protect preterm infants against ROP.

Although these results need cautious interpretation and cannot be immediately applied to prevention of ROP in babies, it raises the question of why vitamin E, a potent antioxidant that can readily be used as a nutritional adjunct, has not consistently been shown to be beneficial in the prevention of ROP. One reason may be that studies have shown that with less than 2% oxygen, in liposomes, bilirubin suppresses the oxidation more than alpha-tocopherol,[2] which is regarded by many as the best nutritional antioxidant of lipid peroxidation.

It is not yet clear how knowledge about bilirubin as an antioxidant can be used to assist in the defense against oxidative stress. At this time, simply based on current knowledge from this study, we should not allow elevated levels in the neonate to persist for an unknown time to protect the infant. We do not know the level at which irreparable harm might be done. Nevertheless, this finding may provide important clues for other avenues of ROP prevention based on the structure and function of the bilirubin molecule and its metabolites.

J. Neu, MD

References

1. Sapieha P, Joyal JS, Rivera JC, et al. Retinopathy of prematurity: understanding ischemic retinal vasculopathies at an extreme of life. *J Clin Invest.* 2010;120: 3022-3032.
2. Stocker R, Yamamoto Y, McDonagh AF, Glazer AN, Ames BN. Bilirubin is an antioxidant of possible physiological importance. *Science.* 1987;235:1043-1046.

Potential Neuronal Repair in Cerebral White Matter Injury in the Human Neonate
Haynes RL, Xu G, Folkerth RD, et al (Harvard Med School, Boston, MA; Brigham and Women's Hosp, Boston, MA; et al)
Pediatr Res 69:62-67, 2011

Periventricular leukomalacia (PVL) in the premature infant represents the major substrate underlying cognitive deficits and cerebral palsy and is characterized as focal periventricular necrosis and diffuse gliosis in the immature cerebral white matter. We have recently shown a significant decrease in the density of neurons in PVL relative to controls throughout the white matter, including the subventricular, periventricular, and subcortical regions. These neurons are likely to be remnants of the subplate and/or GABAergic neurons in late migration to the cerebral cortex, both of which are important for proper cortical circuitry in development and throughout adulthood. Here, we tested the hypothesis that intrinsic repair occurs in PVL to attempt to compensate for the deficits in white matter neurons. By using doublecortin (DCX) immunopositivity as a marker of postmitotic migrating neurons, we found significantly increased densities ($p < 0.05$) of DCX-immunopositive cells in PVL cases ($n = 9$) compared with controls ($n = 7$) in the subventricular zone (their presumed site of origin), necrotic foci, and subcortical white matter in the perinatal time-window, *i.e.* 35– 42 postconceptional weeks. These data provide the first evidence suggestive of an attempt at neuronal repair or regeneration in human neonatal white matter injury.

▶ Lesions of the intracranial white matter represent the common final pathway of many types of perinatal brain injury. The form of neonatal white matter injury commonly called periventricular leukomalacia (PVL) is highly associated with later neurodevelopmental deficits, including cerebral palsy. To date, we have assumed that PVL is irreversible and its associated white matter injury inevitably becomes more evident as the baby grows and neurodevelopment becomes increasingly dependent on myelination of white matter tracts. In this pathological study, Dr Haynes and colleagues examined brains of 9 infants with PVL (mean gestational age 36 weeks) and 7 control infants (median age 38 weeks) who died of a variety of causes, including congenital heart disease, sepsis, and necrotizing enterocolitis. These investigators found what appears to be the first documented evidence of attempted neuronal repair at sites of neonatal white matter injury. Using doublecortin (DCX) immunopositivity as a marker of postmitotic migrating neurons, the investigators found significantly increased numbers of DCX immunopositive cells in PVL subjects in the regions of injury: subventricular zone, necrotic foci, and subcortical white matter. Although most of the infants in this study were born at or near full-term gestation, if replicated, these findings will open the door to a potentially revolutionary new field of study that someday might offer the potential of biologically manipulating the white matter repair process and thereby eliminate or ameliorate the neurodevelopmental sequelae of perinatal brain injury.

L. J. Van Marter, MD, MPH

Serial MRI and Neurodevelopmental Outcome in 9- to 10-Year-Old Children with Neonatal Encephalopathy

van Kooij BJM, van Handel M, Nievelstein RAJ, et al (Univ Med Ctr, Utrecht, The Netherlands)
J Pediatr 157:221-227, 2010

Objective.—To assess the relation between patterns of brain injury on neonatal and childhood magnetic resonance imaging (MRI) and long-term neurodevelopmental outcome.

Study Design.—Neonatal (n = 34) and childhood MRIs (n = 77) were analyzed for 80 children with neonatal encephalopathy and for 51 control subjects during childhood. MRIs were graded as normal, mildly abnormal (white matter lesions), or moderately/severely abnormal (watershed injury, lesions in basal ganglia/thalamus or focal infarction). Severity of brain injury was related to different aspects of neurologic outcome: Total impairment score of the Movement Assessment Battery for Children, intelligence quotient score, cerebralpalsy, postneonatal epilepsy, and need for special education. Seven children with neonatal encephalopathy required extracorporeal membrane oxygenation treatment.

Results.—Neonatal and childhood MRI were comparable in 25/33 children (75.8%, P < .001). Children with moderate/severe lesions on neonatal or childhood MRI more often had a total impairment score ≤15th percentile, an intelligence quotient ≤85, and cerebral palsy, and attended special education.

Conclusion.—Different patterns of injury seen on neonatal MRI after neonatal encephalopathy can still be recognized on childhood MRI.

Children with moderate to severe brain lesions on neonatal or childhood MRI significantly more often have impaired motor and cognitive outcomes.

▶ Although only 80 of the 122 surviving infants with hypoxic-ischemic encephalopathy (HIE) are included in this observational study, several of the findings are notable. The first is that none of the infants with severe HIE survived the neonatal period. The second relates to the importance of including a matched control group when conducting research related to neurodevelopmental outcomes. The mean estimated IQ score for children with mild HIE without cerebral palsy was within the normal range (99 ± 14); however, it was significantly lower than the mean estimated IQ score of 109 ± 12 in the control group ($P = .019$). Additionally, 12% attended special education compared with none of the control group and 9% had impairments in motor coordination. Although several studies have shown that children with mild HIE are not at increased risk of severe neurodevelopmental impairment, the results of the current study indicate that children with mild HIE experience more motor and cognitive difficulties than expected.

L. A. Papile, MD

The spectrum of associated brain lesions in cerebral sinovenous thrombosis: relation to gestational age and outcome
Kersbergen KJ, Groenendaal F, Benders MJNL, et al (Univ Med Centre, Utrecht, The Netherlands; et al)
Arch Dis Child Fetal Neonatal Ed 2011 [Epub ahead of print]

Objective.—To describe different patterns of associated brain lesions in preterm and full-term infants with cerebral sinovenous thrombosis (CSVT) and to assess whether these different patterns are related to gestational age at onset.

Design.—Magnetic resonance scans of all neonates (six preterm, 24 full term) with suspected CSVT, collected over a 7-year period in two neonatal intensive care units, were evaluated to assess patterns of associated brain lesions. Comparisons between the two gestational age groups were made.

Results.—CSVT was confirmed on magnetic resonance venography in 26 of 30 neonates (six preterm, 20≥36 weeks' gestational age). The straight (85%) and superior sagittal (65%) sinus were most often affected. Several sinuses were involved in 81% of infants. White matter damage affecting the entire periventricular white matter was seen in fi ve of six preterm infants. Intraventricular haemorrhage (IVH) was common in both groups (4/6 preterm, 16/20 full term). Frontal punctate white matter lesions with restricted diffusion (15/20) and thalamic haemorrhage associated with IVH (11/20) were the most frequent lesions in full-term infants. Focal arterial infarction was present in four of 20 full-term infants. Six infants died in the neonatal period (four preterm, two full term). Follow-up MRIs at 3 months in all survivors showed evolution of the lesions with frontal atrophy in 13 of 20 (12 full term) and delayed myelination in seven of 20 (six full term).

Conclusions.—Preterm and full-term neonates show different patterns of associated brain lesions. Extensive white matter damage is the predominant pattern of injury in the preterm infant, while an IVH associated with a thalamic haemorrhage and punctate white matter lesions are more common in the full-term infant.

▶ Although most periventricular, intraventricular hemorrhages (PIVHs) in preterm infants are thought to arise from hemorrhage in the subependymal germinal matrix or obstruction of the veins draining the lateral cerebral ventricles, this case series is a reminder that thromboses of the cerebral sinuses may also result in PIVH. The mean gestational age of the affected preterm infants was 32 weeks (range 30 + 0 to 35 + 1 weeks) and the onset of clinical signs was at a mean age of 9 days (range 1−28 days). The most common finding among the preterm cohort was extensive white matter lesions affecting the entire periventricular white matter (5/6 infants) with an associated intraventricular hemorrhage noted in 4 infants. The lesions were not noted on cranial ultrasound until after 7 days of age in 3 of the 6 preterm infants. Only 2 infants survived the neonatal period and both were noted to have severe psychomotor retardation on follow-up evaluation. Their magnetic resonance imaging studies at 3 to 7 months of age showed multicystic leukomalacia in one and frontal atrophy with a delay in myelination in the other. These results suggest that cerebral sinovenous thrombosis needs to be considered in preterm infants presenting with late-onset bilateral white matter injury associated with an intraventricular hemorrhage.

L. A. Papile, MD

Tract-Based Spatial Statistics of Magnetic Resonance Images to Assess Disease and Treatment Effects in Perinatal Asphyxial Encephalopathy
Porter EJ, Counsell SJ, Edwards AD, et al (Imperial College London, UK)
Pediatr Res 68:205-209, 2010

Biomarkers are required for efficient trials of neuroprotective interventions after perinatal asphyxia. This study aimed to determine whether diffusion tensor imaging (DTI) analyzed by tract-based spatial statistics (TBSS) may be a suitable biomarker of disease and treatment effects after perinatal asphyxia in small groups of patients. We performed TBSS from DTI obtained at 3 T from eight healthy control infants, 10 untreated and 10 hypothermia-treated infants with neonatal encephalopathy. Median (range) postnatal age at scan was 1 d (1−21) in the healthy infants, 6 d (4−20) in the cooled, and 7 d (4−18) in noncooled infants. Compared with the control group, fractional anisotropy (FA) was significantly reduced not only in several white matter tracts in the noncooled infants but also in the internal capsule in the cooled group. Noncooled infants had significantly lower FA than the cooled treated infants, indicating more extensive damage, in the anterior and posterior limbs of the internal capsule, the corpus callosum, and optic radiations. We conclude that perinatal hypoxic ischemic encephalopathy is associated with widespread white matter abnormalities that are reduced by moderate hypothermia. DTI analyzed by TBSS detects this treatment effect and is therefore a qualified biomarker for the early evaluation of neuroprotective interventions.

▶ Several large randomized clinical trials have demonstrated that therapeutic hypothermia increases survival without neurologic deficit at 18 months of age. Although these trials indicate that neuronal rescue therapy is possible, the treatment effect is modest. In experimental studies, a large number of other interventions also have neuroprotective effects after hypoxia-ischemia and some may have synergistic effects when added to therapeutic hypothermia. Biomarkers are needed to translate these promising results to human studies. Given the high financial cost of large, randomized, clinical trials and the need for longer-term follow-up of children enrolled in these trials, a biomarker that accurately demonstrates biologic effects in small groups of infants would be particularly useful to assess promising therapies quickly and efficiently and to target therapies that subsequently could be evaluated in large, randomized, clinical trials. MR imaging is a candidate biomarker; however, it has not been shown to detect treatment effects in small samples.

Tract-based spatial statistics (TBSS) is a fully automated process that enables voxel-wise and group-wise comparison of (MR) diffusion tensor images (DTI) fractional anisotropy values across all white matter tracts. Because the technique is observer-independent, it avoids the subjective bias inherent in previous DTI studies that have used a region-of-interest approach. In this study, the authors were able to demonstrate widespread microstructure abnormalities in white matter tracts in term infants after perinatal asphyxia that were reduced after therapeutic hypothermia. These data suggest that TBSS can provide a quantifiable, qualified biomarker of neurologic injury and treatment effect in hypoxic ischemic encephalopathy and is a suitable biomarker for early phase trials of novel neuroprotectants.

L. A. Papile, MD

Ultrasonically detectable cerebellar haemorrhage in preterm infants
McCarthy LK, Donoghue V, Murphy JFA (The Natl Maternity Hosp, Dublin, Ireland)
Arch Dis Child Fetal Neonatal Ed 96:F281-F285, 2011

Objective.—To determine the frequency and pattern of cerebellar haemorrhage (CBH) on routine cranial ultrasound (cUS) imaging in infants of ≤32 weeks gestation, and to investigate how extremely preterm infants with CBH differ from those with severe intraventricular haemorrhage (IVH).

Methods.—672 infants of ≤32 weeks gestation were prospectively examined for CBH on serial cUS imaging. In a separate case–control analysis, the clinical features, ultrasound findings and outcome of preterm infants with CBH were compared to those of infants with isolated severe IVH (grade III–IV).

Results.—Nine cases of CBH were identified among 53 infants with severe IVH. The incidence of CBH in infants of ≤32 weeks gestation was 1.3%. Five infants had bilateral CBH involving both hemispheres, three had unilateral left sided CBH and one had a right hemispheric lesion. Infants with CBH were male, significantly more preterm (24.4 vs 27.0 weeks) and of lower birth weight (692 g vs 979 g). Vaginal births predominated in the CBH group (89% vs 50%). The median time to identification of haemorrhage for both groups was 3 days. Mortality in the CBH group was 100% (9/9) compared to 43% (19/44) in the severe IVH group.

Conclusions.—Extensive CBH in preterm infants is rare and devastating. It appears to be confined to very preterm, extremely low birthweight infants and may have a male predominance. The co-existence of severe IVH and extensive CBH on routine cot-side cUS in the early neonatal period is an ominous finding.

▶ Older reports of cerebellar hemorrhage detected by cranial ultrasound (cUS) noted a frequency of 2% to 3% and suggested that in approximately one-third of infants it is an isolated finding. In this study, the frequency was 1.3%, approximately half of that previously reported. Moreover, in none of the cases was cerebellar hemorrhage an isolated finding; all of the infants also had a concomitant severe intraventricular hemorrhage (IVH). The frequency of cerebellar hemorrhage among infants with severe IVH was 17%. The majority of cerebellar hemorrhages were identified on the second day cUS and all were detected by 7 days of age.

Routine screening with cUS is not sufficiently sensitive to detect cerebellar hemorrhage. Additional views through the mastoid fontanelle are needed to adequately visualize the posterior fossa. Should these additional views be added to routine cUS screening? The data presented suggest that the yield from posterior fossa views is highest when a severe IVH is identified.

L. A. Papile, MD

Vulnerability of the fetal primate brain to moderate reduction in maternal global nutrient availability

Antonow-Schlorke I, Schwab M, Cox LA, et al (Friedrich Schiller Univ, Jena, Germany; Southwest Foundation for Biomed Res, San Antonio, TX; et al)
Proc Natl Acad Sci U S A 108:3011-3016, 2011

Moderate maternal nutrient restriction during pregnancy occurs in both developing and developed countries. In addition to poverty, maternal dieting, teenage pregnancy, and uterine vascular problems in older mothers are causes of decreased fetal nutrition. We evaluated the impact of global 30% maternal nutrient reduction (MNR) on early fetal baboon brain maturation. MNR induced major cerebral developmental disturbances without fetal growth restriction or marked maternal weight reduction. Mechanisms evaluated included neurotrophic factor suppression, cell proliferation and cell death imbalance, impaired glial maturation and neuronal process formation, down-regulation of gene ontological pathways and related gene products, and up-regulated transcription of cerebral catabolism. Contrary to the known benefits from this degree of dietary reduction on life span, MNR in pregnancy compromises structural fetal cerebral

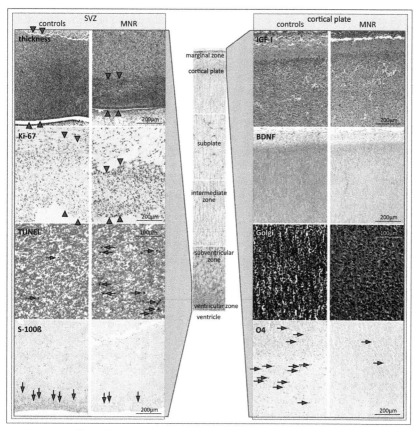

FIGURE 2.—Effects of MNR in the proliferative SVZ and in the cortical plate. SVZ: MNR reduced SVZ thickness (arrowheads), increased the density of proliferative Ki-67+ cells (brown precipitate, arrowheads mark the SVZ), increased apoptotic TUNEL+ cells (dark cells marked by arrows), and reduced glial S-100β IR (brown precipitate, arrows). Cortical plate: MNR decreased local IGF-I and BDNF IR (brown precipitate), density of the neuronal network (Golgi silver impregnation, arrowheads), and O4+ preoligodendrocytes (brown precipitate, arrows) reflecting impaired cerebral myelinogenesis. For interpretation of the references to color in this figure legend, the reader is referred to web version of this article. (Reprinted from Antonow-Schlorke I, Schwab M, Cox LA, et al. Vulnerability of the fetal primate brain to moderate reduction in maternal global nutrient availability. *Proc Natl Acad Sci U S A.* 2011;108:3011-3016. Copyright © 2011 National Academy of Sciences, U.S.A.)

development, potentially having an impact on brain function throughout life (Fig 2).

▶ In developing countries, poverty leads to maternal nutrient reduction during pregnancy, whereas in developed countries, dieting for cosmetic purposes is an important component. It is commonly thought that maternal adaptations under such conditions during pregnancy spare brain growth in the fetus. This very disturbing study suggests otherwise. Using baboons comparable in age to 25- to 29-year-old humans, the impact of global 30% maternal nutrient reduction was evaluated on early brain maturation. This reduction in nutrients induced major cerebral developmental disturbances without fetal growth restriction or marked maternal weight reduction. Examination of gross morphology of the developing fetal brain showed subtle changes in the subventricular proliferation zone (Fig 2) that was also associated with alterations in neuronal and glial maturation. Whole genome profiling found decreased growth factors and complex alterations of pathways related to early brain development associated with a decrease of growth factors, such as circulating insulin growth factor 1 (IGF-I) bioavailability and decreased cerebral IGF-I, brain-derived neurotrophic factor, and glial neurotrophic factor S-100β.

What is most concerning about this study is that it shows that these effects occur even with only marginal effects on maternal weight. Thus, although some studies are suggesting greater longevity with dietary reduction, when it comes to brain development of the fetus that could have life-long lasting effects, early pregnancy is not the right time to restrict nutrients.

J. Neu, MD

Whole-Body Hypothermia for Term and Near-Term Newborns With Hypoxic-Ischemic Encephalopathy: A Randomized Controlled Trial

Jacobs SE, for the Infant Cooling Evaluation Collaboration (Royal Women's Hosp, Melbourne, Victoria, Australia; et al)
Arch Pediatr Adolesc Med 2011 [Epub ahead of print]

Objective.—To determine the effectiveness and safety of moderate whole-body hypothermia in newborns with hypoxic-ischemic encephalopathy born in hospitals with and without newborn intensive care facilities or complicated hypothermia equipment.

Design.—Multicenter, international, randomized controlled trial.

Setting.—Neonatal intensive care units in Australia, New Zealand, Canada, and the United States (N = 28) from February 2001 through July 2007.

Participants.—Newborns of 35 weeks' gestation or more, with indicators of peripartum hypoxia-ischemia and moderate to severe clinical encephalopathy, randomly allocated to hypothermia (n = 110) or standard care (n = 111).

Intervention.—Whole-body hypothermia to 33.5°C for 72 hours or standard care (37°C). Infants who received hypothermia were treated at ambient environmental temperature by turning off the radiant warmer and then applying refrigerated gel packs to maintain rectal temperature at 33°C to 34°C.

Main Outcome Measures.—Death or major sensorineural disability at 2 years of age.

Results.—Therapeutic hypothermia reduced the risk of death or major sensorineural disability at 2 years of age: 55 of 107 infants (51.4%) in the hypothermia group and 67 of 101 infants (66.3%) in the control group died or had a major sensorineural disability at 2 years (risk ratio, 0.77 [95% confidence interval, 0.62-0.98]; $P = .03$). The mortality rate decreased, and the survival rate free of any sensorineural disability increased. Adverse effects of hypothermia were minimal.

Conclusions.—Whole-body hypothermia is effective and appears to be safe when commenced within 6 hours of birth at the hospital of birth in term and near-term newborns with hypoxic-ischemic encephalopathy. This simple method of hypothermia could be used within strict protocols with appropriate training on correct diagnosis and application of hypothermia in nontertiary neonatal settings while awaiting retrieval and transport to the regional neonatal intensive care unit.

Trial Registration.—anzctr.org.au Identifier: ACTRN12606000036516.

▶ Recruitment for the Infant Cooling Evaluation (ICE) trial was halted by the steering committee in 2007 after the enrollment of 211 of the planned 300 infants. The committee concluded that clinical equipoise within the neonatal medical community was lost after the publication in 2007 of several systematic reviews favoring therapeutic hypothermia. As a result, the power of the study was reduced from 80% to 61% and may partly explain why the study was not published sooner. Nonetheless, the study contributes valuable information.

Unlike prior studies, the ICE trial used a simple method of therapeutic cooling that consisted of exposing infants to ambient temperature and applying refrigerated gel packs if passive cooling did not lower rectal temperature sufficiently. For infants born outside the treating center, this method of cooling was initiated at the referral nursery by the transport team. Although outborn infants had higher temperatures before cooling, on average they achieved the target temperature of 33 to 34°C sooner than inborn infants. The primary outcome, death or major sensorineural disability at 2 years of age, was similar for the outborn and inborn cohorts.

In the ICE trial, 19% of enrolled infants did not have moderate to severe encephalopathy. This occurred in spite of providing education to referring nurseries and the transport team. It is incumbent on treating centers to develop standardized neurologic assessment protocols to be used in referring centers, provide outreach education and, if passive cooling is initiated in the field, ensure that the transport team can accurately identify infants with moderate to severe encephalopathy.

L. A. Papile, MD

A Clinical Prediction Model to Stratify Retinopathy of Prematurity Risk Using Postnatal Weight Gain

Binenbaum G, the Premature Infants in Need of Transfusion Study Group (Children's Hosp of Philadelphia, PA; et al)
Pediatrics 127:e607-e614, 2011

Objective.—To develop an efficient clinical prediction model that includes postnatal weight gain to identify infants at risk of developing severe retinopathy of prematurity (ROP). Under current birth weight (BW) and gestational age (GA) screening criteria, <5% of infants examined in countries with advanced neonatal care require treatment.

Patients and Methods.—This study was a secondary analysis of prospective data from the Premature Infants in Need of Transfusion Study, which enrolled 451 infants with a BW <1000 g at 10 centers. There were 367 infants who remained after excluding deaths (82) and missing weights (2). Multivariate logistic regression was used to predict severe ROP (stage 3 or treatment).

Results.—Median BW was 800 g (445−995). There were 67 (18.3%) infants who had severe ROP. The model included GA, BW, and daily weight gain rate. Run weekly, an alarm that indicated need for eye examinations occurred when the predicted probability of severe ROP was >0.085. This identified 66 of 67 severe ROP infants (sensitivity of 99% [95% confidence interval: 94%−100%]), and all 33 infants requiring treatment. Median alarm-to-outcome time was 10.8 weeks (range: 1.9−17.6). There were 110 (30%) infants who had no alarm. Nomograms were developed to determine risk of severe ROP by BW, GA, and postnatal weight gain.

Conclusion.—In a high-risk cohort, a BW-GA-weight-gain model could have reduced the need for examinations by 30%, while still identifying all infants requiring laser surgery. Additional studies are required to determine whether including larger-BW, lower-risk infants would reduce examinations further and to validate the prediction model and nomograms before clinical use.

▶ Both the progressive growth in the numbers of extremely preterm infants at risk of retinopathy of prematurity (RoP) and the medical-legal risk inherent in caring for these babies has created a relative shortage in ophthalmologists available to provide optimal schedules of preventive screening. In some geographic regions, this has been ameliorated by a network approach that capitalizes on the recent ability to capture and submit for centralized expert review at scheduled intervals digital images of retinal vasculature. The cost of missing the opportunity to intervene in a case of threshold RoP can be devastating. For this reason, screening criteria have been kept sufficiently broad to minimize to as close to zero as possible the risk of such an occurrence. The study by Binenbaum and colleagues within the Premature Infants in Need of Transfusion (PINT) Study Group reexamines current assumptions concerning screening criteria, assessing predictors of RoP progression in an effort to narrow the population for whom retinal screening is indicated. In a secondary analysis of data from the PINT study that examined 351 survivors of the 451 infants born below 1000 g birth weight at 10 units in Canada and the United States, the group developed nomograms of baparietal diameter risk using 3 factors: birth weight, gestational age, and postnatal weight gain. Run weekly, the nomogram signaled "alarm" when the predicted probability of severe RoP exceeded 0.085, indicating the need for an eye examination. Thirty percent of infants had no nomogram-generated alarm events, suggesting that this is the proportion of infants for whom screening might not be required. The nomogram missed 1 infant with severe RoP but none who required laser surgery. This is an initial study that, although conducted in a diverse multicenter population, would require validation before adoption into widespread use. Still, I found it intriguing from at least 2 viewpoints. First, the importance of postnatal weight gain as a "protective" factor is interesting. Is it simply a reflection of a neonatal intensive care unit course less burdened by complications of prematurity? Does it underscore the importance of early and adequate nutrition in the general sense? Might it be a surrogate for the provision of 1 or more specific nutrients facilitating normal retinal development? I was also intrigued by the possibility that this approach might greatly help those struggling with appropriate use of scarce ophthalmological services in resource-poor settings.

L. J. Van Marter, MD, MPH

A Pilot Study of Novel Biomarkers in Neonates With Hypoxic-Ischemic Encephalopathy
Douglas-Escobar M, Yang C, Bennett J, et al (Baylor College of Medicine, Houston, TX; Univ of Florida, Gainesville)
Pediatr Res 68:531-536, 2010

Severe hypoxic-ischemic encephalopathy (HIE) is a devastating condition that can lead to mortality and long-term disabilities in term newborns. No rapid and reliable laboratory test exists to assess the degree of neuronal injury in these patients. We propose two possible biomarkers: 1) phosphorylated axonal neurofilament heavy chain (pNF-H) protein, one of the major subunits of neurofilaments, found only in axonal cytoskeleton of neurons and 2) Ubiquitin C-terminal hydrolase 1 (UCHL1 protein) that is heavily and specifically concentrated in neuronal perikarya and dendrites. High-serum pNF-H and UCHL1 levels are reported in subarachnoid hemorrhage and traumatic brain injury, suggesting that they are released into blood following neuronal injury. We hypothesized that serum pNF-H and UCHL1 were higher in neonates with moderate-to-severe HIE than in healthy neonates. A time-limited enrollment of 14 consecutive patients with HIE and 14 healthy controls was performed. UCHL1 and pNF-H were correlated with clinical data and brain MRI. UCHL1 and pNF-H serum levels were higher in HIE versus controls. UCHL1 showed correlation with the 10-min Apgar score, and pNF-H showed correlation with abnormal brain MRI. Our findings suggest that serum UCHL1 and pNF-H could be explored as diagnostic and prognostic tools in neonatal HIE.

▶ Hypoxic-ischemic events are among the greatest scourges of perinatal medicine, and none is of greater significance than the hypoxic-ischemic brain injury that deprives many otherwise normal infants of the opportunity to live healthy, productive lives. Improvements in perinatal and neonatal care have made an impact on prevention but have failed to eradicate hypoxic-ischemic encephalopathy (HIE). Initial excitement accompanying the publication of results of landmark clinical trials of therapeutic hypothermia (TH)[1,2] showing improved health and neurodevelopmental outcomes among infants with HIE treated with brain or whole body cooling was followed by the grim recognition that therapeutic hypothermia (TH) did not benefit all affected infants. Recent efforts have focused on identifying methods of better quantitating brain injury and identifying the populations of infants most and least likely to benefit from TH. In this study, Dr. Douglas-Escobar and colleagues found an association between 2 novel biomarkers, ubiquitin C-terminal hydrolalse 1 (UCHL1) protein and phosphorylated axonal neurofilament heavy chain (pNF-H) protein and the 10-minute Apgar score, HIE, and early MRI abnormalities. These proteins might serve as useful biomarkers of severity of HIE and potentially other forms of neonatal brain injury. In a clinical study of 85 consecutive infants hospitalized at the University of Michigan in Ann Arbor who received TH for HIE, Sarkar and colleagues attempted to identify factors preceding TH that predicted later death.[3] Thirteen of the 85 TH-treated infants died during 9 to 18 months of follow-up. In multivariate analysis, only an Apgar score of zero at 10 minutes predicted death following TH. In this cohort, 12 infants had no detectable heart rate at 10 minutes or beyond, and all died or had severe impairments: 9 died with HIE, 2 had quadriparesis and global delay at 18 to 24 months, and 1 had extensive encephalomalacia on brain MRI at follow-up. These results add to those of others seeking to predict outcomes of HIE following TH, such as a recent meta-analysis of 3 large studies of TH that found that severity of HIE did not predict response to TH.[4] Additional multicenter studies are necessary to lend further insight into predictors of outcomes following TH among infants with HIE. In an ideal world, such studies would provide improved predictive data with which parents could be fully informed and lead to modifications of treatment protocols that could be tested in clinical trials with the aim of finding strategies to improve outcomes among a broader range of affected infants. In the short term, these studies underscore the importance of conducting additional biomarker and clinical studies and of ongoing assessment of biological, clinical, and ethical dimensions of TH.

L. J. Van Marter, MD, MPH

References

1. Jacobs S, Hunt R, Tarnow-Mordi W, Inder T, Davis P. Cooling for newborns with hypoxic ischaemic encephalopathy. *Cochrane Database Syst Rev.* 2007;(4). CD003311.
2. Shah PS, Ohlsson A, Perlman M. Hypothermia to treat neonatal hypoxic ischemic encephalopathy: systematic review. *Arch Pediatr Adolesc Med.* 2007;161:951-958.

3. Sarkar S, Bhagat I, Dechert RE, Barks JD. Predicting death despite therapeutic hypothermia in infants with hypoxic-ischaemic encephalopathy. *Arch Dis Child Fetal Neonatal Ed.* 2010;95:F423-F428.
4. Edwards AD, Brocklehurst P, Gunn AJ, et al. Neurological outcomes at 18 months of age after moderate hypothermia for perinatal hypoxic ischemic encephalopathy: synthesis and meta-analysis of trial data. *BMJ.* 2010;340:c363.

Patterns of cerebral white matter damage and cognitive impairment in adolescents born very preterm

Soria-Pastor S, Gimenez M, Narberhaus A, et al (Univ of Barcelona, Spain)
Int J Dev Neurosci 26:647-654, 2008

There is increasing evidence about the presence of white matter damage in subjects with a history of premature birth, even in those classified as good outcome because of an apparently normal development. Although intellectual performance is within normal limits in premature children it is significantly decreased compared to paired controls. The purpose of this study was to investigate the relationship between a lower performance intelligence quotient and white matter damage in preterm adolescents. The sample comprised 44 adolescents (mean age ± S.D.: 14.4 ± 1.6 years) born before 32 weeks of gestational age and 43 term-born adolescents (14.5 ± 2.1 years). Individual voxel-based morphometry analyses demonstrated that 35/44 (80%) preterm subjects had white matter abnormalities. The centrum semiovale and the posterior periventricular regions were the most frequently affected areas. Correlation analysis showed that in preterms the performance intelligence quotient correlated with the whole-brain white matter volume (r=0.32; P=0.036) but not with grey matter volume. Complementary analysis showed that low scores in the Digit Symbol subtest, a measure of processing speed, in the preterm group correlated with reductions in white matter concentration. These results suggest that white matter damage is highly common and that it persists until adolescence. Hence, diffuse white matter loss may be responsible for performance intelligence quotient and processing speed decrements in subjects with very preterm birth.

▶ Increasingly sophisticated MRI techniques (voxel-based morphometry) allow for the identification and quantification of gray and white matter concentration and regional abnormalities in the brain of infants with periventricular leukomalacia (PVL).[1] Inder et al[2] in 1999 first showed that the neuropathology associated with PVL in preterm infants is not exclusive to white matter and that gray matter volume is also decreased at term. Compared with full-term children, preterm infants with PVL have gray matter reductions bilaterally in the temporal lobe, as well as the left parietal and right frontal lobe. White matter alterations in preterm infants with PVL include decrements in the corpus callosum, around the posterior horns of the lateral ventricles and the basal ganglia. These findings persist through adolescence.[3] There is a complex interaction of gestational age, cortical and subcortical connections, and compensatory mechanisms that are ultimately responsible for the motor, cognitive, and neurodevelopmental deficits seen in children with PVL. Radiological studies are limited per se, as they are manifestations of the end result of complex cellular mechanisms of brain damage and repair, but MR images do highlight the likelihood of a close relationship between cortical and subcortical processes as well as selective vulnerability to brain damage in different brain regions.

The authors acknowledge the limitations of their methodology that requires multiple steps of an automated algebraic-based algorithm as well as a small sample with limited statistical power. However, their findings are similar to those of others, and the importance of this article is that the application of this technology might improve the prediction of cognitive defects in infants with PVL.

H. M. Towers, MBBCh, FRCPI

References

1. Peterson BS, Vohr B, Staib LH, et al. Regional brain volume abnormalities and long-term cognitive outcome in preterm infants. *JAMA*. 2000;284:1939-1947.
2. Inder TE, Huppi PS, Warfield S, et al. Periventricular white matter injury in the premature infant is followed by reduced cerebral cortical gray matter volume at term. *Ann Neurol*. 1999;46:755-760.
3. Nosarti C, Giouroukou E, Healy E, et al. Grey and white matter distribution in very preterm adolescents mediates neurodevelopmental outcome. *Brain*. 2008; 131:205-217.

Hypocarbia and Adverse Outcome in Neonatal Hypoxic-Ischemic Encephalopathy

Pappas A, for the Eunice Kennedy Shriver National Institute of Child Health and Human Development Neonatal Research Network (Wayne State Univ School of Medicine, Detroit, MI; et al)

J Pediatr 158:752-758, 2011

Objective.—To evaluate the association between early hypocarbia and 18- to 22-month outcome among neonates with hypoxic-ischemic encephalopathy.

Study Design.—Data from the National Institute of Child Health and Human Development Neonatal Research Network randomized, controlled trial of whole-body hypothermia for neonatal hypoxic-ischemic encephalopathy were used for this secondary observational study. Infants (n = 204) had multiple blood gases recorded from birth to 12 hours of study intervention (hypothermia versus intensive care alone). The relationship between hypocarbia and outcome (death/disability at 18 to 22 months) was evaluated by unadjusted and adjusted analyses examining minimum PCO_2 and cumulative exposure to PCO_2 <35 mm Hg. The relationship between cumulative PCO_2 <35 mm Hg (calculated as the difference between 35 mm Hg and the sampled PCO_2 multiplied by the duration of time spent <35 mm Hg) and outcome was evaluated by level of exposure (none-high) using a multiple logistic regression analysis with adjustments for pH, level of encephalopathy, treatment group (±hypothermia), and time to spontaneous respiration and ventilator days; results were expressed as odds ratios and 95% confidence intervals. Alternative models of CO_2 concentration were explored to account for fluctuations in CO_2.

Results.—Both minimum PCO_2 and cumulative PCO_2 <35 mm Hg were associated with poor outcome ($P < .05$). Moreover, death/disability increased with greater cumulative exposure to PCO_2 <35 mm Hg.

Conclusions.—Hypocarbia is associated with poor outcome after hypoxic-ischemic encephalopathy.

▶ Early unintentional hypocarbia following neonatal hypoxic-ischemic encephalopathy (HIE) may modulate neuronal injury and contribute to adverse long-term neurodevelopmental outcome. Although hyperventilation-mediated experimental hypocarbia can prevent further damage in patients with brain injury by restoring cerebral autoregulation, low partial pressure of carbon dioxide (P_{CO_2}) levels are known to contribute to detrimental effects of cerebral vasoconstriction, decreased partial pressure of oxygen, decreased oxygen release from hemoglobin, and excessive neuronal excitability due to increased oxygen demands. Moreover, animal data suggest that hypocarbia is associated with nuclear DNA fragmentation, decreased levels of high-energy phosphates, and neuronal and mitochondrial alterations that lead to apoptotic cell death. In this article, Pappas et al present their secondary analysis of the National Institute of Child Health and Human Development Neonatal Research Network trial of whole-body cooling evaluating the association between early hypocarbia and 18- to 24-month outcome (death/disability) among neonates with HIE. They found that both minimum P_{CO_2} and cumulative exposure to P_{CO_2} < 35 mm Hg within the first 16 hours of birth were associated with poor outcomes at 18 to 22 months of age. Furthermore, death/disability increased with greater cumulative exposure to P_{CO_2} < 35 mm Hg. Similarly, Klinger et al[1] reported that hypocarbia and hyperoxia within 2 hours of life following HIE were associated with an increased risk of death or disability, with risk of death/disability being highest among infants with both hypocarbia and hyperoxia. These studies raise important questions regarding the complexity of resuscitation and early postnatal ventilatory management of neonates with HIE. Is hypocarbia a modifiable risk factor or simply a marker of poor outcome? Should the initial ventilator settings to maintain normocarbia be lower or weaning be more rapid in infants undergoing hypothermia for HIE in view of lower metabolic rate and consequent lower carbon dioxide production? Will avoidance of early hypocarbia improve outcome in infants with HIE? The answers to these questions will certainly alter the way clinicians treat neonates with HIE in the future.

R. Sahni, MBBS

Reference

1. Klinger G, Beyene J, Shah P, Perlman M. Do hyperoxaemia and hypocapnia add to the risk of brain injury after intrapartum asphyxia? *Arch Dis Child Fetal Neonatal Ed.* 2005;90:F49-F52.

The relationship between early concentrations of 25 blood proteins and cerebral white matter injury in preterm newborns: the ELGAN study

Leviton A, Kuban K, O'Shea TM, et al (Harvard Med School, Boston, MA)
J Pediatr 158:897-903, 2011

Objective.—To evaluate whether concentrations of inflammation-related proteins are elevated in the blood of preterm newborns who develop cerebral white matter damage.

Study Design.—We measured 25 proteins in blood collected on days 1, 7, and 14 from 939 infants born before the 28th week of gestation. Brain ultrasound scans were read by at least two sonologists, who agreed on the presence or absence of lesions. A protein concentration was considered elevated if it was in the highest quartile for gestational age and the day on which the specimen was collected.

Results.—In time-oriented models, elevated concentrations of vascular endothelial growth factor receptor 1, serum amyloid A, and macrophage inflammatory protein 1β on day 1 and interleukin-8 on day 7 were associated with increased risk of ventriculomegaly. Elevated concentrations of macrophage inflammatory protein 1β on day 1 and intercellular adhesion molecule 1 on day 7 were associated with increased risk of an echolucent lesion. Infants with elevated concentrations of inflammation-related proteins on two separate days were at significantly increased risk for ventriculomegaly, but at only modestly increased risk for an echolucent lesion.

Conclusions.—Concentrations of inflammation-related proteins in the circulation in the first days after preterm birth provide information about the risk of sonographic white matter damage. The inflammatory process might begin in utero.

▶ Advances in perinatal and neonatal care have dramatically improved the survival of extremely low gestational age newborns. The increased survival rate has been associated with cerebral white matter injury in these infants, which is characterized by adverse motor and cognitive outcomes. Cerebral white matter injury identified by cranial ultrasound scan is a powerful prediction of cerebral palsy in low birth weight infants.

In this large prospective, multicenter study, Leviton et al showed that elevated concentrations of inflammation-related proteins in the blood of extremely low gestational age newborns during postnatal days 1 to 14, predicted the presence of both ventriculomegaly and an echolucent lesion evident on cranial ultrasound scans (Level of Evidence B). This study supports the hypothesis that inflammation contributes to cerebral white matter damage in premature infants. Moreover, the data suggest that inflammation begins in utero and that monocytes play a key role in white matter damage.

The role of inflammation in medicating brain injury in preterm infants remains controversial. While it is clear that cytokine concentrations are increased in infants who develop white matter injury, numerous investigators have failed to demonstrate a relationship between histologic chorioamnionitis and cerebral palsy.[1] Prior reports from the ELGAN database have shown a relationship between positive culture results from the placenta and ventriculomegaly.[2] Other studies suggest that elevated concentrations of cytokines on cerebrospinal fluid may be a better predictor of white matter injury than systemic cytokine levels.[3] This study shows the linkage between elevation of inflammatory proteins and white matter damage and suggests that determination of inflammatory proteins in the first 2 weeks might predict white matter damage.

F. Akita, MB, ChB

References

1. Nelson KB, Grether JK, Dambrosia JM, et al. Neonatal cytokines and cerebral palsy in very preterm infants. *Pediatr Res.* 2003;53:600-607.
2. Leviton A, Allred EN, Kuban KC, et al. Microbiologic and histologic characteristics of the extremely preterm infant's placenta predict white matter damage and later cerebral palsy. the ELGAN study. *Pediatr Res.* 2010;67:95-101.
3. Viscardi RM, Muhumuza CK, Rodriguez A, et al. Inflammatory markers in intrauterine and fetal blood and cerebrospinal fluid compartments are associated with adverse pulmonary and neurologic outcomes in preterm infants. *Pediatr Res.* 2004;55:1009-1017.

4 Epidemiology and Pregnancy Complications

17-alpha-hydroxyprogesterone caproate for the prevention of preterm birth in women with prior preterm birth and a short cervical length

Berghella V, for the Vaginal Ultrasound Trial Consortium (Thomas Jefferson Univ, Philadelphia, PA; et al)
Am J Obstet Gynecol 202:351.e1-351.e6, 2010

Objective.—We sought to evaluate 17-alpha-hydroxyprogesterone caproate (17P) for prevention of preterm birth (PTB) in women with prior spontaneous PTB (SPTB) and cervical length (CL) <25 mm.

Study Design.—We conducted planned secondary analysis of the *Eunice Kennedy Shriver* National Institute of Child Health and Human Development-sponsored randomized trial evaluating cerclage for women with singleton gestations, prior SPTB (17-33 6/7 weeks), and CL <25 mm between 16-22 6/7 weeks. Women were stratified at randomization to intent to use or not use 17P. The effect of 17P was analyzed separately for cerclage and no-cerclage groups. Primary outcome was PTB <35 weeks.

Results.—In 300 women, 17P had no effect on PTB <35 weeks in either cerclage (P =.64) or no-cerclage (P =.51) groups. Only PTB <24 weeks (odds ratio, 0.08) and perinatal death (odds ratio, 0.14) were significantly lower for those with 17P in the no-cerclage group.

Conclusion.—17P had no additional benefit for prevention of PTB in women who had prior SPTB and got ultrasound-indicated cerclage for CL <25 mm. In women who did not get cerclage, 17P reduced previable birth and perinatal mortality.

▶ In 2003, Meis[1] demonstrated that treatment with 17 alpha-hydroxyprogesterone caproate (17OHP), a synthetic progestin, initiated before 21 weeks' gestation reduced the risk of preterm births at less than 37 weeks of gestation in women who previously had a spontaneous preterm delivery (incidence, 36.3% in the progesterone group vs 54.9% in the placebo group; delivery at less than 35 weeks of gestation [incidence, 20.6% vs 30.7%]; and delivery at less than 32 weeks of gestation [incidence, 11.4 % vs 19.6 %]). Although the study was not powered to show the benefit of preventing prematurity-associated infant deaths, the drug did reduce the risks of several serious medical complications in preterm infants. 17OHP is currently widely available as a prescription product at compounding pharmacies. "Moreover, it is inexpensive — about $15 per 250-mg injection or about $300 for a 20-week treatment course, according to Aetna claims data for 2010."[2] This situation nearly changed dramatically when, after US Food and Drug Administration approval for the drug named Makena, the proposed price was to be $1440 per injection for 20 weeks or nearly $40 000. However, with Congress intervening and cooler heads prevailing, a more reasonable cost structure has been agreed upon, and home pharmacies that continue to make the compound will no longer be jeopardized. (There was the possibility of huge fines and even incarceration if they manufactured the compound.)[2] Of the 4.2 million live births in the United States each year, it is estimated that about 139 000 (3.3%) are to women who are candidates for 17OHP therapy.[3] Furthermore, women receiving 17OHP prophylaxis remain at an increased risk for preterm labor (PTL) and preterm birth. Patient education and surveillance for PTL symptoms is mandatory after commencing 17OHP therapy.

The trial by Berghella is 1 of 3 articles documenting the restricted value of 17OHP. It is somewhat disappointing to learn that 17OHP had no additional benefit for the prevention of preterm birth in women who had prior spontaneous preterm birth and got ultrasound-indicated cerclage for cervical length less than 25 mm. However, in women who did not get cerclage, 17OHP reduced previable birth and perinatal mortality. Similarly, the supplementation omega-3 long-chain polyunsaturated fatty acid offered no benefit in reducing preterm birth among women receiving 17OHP who had a history of preterm delivery. Almost 40% of both the treated and control group delivered prematurely.[4] In a randomized trial of 39 twin pregnancies, Briery[5] concluded that progesterone does not prevent preterm births in women with twins.

Although the preterm birth rate in the United States has started to decline, it is still too high; and the biggest immediate impact will come from the prevention of unnecessary, unindicated late preterm deliveries. It remains important to judiciously use tocolytics such as magnesium to delay preterm births long enough for a full course of antenatal corticosteroids to be administered.

A. A. Fanaroff, MD, FRCPE, FRCP&CH

References

1. Meis PJ, Klebanoff M, Thom E, et al. Prevention of recurrent preterm delivery by 17 alpha-hydroxyprogesterone caproate. *N Engl J Med.* 2003;348:2379-2385.
2. Armstrong J. Unintended consequences—the cost of preventing preterm births after FDA approval of a branded version of 17OHP. *N Engl J Med.* 2011;364: 1689-1691.
3. Petrini JR, Callaghan WM, Klebanoff M, et al. Estimated effect of 17 alpha-hydroxyprogesterone caproate on preterm birth in the United States. *Obstet Gynecol.* 2005;105:267-272.
4. Harper M, Thom E, Klebanoff MA, et al. Eunice Kennedy Shriver National Institute of Child Health and Human Development Maternal-Fetal Medicine Units Network. Omega-3 fatty acid supplementation to prevent recurrent preterm birth: a randomized controlled trial. *Obstet Gynecol.* 2010;115:234-242.
5. Briery CM, Veillon EW, Klauser CK, et al. Progesterone does not prevent preterm births in women with twins. *South Med J.* 2009;102:900-904.

Cerclage for Short Cervix on Ultrasonography in Women With Singleton Gestations and Previous Preterm Birth: A Meta-Analysis

Berghella V, Rafael TJ, Szychowski JM, et al (Jefferson Med College of Thomas Jefferson Univ, Philadelphia, PA; Univ of Alabama, Birmingham; Lehigh Valley Hosp and Health Network, Allentown, PA)

Obstet Gynecol 117:663-671, 2011

Objective.—To estimate if cerclage prevents preterm birth and perinatal mortality and morbidity in women with previous preterm birth, singleton gestation, and short cervical length in a meta-analysis of randomized trials.

Data Sources.—MEDLINE, PUBMED, EMBASE, and the Cochrane Library were searched using the terms "cerclage," "short cervix," "ultrasound," and "randomized trial."

Methods of Study Selection.—We included randomized trials of cerclage in women with short cervical length on transvaginal ultrasonography, limiting the analysis to women with previous spontaneous preterm birth and singleton gestation.

Tabulation, Integration, and Results.—Patient-level data abstraction and analysis were accomplished by two independent investigators. Five trials met inclusion criteria. In women with a singleton gestation, previous spontaneous preterm birth, and cervical length less than 25 mm before 24 weeks of gestation, preterm birth before 35 weeks of gestation was 28.4% (71/250) in the cerclage compared with 41.3% (105/254) in the no cerclage groups (relative risk 0.70, 95% confidence interval 0.55–0.89). Cerclage also significantly reduced preterm birth before 37, 32, 28, and 24 weeks of gestation. Composite perinatal mortality and morbidity were significantly reduced (15.6% in cerclage compared with 24.8% in no cerclage groups; relative risk 0.64, 95% confidence interval 0.45–0.91).

Conclusion.—In women with previous spontaneous preterm birth, singleton gestation, and cervical length less than 25 mm, cerclage significantly prevents preterm birth and composite perinatal mortality and morbidity (Table 3).

▶ In 1976, Fuchs[1] wrote "only about 8 per cent of pregnancies end prematurely, as much as 75 per cent of perinatal deaths are due to prematurity. Since it is difficult to identify the predisposing factors in individual cases and to prevent the premature onset of labor, it is necessary to try to arrest such labor when it occurs." He proposed 4 possible points of attack: (1) replacement of progesterone to reduce the myometrial sensitivity to oxytocin, (2) administration of beta-mimetic agents to relax the uterus and make it unresponsive to stimuli, (3) administration of ethanol to block oxytocin secretion, and (4) administration of anti-inflammatory drugs to inhibit prostaglandin synthesis. These broad principles apply today and have been successful in limited cases. We have of course been spared the horrendous vomiting and intoxication induced by alcohol to inhibit oxytocin.

TABLE 3.—Selected Outcomes in Women With Previous Preterm Birth, Singleton Gestation, and Short Cervical Length Comparing Those With Cerclage and Those With No Cerclage

Population	Outcome	Cerclage	No Cerclage	RR (95% CI)
Singleton gestation, previous PTB at less than 37 wk, short CL before 24 wk				
CL less than 25 mm	PTB less than 37 wk	105/250 (42)	154/254 (60.6)	**0.70 (0.58−0.83)**
	PTB less than 35 wk	71/250 (28.4)	105/254 (41.3)	**0.70 (0.55−0.89)**
	PTB less than 32 wk	48/250 (19.2)	75/254 (29.5)	**0.66 (0.48−0.91)**
	PTB less than 28 wk	32/250 (12.8)	51/254 (20.1)	**0.64 (0.43−0.96)**
	PTB less than 24 wk	13/250 (5.2)	28/254 (11)	**0.48 (0.26−0.90)**
	Perinatal mortality	22/250 (8.8)	35/254 (13.8)	0.65 (0.40−1.07)
CL 16−24.9 mm	PTB less than 37 wk	67/170 (39.4)	98/180 (54.4)	**0.74 (0.59−0.93)**
	PTB less than 35 wk	43/170 (25.3)	62/180 (34.4)	0.77 (0.55−1.06)
	PTB less than 32 wk	30/170 (17.6)	42/180 (23.3)	0.80 (0.53−1.21)
	PTB less than 28 wk	18/170 (10.6)	25/180 (13.9)	0.77 (0.44−1.35)
	PTB less than 24 wk	5/170 (2.9)	16/180 (8.9)	**0.38 (0.15−0.94)**
	Perinatal mortality	11/170 (6.5)	19/180 (10.6)	0.63 (0.31−1.26)
CL 15.9 mm or less	PTB less than 37 wk	38/80 (47.5)	56/74 (75.7)	**0.62 (0.48−0.80)**
	PTB less than 35 wk	28/80 (35)	43/74 (58.1)	**0.59 (0.42−0.83)**
	PTB less than 32 wk	18/80 (22.5)	33/74 (44.6)	**0.50 (0.32−0.78)**
	PTB less than 28 wk	14/80 (17.5)	26/74 (35.1)	**0.47 (0.28−0.79)**
	PTB less than 24 wk	8/80 (10)	12/74 (16.2)	0.53 (0.24−1.16)
	Perinatal mortality	11/80 (13.8)	16/74 (21.6)	0.59 (0.31−1.14)
Singleton gestation, previous PTB at less than 37 wk, CL less than 25 mm before 20 wk	PTB less than 35 wk	42/132 (31.8)	63/120 (52.5)	**0.61 (0.45−0.83)**
	Perinatal mortality	15/132 (11.4)	28/120 (23.3)	**0.49 (0.27−0.87)**
Singleton gestation, previous PTB at less than 24 wk, CL less than 25 mm before 24 wk	PTB less than 35 wk	43/140 (30.7)	54/119 (45.4)	**0.71 (0.52−0.96)**
	Perinatal mortality	12/140 (8.6)	21/119 (17.6)	**0.52 (0.27−0.99)**

RR, relative risk; CI, confidence interval; PTB, preterm birth; CL, cervical length.
Data are n/N (%) unless otherise indicated.
Significant results are in bold.

Nonetheless, despite major research efforts, more than 10 million births before 37 weeks of gestation occur annually worldwide, and more than 1 million infants die from this common complication of pregnancy (5%-12% incidence).[2]

A short cervical length detected by transvaginal ultrasonography before 24 weeks of gestation has long been shown to be one of the best predictors for preterm birth.[3] The next step after identifying a risk factor is to develop a remedy.

Easier said than done.

Cervical cerclage refers to a variety of surgical procedures in which sutures, wires, or synthetic tape are used to reinforce the cervix. It is used for the treatment of cervical incompetence or insufficiency. Berghella et al, in this excellent meta-analysis, prove beyond a reasonable shadow of doubt that for a specific population (women with a cervical length of < 25 mm with a previous spontaneous birth and single gestation) cervical cerclage reduces preterm birth and substantially decreases perinatal morbidity and mortality (Table 3). These women represent but a small proportion of those who deliver preterm; however, it is a step in the right direction, and there is an evidence-based intervention.

A. A. Fanaroff, MD, FRCPE, FRCP&CH

References

1. Fuchs F. Prevention of prematurity. *Am J Obstet Gynecol.* 1976;126:809-820.
2. Harris-Requejo J, Merialdi M. The global impact of preterm birth. In: Berghella V, ed. *Preterm birth: prevention and management.* Oxford, UK: Wiley-Blackwell; 2010:1-7.
3. Iams JD, Goldenberg RL, Meis PJ, et al. The length of the cervix and the risk of spontaneous premature delivery. National Institute of Child Health and Human Development Maternal Fetal Medicine Unit Network. *N Engl J Med.* 1996;334: 567-572.

Clinical Significance of Borderline Amniotic Fluid Index and Oligohydramnios in Preterm Pregnancy

Petrozella LN, Dashe JS, McIntire DD, et al (Univ of Texas Southwestern Med Ctr, Dallas, TX)
Obstet Gynecol 117:338-342, 2011

Objective.—To estimate pregnancy and neonatal outcomes in women with decreased amniotic fluid index (AFI) between 24 and 34 weeks of gestation, compared with outcomes in those with normal AFI.

Methods.—This is a review of singleton pregnancies that received ultrasound examinations at 24—34 weeks from 1997 to 2008. If more than one ultrasound examination was performed, the lowest AFI was used for analysis. An AFI 5 cm or less was considered oligohydramnios, 5—8 cm was considered borderline, and more than 8 cm to 24 cm was considered normal. Women with hydramnios or ruptured membranes at time of ultrasound examination were excluded.

Results.—A total of 28,555 pregnancies met inclusion criteria. Ultrasound examination had been performed to estimate gestational age or evaluate fetal growth in 78%. Major malformations were more common in pregnancies with oligohydramnios and borderline AFI than in those with normal fluid—25%, 10%, and 2%, respectively, $P < .001$. Among nonanomalous fetuses, complications that occurred more often in pregnancies with oligohydramnios and borderline AFI than in those with normal fluid included preterm birth (62%, 37%, 8%), either indicated (20%, 13%, 2%) or resulting from spontaneous preterm labor (42%, 24%, 6%); cesarean delivery for nonreassuring fetal status (9%, 9%, 4%), and birth weight below the third percentile (37%, 21%, 4%), all $P < .001$.

Conclusion.—Pregnancies with decreased AFI between 24 and 34 weeks, including borderline AFI as well as oligohydramnios, were significantly more likely to be associated with major fetal malformations, and in the absence of malformations, to be complicated by fetal growth restriction and preterm birth.

▶ For more than 2 decades, maternal fetal specialists have been more precisely monitoring amniotic fluid volumes by means of the amniotic fluid index (AFI). Whereas everyone is familiar with the increase in amniotic fluid associated with

gastrointestinal obstruction, neurologic anomalies, and pregnancies complicated by hydrops fetalis, multiple gestation, and diabetes, the role of the
placenta and membranes in regulating amniotic fluid is unclear. It is known
that the permeability of the human placenta increases with advancing gestation.
Indirect evidence has also proposed that aquaporins (AQPs) may be involved in
the regulation of placental water flow but the mechanisms are poorly understood. Five AQPs have been found in the human placenta and fetal membranes
(AQP1, 3, 4, 8, and 9); however, the physiological function(s) and the regulation of these proteins remain unknown. The AQPs in the fetal membranes may
have a role in intramembranous amniotic fluid water regulation and alterations
in their expression can be related to polyhydramnios and oligohydramnios.[1]

Magann et al[2] reviewed 2597 pregnancies with a normal AFI (2.5-97.5th
percentile): 73 with hydramnios (AFI > 97.5th percentile) and 72 with oligohydramnios (AFI < 2.5th percentile). Abnormal fetal heart rates influencing
delivery, cesarean deliveries for fetal labor intolerance, low 5-minute Apgar
scores, increased neonatal birth weight, and newborn intensive care unit admissions were more common with polyhydramnios. The fetuses of pregnancies
complicated by oligohydramnios had a greater risk of labor induction, intrauterine growth restriction, and preterm delivery. So both polyhydramnios and
oligohydramnios adversely influenced different pregnancy outcomes.

As noted in the abstract, Petrozella et al reported that pregnancies with
decreased AFI between 24 and 34 weeks, including borderline AFI and oligohydramnios, were significantly more likely to be associated with major fetal
malformations, and in the absence of malformations, to be complicated by
fetal growth restriction and preterm birth.

The fetus does best when surrounded by the normal amount of amniotic
fluid.

A. A. Fanaroff, MD, FRCPE, FRCP&CH

References

1. Damiano AE. Review: water channel proteins in the human placenta and fetal
   membranes. *Placenta*. 2011;32:S207-S211.
2. Magann EF, Doherty DA, Lutgendorf MA, Magann MI, Chauhan SP, Morrison JC.
   Peripartum outcomes of high-risk pregnancies complicated by oligo- and polyhydramnios: a prospective longitudinal study. *J Obstet Gynaecol Res*. 2010;36:
   268-277.

**Effects of the September 11, 2001 disaster on pregnancy outcomes:
a systematic review**
Ohlsson A, the Knowledge Synthesis Group of Determinants of Preterm/LBW
births (Univ of Toronto, Canada)
Acta Obstet Gynecol Scand 90:6-18, 2011

Background.—The terrorist explosions of the World Trade Center in
New York City and the other events on the Pentagon and in Pennsylvania
on 11 September 2001 were stressful events that affected people around

the world. Pregnant women and their offspring are especially vulnerable during and after such a terrorist attack. The objective was to systematically review the risks of adverse pregnancy outcomes after the terrorist attacks on Sept 11, 2001.

Methods.—The Meta-analysis of Observational Studies in Epidemiology (MOOSE) criteria were used for reporting of this review. Statistical analyses were performed using RevMan 5.0.

Results.—Ten reports of low-to-moderate risk of methodological bias were included. There was increased risks of infants with birthweight of 1,500 g—1,999 g (adjusted odds ratio [AOR] 1.67 [*95%*CI 1.11—2.52]) and small-for-gestational age births (AOR 1.90; 95%CI 1.05-3.46) in New York. There was increased risks of low birthweight (relative risk 2.25; 95%CI 1.29—3.90) and preterm births (relative risk 1.50; 95%CI 1.06—2.14) among ethnically Arabic women living in California There was a reduction in birthweight by 276 g and in head circumference by 1 cm when DNA adducts, a marker for environmental toxin exposure, were doubled in maternal blood. In Holland, a 48-g reduction in birthweight was reported.

Conclusions.—The World Trade Center disaster influenced pregnancy outcomes in New York, among ethnically Arab women living in California and among Dutch women. The adverse outcomes are likely due to environmental pollution and stress in New York, ethnic harassment in California and communal bereavement and stress in Holland.

▶ It is perhaps fortuitous that I discovered this article on the day we learned that Osama Bin Laden had been killed in a daring raid in Pakistan. The science is not as strong as it might be, but watching and reading the national news rekindled all the feelings related to the horror of 9/11. They compelled me to include this report since it demonstrates the far-reaching consequences of this life-changing event. Not only did almost 3000 individuals lose their lives, but even unborn babies were harmed.

It is a decade since the tumbling of the Twin Towers, and Arne Ohlsson, Prakesh S. Shah, and the Knowledge Synthesis Group of Determinants of Preterm/LBW systematically review the risks of adverse pregnancy outcomes after the terrorist attacks on September 11, 2001. All studies included in the review used controls born before or after the event. To cut to the chase the systematic review, with low to moderate overall risk of bias, demonstrated that the terrorist attack affected pregnancy and birth outcomes adversely in and around the disaster area in New York, among Arabic women in California, and in a cohort of women in Holland. The most consistent finding was reduction in birth weight and an increase in small for gestational age births. In New York, a doubling of adducts (which are compounds formed by direct combination of two or more compounds or elements) in environmental tobacco smoke—exposed mothers resulted in an estimated average 276 g (8%) (95% confidence interval 31—480 g) reduction in birth weight (*P* = .03). Whereas women of Arabic origin in California were affected, the findings were not duplicated in women of Arabic origin in Michigan, for reasons that are not entirely clear.

The recently documented increase in male fetal loss in the United States following the World Trade Center (WTC) disaster supports the notion of impact of the WTC disaster on birth outcomes.

At the WTC site and its surroundings, a toxic atmospheric plume was released that contained soot, benzene, polycyclic aromatic hydrocarbons (PAHs), polychlorinated biphenyls, polychlorinated furans, dioxins, heavy metals, pulverized glass, cement, asbestos, lead, and alkaline particulates. Particulate levels in the air were very high immediately after the disaster and decreased sharply with increasing distance from the WTC. This increased pollution may have affected birth outcomes among pregnant women who were directly exposed. In the vicinity of the WTC, it is likely the effect on fetal growth was a combination of pollution and psychological stress, whereas in Holland stress only ("communal bereavement") has been implicated. The long-term affects on the offspring are unavailable at this time, but there are concerns that intellect and verbal communicating skills may be impaired.

The authors suggest population-based registration such as is available in Nordic countries and measurement of stress and markers of pollution in cord blood following manmade and natural disasters. The tsunami/earthquake in Japan unfortunately immediately provides the opportunity to test these techniques.

A. A. Fanaroff, MD, FRCPE, FRCP&CH

Intake of artificially sweetened soft drinks and risk of preterm delivery: A prospective cohort study in 59,334 Danish pregnant women
Halldorsson TI, Strøm M, Petersen SB, et al (Statens Serum Institut, Copenhagen, Denmark)
Am J Clin Nutr 92:626-633, 2010

Background.—Sugar-sweetened soft drinks have been linked to a number of adverse health outcomes such as high weight gain. Therefore, artificially sweetened soft drinks are often promoted as an alternative. However, the safety of artificial sweeteners has been disputed, and consequences of high intakes of artificial sweeteners for pregnant women have been minimally addressed.

Objective.—We examined the association between intakes of sugar-sweetened and artificially sweetened soft drinks and preterm delivery.

Design.—We conducted prospective cohort analyses of 59,334 women from the Danish National Birth Cohort (1996–2002). Soft drink intake was assessed in midpregnancy by using a food-frequency questionnaire. Preterm delivery (<37 wk) was the primary outcome measure. Covariate information was assessed by telephone interviews.

Results.—There was an association between intake of artificially sweetened carbonated and noncarbonated soft drinks and an increased risk of preterm delivery (P for trend: ≤0.001, both variables). In comparison with women with no intake of artificially sweetened carbonated soft drinks, the adjusted odds ratio for women who consumed ≥1 serving of artificially sweetened carbonated soft drinks/d was 1.38 (95% CI: 1.15, 1.65). The corresponding odds ratio for women who consumed ≥4 servings of artificially sweetened carbonated soft drinks/d was 1.78 (95% CI: 1.19, 2.66). The association was observed for normal-weight and overweight women. A stronger increase in risk was observed for early preterm and moderately preterm delivery than with late-preterm delivery. No association was observed for sugar-sweetened carbonated soft drinks (*P* for trend: 0.29) or for sugar-sweetened noncarbonated soft drinks (*P* for trend: 0.93).

Conclusions.—Daily intake of artificially sweetened soft drinks may increase the risk of preterm delivery. Further studies are needed to reject or confirm these findings.

▶ There is a lot of concern about optimal weight gain, diet, and nutrition during pregnancy. One of these concerns is regarding artificial sweeteners and their use during pregnancy. Many women will cut sugar out of their diet, only to replace it with foods and drinks that are artificially sweetened. Is this practice safe? Firstly, there is limited research on the safety and use of non-nutritive sweeteners during pregnancy. The following artificial sweeteners have been deemed safe for use in pregnancy by the US Food and Drug Administration (FDA): rebaudioside A (Stevia), acesulfame potassium (Sunett), aspartame (Equal or NutraSweet), and sucralose (Splenda). However, the FDA emphasized they should be "used in moderation" or "it is recommended to limit consumption to a moderate level." Aspartame should not be used by anyone with PKU, rare liver disease, or by pregnant women who have high levels of phenylalanine in their blood. Phenylalanine is a component of aspartame and it may not metabolize correctly in anyone who has these conditions. Saccharin (Sweet'N Low) crosses the placenta and may remain in fetal tissues and is not recommended by some providers for pregnant women, whereas cyclamates were linked to cancer, have been banned in the United States, and are not considered safe for anyone, certainly not pregnant women.

Halldorsson et al add more fuel to the discussion with their large data set. In this large prospective cohort of pregnant women, they observed a positive association between the intake of artificially sweetened soft drinks and the risk of preterm delivery. No association was observed for sugar-sweetened soft drinks. The associations for the artificially sweetened soft drinks were robust to stratification by prepregnancy body mass index and were primarily driven by medically induced preterm delivery rather than spontaneous delivery. They were of the opinion that the finding was unrelated to preeclampsia or hypertensive disorders in pregnancy since artificial sweeteners may raise blood pressure.

There was an interesting discussion on potential mechanisms, and the presumed culprit is methanol, which is a break down product of aspartame. It has been blamed for the headaches associated with aspartame, and methanol exposure (even to vapors) shortens gestation in animals. As is inevitable, the article concludes with the clarion call for more studies: "However, the replication of our findings in another experimental setting is warranted." This is a very reasonable conclusion.

A. A. Fanaroff, MD, FRCPE, FRCP&CH

Knowledge and Practice of Prechewing/Prewarming Food by HIV-Infected Women

Gaur AH, Freimanis-Hance L, Dominguez K, et al (St Jude Children's Res Hosp, Memphis, TN; Westat, Rockville, MD; Ctrs for Disease Control and Prevention, Atlanta, GA; et al)
Pediatrics 127:e1206-e1211, 2011

Objective.—HIV transmission has been associated with offering a child food prechewed by an HIV-infected caregiver. We assessed awareness of prechewing and oral prewarming of food by an adult before offering it to a child among HIV-infected pregnant women and clinical investigators in 3 Latin American countries.

Methods.—HIV-infected pregnant women at 12 sites (Eunice Kennedy Shriver National Institute of Child Health and Human Development International Site Development Initiative Perinatal Longitudinal Study in Latin American Countries, a prospective cohort trial) in Argentina, Brazil, and Peru were administered a screening survey about prechewing/prewarming of infant foods and cautioned against these feeding practices. Survey responses were analyzed, overall, and stratified according to country.

Results.—Of the 401 HIV-infected pregnant women interviewed, 34% had heard about prechewing (50% from Argentina, 32% from Brazil, and 36% from Peru), 23% knew someone who prechewed food for infants, and 4% had prechewed food in the past. Seventeen percent had heard about oral prewarming of food, 13% knew someone who prewarmed food for infants, and 3% had prewarmed food for an infant in the past. Women who reported knowing someone who prechewed were more likely to also know someone who prewarmed food ($P < .0001$). Few site investigators anticipated that their patients would be aware of these practices.

Conclusions.—Prechewing food, a potential risk factor for HIV transmission, and orally prewarming food, which has not been associated with HIV transmission but might expose a child to blood from an HIV-infected adult, are not uncommon practices in Latin America. Both practices should be further investigated. Site investigator responses underscore that health care providers could be missing information about cultural practices that patients may not report unless specifically asked.

▶ Premastication (prechewing) of foods for infants is a common practice that provides an alternative to blending foods for infants or sometimes buying expensive baby foods. It may even play a role in supporting infant health.[1] Prior to this study, the authors reported 3 cases of HIV infection associated with providing premasticated food to a child. The source of blood in the saliva of the person prechewing the food for the child likely was the source of the infection in the children. In this article, it was found that HIV almost certainly was transmitted from mothers or other caregivers to children through prechewed food. The authors thus undertook this broader study where they administered a survey to a cohort of pregnant women with HIV from 3 countries in

Latin America (Peru, Argentina, and Brazil) to determine the prevalence of this practice. Of 401 pregnant women with HIV interviewed, 34% had heard about prechewing, but only 4% said they had prechewed food for their infants in the past. Even though most of these mothers stated they did not premasticate food for their infants, the fact that such a large number know of people who did, suggests a relatively high prevalence of this practice. Although this practice and its relationship to HIV has not been broadly studied, it suggests that it is reasonable that HIV-infected mothers or other caregivers should be warned against giving infants prechewed food and directed toward safer feeding options. Beyond the mothers with HIV, this practice is intriguing and may actually provide some benefits in societies where access to baby foods as we know them are not readily available.

J. Neu, MD

Reference

1. Pelto GH, Zhang Y, Habicht JP. Premastication: the second arm of infant and young child feeding for health and survival? *Matern Child Nutr.* 2010;6:4-18.

Neonatal Abstinence Syndrome after Methadone or Buprenorphine Exposure

Jones HE, Kaltenbach K, Heil SH, et al (Johns Hopkins Univ School of Medicine, Baltimore, MD; Thomas Jefferson Univ, Philadelphia, PA; Univ of Vermont, Burlington; et al)
N Engl J Med 363:2320-2331, 2010

Background.—Methadone, a full mu-opioid agonist, is the recommended treatment for opioid dependence during pregnancy. However, prenatal exposure to methadone is associated with a neonatal abstinence syndrome (NAS) characterized by central nervous system hyperirritability and autonomic nervous system dysfunction, which often requires medication and extended hospitalization. Buprenorphine, a partial mu-opioid agonist, is an alternative treatment for opioid dependence but has not been extensively studied in pregnancy.

Methods.—We conducted a double-blind, double-dummy, flexible-dosing, randomized, controlled study in which buprenorphine and methadone were compared for use in the comprehensive care of 175 pregnant women with opioid dependency at eight international sites. Primary outcomes were the number of neonates requiring treatment for NAS, the peak NAS score, the total amount of morphine needed to treat NAS, the length of the hospital stay for neonates, and neonatal head circumference.

Results.—Treatment was discontinued by 16 of the 89 women in the methadone group (18%) and 28 of the 86 women in the buprenorphine group (33%). A comparison of the 131 neonates whose mothers were followed to the end of pregnancy according to treatment group (with 58 exposed to buprenorphine and 73 exposed to methadone) showed that the former group required significantly less morphine (mean dose, 1.1 mg vs. 10.4 mg; P<0.0091), had a significantly shorter hospital stay (10.0 days vs. 17.5 days, P<0.0091), and had a significantly shorter duration of treatment for the neonatal abstinence syndrome (4.1 days vs. 9.9 days, P<0.003125) (P values calculated in accordance with prespecified thresholds for significance). There were no significant differences between groups in other primary or secondary outcomes or in the rates of maternal or neonatal adverse events.

Conclusions.—These results are consistent with the use of buprenorphine as an acceptable treatment for opioid dependence in pregnant women. (Funded by the National Institute on Drug Abuse; ClinicalTrials. gov number, NCT00271219.)

▶ In 2009 in the United States, medical costs associated with the treatment of neonates exposed to opioids were estimated at $70.6 million to $112.6 million. Much of the cost is related to the treatment of neonatal abstinence syndrome (NAS), a clinical condition characterized by hyperirritability of the central nervous system and dysfunction in the autonomic nervous system, gastrointestinal tract, and respiratory system.

The recommended standard of care for opioid-dependent pregnant women is methadone, a mu-opioid agonist. However, maternal methadone treatment is associated with a more severe and prolonged course of NAS compared with heroin exposure. This issue has encouraged the development of other synthetic opioids as alternative treatments to methadone. In this study, the investigators compared the safety and efficacy of buprenorphine, a partial mu-opioid agonist, with that of methadone. The number of infants requiring NAS treatment and the peak NAS scores were not different for the 2 cohorts of infants, but the total amount of morphine needed to treat NAS and the length of hospital stay were significantly less for infants who had prenatal exposure to buprenorphine. These results suggest that buprenorphine has some advantages to methadone as a treatment for opioid dependence in pregnant women. The high discontinuation rate among women in the buprenorphine group is concerning and implies that buprenorphine may not be the optimal treatment for all pregnant women with dependence on opioids and will likely limit its use to a select group of women.

L. A. Papile, MD

Neonatal Outcomes After Demonstrated Fetal Lung Maturity Before 39 Weeks of Gestation
Bates E, Rouse DJ, Mann ML, et al (Univ of Alabama at Birmingham; Warren Alpert Med School of Brown Univ, Providence, RI)
Obstet Gynecol 116:1288-1295, 2010

Objective.—To compare outcomes among neonates delivered after documentation of fetal lung maturity before 39 weeks and those delivered at 39 or 40 weeks.

Methods.—This was a retrospective cohort study of women with singleton pregnancy delivered at 36 0/7 to 38 6/7 weeks after positive fetal lung maturity testing (based on amniotic fluid lecithin to sphingomyelin ratio) or at 39 0/7 to 40 6/7 weeks (without maturity testing) at our center from 1999 to 2008. Women with fetuses with major congenital anomalies, cord prolapse, nonreassuring antepartum testing, placental abruption, or oligohydramnios were excluded. A primary composite neonatal outcome included death, adverse respiratory outcomes, hypoglycemia, treated hyperbilirubinemia, generalized seizures, necrotizing enterocolitis, hypoxic ischemic encephalopathy, periventricular leukomalacia, and suspected or proven sepsis.

Results.—There were 459 neonates delivered at 36 to 38 weeks and 13,339 delivered at 39 to 40 weeks; mean birth weight was $3,107 \pm 548$ g and $3,362 \pm 439$ g, respectively. The risk of the composite adverse neonatal outcome was 6.1% for the 36- to 38-week group compared with 2.5% for the 39- to 40-week group (relative risk 2.4; confidence interval [CI] 1.7–3.5). After multivariable adjustment, early delivery remained significantly associated with an increased risk of the composite outcome (adjusted odds ratio [OR]1.7; CI 1.1–2.6) as well as several individual outcomes, including respiratory distress syndrome (adjusted OR 7.6; CI 2.2–26.6), treated hyperbilirubinemia (adjusted OR 11.2; CI 3.6–34), and hypoglycemia (adjusted OR 5.8; CI 2.4–14.3).

Conclusion.—Neonates delivered at 36 to 38 weeks after confirmed fetal lung maturity are at higher risk of adverse outcomes than those delivered at 39 to 40 weeks.

▶ This retrospective cohort study reminded me of that old television commercial, which chided "It's not nice to fool Mother nature." The investigators compared short-term outcomes of infants born prior to 39 weeks with documented fetal lung maturity with outcomes of infants born after 39 weeks without lung maturity testing. Although subject to the usual limitations of study methodology, there are 2 strong messages that we should heed. First, fetal lung maturity does not connote neonatal maturity. The lecithin:sphingomyelin ratio may give us information about the presence or absence of surfactant, but it doesn't tell us whether other necessary elements of fetal-to-neonatal transition are going to work. Odds ratios for most adverse respiratory outcomes were significantly higher in the less mature infants, including the use of surfactant, ventilator support, and respiratory distress syndrome. Second, there are significant economic consequences of earlier delivery, including admission to the neonatal intensive care unit and hospitalization longer than 4 days. Our obstetrical colleagues would be wise to heed the conclusions of this study.

S. M. Donn, MD

Obstetric outcomes after treatment of periodontal disease during pregnancy: systematic review and meta-analysis

Polyzos NP, Polyzos IP, Zavos A, et al (Panhellenic Association for Continual Med Res (PACMeR), Athens, Greece; Univ of Manchester, UK; Univ of Thessalia, Larisa, Greece; et al)
BMJ 341:c7017, 2010

Objective.—To examine whether treatment of periodontal disease with scaling and root planing during pregnancy is associated with a reduction in the preterm birth rate.

Design.—Systematic review and meta-analysis of randomised controlled trials.

Data Sources.—Cochrane Central Trials Registry, ISI Web of Science, Medline, and reference lists of relevant studies to July 2010; hand searches in key journals.

Study Selection.—Randomised controlled trials including pregnant women with documented periodontal disease randomised to either treatment with scaling and root planing or no treatment.

Data Extraction.—Data were extracted by two independent investigators, and a consensus was reached with the involvement a third. Methodological quality of the studies was assessed with the Cochrane's risk of bias tool, and trials were considered either high or low quality. The primary outcome was preterm birth (<37 weeks). Secondary outcomes were low birthweight infants (<2500 g), spontaneous abortions/stillbirths, and overall adverse pregnancy outcome (preterm birth <37 weeks and spontaneous abortions/stillbirths).

Results.—11 trials (with 6558 women) were included. Five trials were considered to be of high methodological quality (low risk of bias), whereas the rest were low quality (high or unclear risk of bias). Results among low and high quality trials were consistently diverse; low quality trials supported a beneficial effect of treatment, and high quality trials provided clear evidence that no such effect exists. Among high quality studies, treatment had no significant effect on the overall rate of preterm birth (odds ratio 1.15, 95% confidence interval 0.95 to 1.40; P=0.15). Furthermore, treatment did not reduce the rate of low birthweight infants (odds ratio 1.07, 0.85 to 1.36; P=0.55), spontaneous abortions/stillbirths (0.79, 0.51 to 1.22; P=0.28), or overall adverse pregnancy outcome (preterm births <37 weeks and spontaneous abortions/stillbirths) (1.09, 0.91 to 1.30; P=0.34).

Conclusion.—Treatment of periodontal disease with scaling and root planing cannot be considered to be an efficient way of reducing the incidence of preterm birth. Women may be advised to have periodical dental examinations during pregnancy to test their dental status and may have treatment for periodontal disease. However, they should be told that such treatment during pregnancy is unlikely to reduce the risk of preterm birth or low birthweight infants.

▶ The hypothesis that there is a possible connection between preterm delivery and periodontal disease in pregnant women emerged in the early 1990s. However, there is still controversy as to whether there is a true correlation among periodontal infection, preterm delivery, and restriction of fetal growth. Wimmer et al[1] noted "Variability among studies in definitions of periodontal disease and adverse pregnancy outcomes as well as widespread inadequate control for confounding factors and possible effect modification make it difficult to base meaningful conclusions on published data. However, while there are indications of an association between periodontal disease and increased risk of adverse pregnancy outcome in some populations, there is no conclusive evidence that treating periodontal disease improves birth outcome." Some study designs were epidemiological, some microbiological, and others interventional. In contrast, Polyzos et al,[2] on the basis of a meta-analysis of randomized controlled trials, concluded that periodontal disease treatment with scaling and/or root planing during pregnancy reduced preterm birth without evidence of harm. There is a consensus that more methodologically rigorous studies are needed in this field. Now these trials have been completed and published and Polyzos et al present the evidence in this systematic review and meta-analysis. Indeed, after reweighting the evidence, they have changed their conclusions. They have divided the trials into those

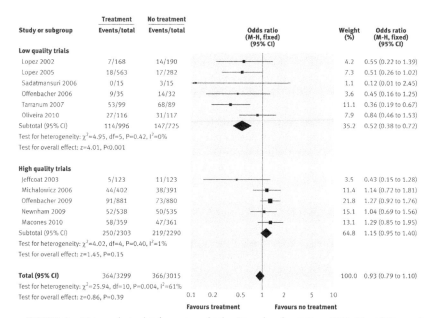

FIGURE 3.—Meta-analysis plot for preterm birth <37 weeks of gestation. M-H=Mantel-Haenszel model. (Reprinted from Polyzos NP, Polyzos IP, Zavos A, et al. Obstetric outcomes after treatment of periodontal disease during pregnancy: systematic review and meta-analysis. *BMJ.* 2010;341:c7017, reproduced with permission from the BMJ Publishing Group Ltd.)

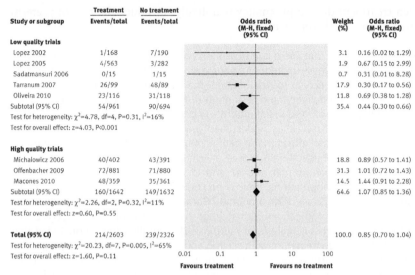

FIGURE 4.—Meta-analysis plot for low birthweight infants (<2500 g). M-H=Mantel-Haenszel model. (Reprinted from Polyzos NP, Polyzos IP, Zavos A, et al. Obstetric outcomes after treatment of peri-odontal disease during pregnancy: systematic review and meta-analysis. *BMJ.* 2010;341:c7017, repro-duced with permission from the BMJ Publishing Group Ltd.)

with low risk of bias (high quality) and those with high risk of bias (low quality; see Figs 3 and 4), with consistently diverse outcomes. Those trials considered to be low quality consistently showed a beneficial effect of the intervention, whereas the high-quality trials showed no such benefit. I am impressed with the quality of the evidence as well as the numbers of patients included in the trials and would concur with the findings that treatment of periodontal disease with scaling and root planning during pregnancy does not reduce the risk of preterm birth and should not be routinely recommended as a measure to prevent preterm birth. Nonetheless, pregnancy must be regarded as a critical opportunity to educate women on the benefits of good oral health and identify and refer women who are in need of dental care for treatment.

A. A. Fanaroff, MD, FRCPE, FRCP&CH

References

1. Wimmer G, Pihlstrom BL. A critical assessment of adverse pregnancy outcome and periodontal disease. *J Clin Periodontol.* 2008;35:380-397.
2. Polyzos NP, Polyzos IP, Mauri D, et al. Effect of periodontal disease treatment during pregnancy on preterm birth incidence: a metaanalysis of randomized trials. *Am J Obstet Gynecol.* 2009;200:225-232.

Placental Infarction and Thrombophilia

Franco C, Walker M, Robertson J, et al (Univ of Toronto, Canada; Mount Sinai Hosp, Toronto, Canada; Sunnybrook Health Sciences Centre, Toronto, Canada)
Obstet Gynecol 117:929-934, 2011

Objective.—To estimate the relative importance of positive maternal thrombophilia testing compared with additional pathological evidence of abnormal placentation with placental infarction.

Methods.—We performed a retrospective cohort study over a 10-year period in 180 singleton high-risk pregnancies (delivery at 22−34 6/7 weeks of gestation) that had histologic evidence of placental infarction. The rate of positive maternal tests for antiphospholipid syndrome, factor V Leiden, and prothrombin gene mutation were compared with the rate of detection of one or more gross or histological features of abnormal placentation (impaired placental development or differentiation, maternal vascular underperfusion, fetal vascular underperfusion, chronic inflammation, or intervillous thrombosis).

Results.—Only 14 of 108 (13.0%) of placentas with documented infarction were associated with a positive maternal thrombophilia result. In contrast, 67 of 108 (62.3%) placentas showed features of abnormal placental development or differentiation and 85 of 108 (78.7%) had evidence of noninfarct-related maternal vascular underperfusion ($P < .001$). Only four of 108 (3.7%) infarcted placentas had no other pathologic lesions.

Conclusion.—Our data indicate that gross and histologic features of abnormal placentation associate strongly with placental infarction in comparison with maternal thrombophilia tests.

Level of Evidence.—II.

▶ Over the past 25 years, the sanctity of the fetus in the uterus has been disturbed to determine fetal growth, well-being, presence or absence of anomalies, or even to correct a few specific birth defects. Fetal outcome is ultimately determined by the composite of genetic risk factors, preexisting or pregnancy-related maternal disease, maternal nutrition, exposure to toxins (with or without recognition that they are indeed toxins), and a host of other injurious extrinsic events. Contemporary thought is that short-term and long-term adverse pregnancy outcomes and even some long-term chronic diseases extending into adult life are at least partly determined by processes occurring during intrauterine life. Redline, from our institution, is a remarkable pediatric pathologist with special interest in the placenta. He refers to the placenta as a "diary of intrauterine life" that has the potential to illuminate many aspects of these processes.[1] He is a master detective at finding all the clues in the diary and has been responsible for helping us make or confirm the diagnosis in many complex cases, merely by examining the placenta. He laments the fact that there has not been general agreement on defining placental lesions. He proposed a simple conceptual framework separating placental patterns of injury and maladaptation into 3 categories of lesions affecting the maternal and fetal vasculature (maldevelopment, obstruction, and disruption) and 2 categories of inflammatory lesions (infectious and idiopathic).[2]

Disorders of the placental circulation, including the release of deleterious mediators to the fetus, are important risk factors for central nervous system complications. Less than 10% of placentas from term infants that later develop cerebral palsy lack any evidence of placental abnormalities potentially related to adverse outcome.[3] In an evaluation of 125 neurologically impaired term infants who were the focus of clinical negligence litigation and 250 consecutive singleton term deliveries, severe fetal placental vascular lesions, including fetal thrombotic vasculopathy, chronic villitis with obliterative fetal vasculopathy, chorioamnionitis with severe fetal vasculitis, and meconium-associated fetal vascular necrosis, were correlated highly with neurologic impairment and cerebral palsy.[4] Their nature, duration, and anatomic location make them strong candidates for the antepartum processes that place fetuses at risk for brain injury during the intrapartum period.

Elevated nucleated red blood cells in the newborn are regarded as evidence of hostile in utero events. Redline et al[5] reported that the number of nucleated red blood cells per 10 high-power fields of villous parenchyma was directly correlated with the nucleated red blood cell count and a threshold of 10 or more nucleated red blood cells predicted a nucleated red blood cell count greater than $2.5 \times 10(3)/mm$. Among individual placental lesions, multiple foci of avascular villi and chronic villitis were significantly associated with an elevated nucleated red blood cell count, whereas meconium-associated vascular necrosis showed a borderline association. Acute chorioamnionitis was the only placental lesion more common in the group without elevated nucleated red blood cell count.

The article abstracted here provides further insight into the role of placental pathology in adverse perinatal outcomes. Rather than finding a strong association between maternal disorders of coagulation and placental infarction, the authors found histopathologic evidence of noninfarct utero-placental (maternal) vascular pathology in 85 of 108 (78.7%) placentas. This is strikingly in contrast with the weak association with detectable maternal thrombophilia in only 14 of 108 (13%) placentas with documented infarction associated with a positive maternal thrombophilia result. The message is to start comprehensively evaluating the placenta with biochemistry, Doppler, and ultrasound early in pregnancy. Evidence of placental dysfunction includes false-positive maternal serum blood test results for trisomy 21, reduced placental size, and reduced utero-placental blood flow. Two or more abnormal test categories of placental function are highly predictive of placental infarction. Trials of heparin therapy in the presence of abnormal placental function are underway and will provide the framework for managing such pregnancies that are likely to be complicated by intrauterine growth restriction, stillbirth, or neurologic injury.

A. A. Fanaroff, MD, FRCPE, FRCP&CH

References

1. Redline RW. Severe fetal placental vascular lesions in term infants with neurologic impairment. *Am J Obstet Gynecol.* 2005;192:452-457.

2. Redline RW. Placental pathology: a systematic approach with clinical correlations. *Placenta.* 2008;29:S86-S91.
3. Redline RW, Minich N, Taylor HG, Hack M. Placental lesions as predictors of cerebral palsy and abnormal neurocognitive function at school age in extremely low birth weight infants (<1 kg). *Pediatr Dev Pathol.* 2007;10:282-292.
4. Redline RW. Clinical and pathological umbilical cord abnormalities in fetal thrombotic vasculopathy. *Hum Pathol.* 2004;35:1494-1498.
5. Redline RW. Elevated circulating fetal nucleated red blood cells and placental pathology in term infants who develop cerebral palsy. *Hum Pathol.* 2008;39: 1378-1384.

Risk of Gestational Diabetes Mellitus in Relation to Maternal Egg and Cholesterol Intake

Qiu C, Frederick IO, Zhang C, et al (Swedish Med Ctr, Seattle, WA; Natl Insts of Health, Bethesda, MD)
Am J Epidemiol 173:649-658, 2011

Higher egg and cholesterol intakes are associated with increased risk of type 2 diabetes mellitus. However, their association with gestational diabetes mellitus (GDM) has not been evaluated. The authors assessed such associations in both a prospective cohort study (1996—2008; 3,158 participants) and a case-control study (1998—2002; 185 cases, 411 controls). A food frequency questionnaire was used to assess maternal diet. Multivariable models were used to derive relative risks and 95% confidence intervals. Compared with no egg consumption, adjusted relative risks for GDM were 0.94, 1.01, 1.12, 1.54, and 2.52 for consumption of ≤1, 2—3, 4—6, 7—9, and ≥10 eggs/week, respectively (*P* for trend = 0.008). Women with high egg consumption (≥7/week) had a 1.77-fold increased risk compared with women with lower consumption (95% confidence interval (CI): 1.19, 2.63). The relative risk for the highest quartile of cholesterol intake (≥294 mg/day) versus the lowest (<151 mg/day) was 2.35 (95% CI: 1.35, 4.09). In the case-control study, the adjusted odds ratio for consuming ≥7 eggs/week versus <7 eggs/week was 2.65 (95% CI: 1.48, 4.72), and the odds of GDM increased with increasing cholesterol intake (*P* for trend = 0.021). In conclusion, high egg and cholesterol intakes before and during pregnancy are associated with increased risk of GDM.

▶ The concern that eating eggs can cause heart attacks and metabolic problems, such as type 2 diabetes, comes from the fact that eggs are one of the most concentrated sources of dietary cholesterol. This study used 2 different cohorts, one prospective and the other a case control study, to evaluate whether higher maternal egg intake was associated with a higher risk of gestational diabetes mellitus. There appeared to be a stepwise increase in adjusted relative risk for gestational diabetes with increasing egg intake in the prospective study. A similar relationship was found in the case control study. This is reminiscent of previous studies that suggested that eating more eggs also increased heart disease. However, skepticism is in order. The Physician's Health Study followed doctors for 20 years and showed no association between eating eggs and heart attacks or strokes. However, the doctors who ate lots of eggs did die earlier than those who avoided eggs, possibly because they also ate more bacon, sausage, and butter.[1]

It is obvious when one looks closely at the data in this study that the women who ate more eggs also had a higher total caloric intake. This probably did not start when these women became pregnant. Statistical correction may take several covariates into account, but this is a complex issue and dietary recall studies may not be able to dissect all the covariates. In this study, the analysis needed to manipulate the data so that all the groups of women who ate less than 7 eggs per week were compared with those who ate more. The risk was 1.77 with confidence intervals of 1.19 and 2.63, which is not terribly impressive. Nevertheless, this study shows a correlation with egg intake (with putative increased cholesterol intake) but does not clearly dissect whether it is the higher egg intake or the baggage that comes with higher egg intake (other eating habits, previous metabolic status, etc) that is causative.

J. Neu, MD

Reference

1. Kritchevsky SB, Kritchevsky D. Egg consumption and coronary heart disease: an epidemiologic overview. *J Am Coll Nutr.* 2000;19:549S-555S.

The Tiniest Babies: A Registry of Survivors With Birth Weight Less Than 400 Grams

Bell EF, Zumbach DK (Univ of Iowa, Iowa City)
Pediatrics 127:58-61, 2011

Objective.—The purpose of this project was to collect information on surviving infants with birth weights of <400 g.

Methods.—A Web-based registry was started in 2000 after searching for published reports of infants who survived to hospital discharge despite being born at <400 g. Fifteen cases were identified from scientific and lay print and Web-based publications. Parents, patients, and health providers were invited to submit data on additional infants. In the case of submissions from parents or patients, the information was confirmed by communication with a treating physician.

Results.—As of September 1, 2010, the Tiniest Babies Registry had compiled data on 110 patients born between 1936 and 2010. The number of infants who survived each year increased since the early 1990s. The infants in the registry weighed between 260 and 397 g at birth and had gestational ages from 21⁶/₇ to 34 weeks. Eighty-three (75%) of the patients are female. The 10 smallest infants are female, and the registry contains only 1 boy who was born weighing <300 g. The patients were born in 10 countries, including 80 (73%) born in the United States. The

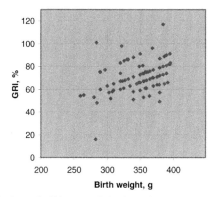

FIGURE 4.—GRI ([birth weight/fifth-percentile birth weight] × 100%) versus birth weight for 108 infants in the Tiniest Babies Registry. Data for 2 patients are not plotted because of lack of sufficiently accurate information about gestational length. (Reproduced with permission from *Pediatrics*, Bell EF, Zumbach DK. The tiniest babies: a registry of survivors with birth weight less than 400 grams. *Pediatrics*. 2011;127:58-61. Copyright © 2011 by the American Academy of Pediatrics.)

information on long-term functional outcome and health outcomes is limited. Many patients have ongoing health and learning concerns, and most of those for whom growth data are available remain short in stature and underweight for their age.

Conclusions.—Survival of infants born weighing <400 g is rare but increasing. The Tiniest Babies Registry provides a repository for information about this remarkable group of infants.

▶ This short report should be required reading for every neonatologist. Although the reported data is essentially anecdotal, it enables a few important conclusions, which are concisely stated by the authors. Reports of survival of infants with birth weights less than 400 g are rare, but these events may be increasing in frequency in the past 2 decades or so. Virtually all such infants are small for dates (Fig 4), so the authors remind us pointedly that these anecdotes should not encourage efforts to save such tiny preterm infants who are appropriately grown and therefore too immature (<20 weeks' gestation) to have any chance of survival to hospital discharge. These cases do provide support for a cautious and circumspect approach to management of fetuses and newborn infants with very severe fetal growth restriction, but data on long-term outcomes are scant. Although 2 instances of apparently satisfactory quality of life are described, the authors note: "Most of the patients have ongoing health and learning concerns, and most of those for whom growth data are available remain short in stature and underweight for their age." Along with Dr Bell and Ms Zumbach, we must "hope the registry does not spur competition to save the smallest infant on record."

W. E. Benitz, MD

5 Ethics

Bereaved Parents' Perceptions of the Autopsy Examination of Their Child
Sullivan J, Monagle P (Univ of Melbourne, Australia)
Pediatrics 127:e1013-e1020, 2011

Objective.—In this study we explored parental views of their child's autopsy, their experiences with autopsy-related processes, and the impact of the examination on their grief.

Methods.—A survey design with a mailed questionnaire was used. The inclusion criteria were that an autopsy had been performed on the child and it was at least 3 months since his or her death. The questionnaire consisted of nonidentifying demographic details about the child, a standardized grief measure (parts A and B of the Texas Revised Inventory of Grief), and 28 questions with response sets and opportunities for comment. Fifty-three parents participated.

Results.—Our findings suggest a complexity of perceptions associated with pediatric autopsy examination. A distinction was identified between the informational and altruistic benefits of autopsy and its supportive qualities. Ninety percent of parents valued autopsy as a means of finding out why their child died, and 77% appreciated its contribution to medical knowledge. The general unequivocal helpfulness for bereaved parents commonly ascribed to autopsy examinations was not found. Parents expressed uncertainty about their perceptions of autopsy. Forty-one percent of the parents felt that it helped them live with their loss and 30% found it a comfort, whereas 42% of the parents felt that their child's autopsy examination added to their grief. The results underscore the necessity for open discussion with parents about the realities of what autopsy can offer them.

Conclusions.—Our results add to the knowledge about the meaning of autopsy for grieving parents and challenge some current beliefs.

▶ This study challenges the notion that an autopsy may be a tool for the resolution of grief for parents by the availability of factual data; it should make everyone who obtains parental consent do so with due circumspection about the potential impact of the autopsy on the parents, particularly in relation to their grief and mourning.

The study strongly confirmed the view that parents need to know why their child died, regardless of predeath circumstances. However, the caveat to this is that although an autopsy may provide a factual cause for the child's death, at least for one-third of the parents, it still does not answer the question in a more existential, spiritual, or philosophical sense as to why their child had died.

Altruism in the advancement of medical knowledge was a strong theme that parents expressed. This was true even in autopsies of those with chronic illness, where consent to autopsy may have reflected parents' sense of giving back to society, thereby highlighting the obligation of the medical profession to disseminate and use autopsy findings. Overall, the study found complex reactions not readily categorized into positive or negative responses. For example, parental views were almost evenly divided on questions of whether the autopsy added to grief, assisted parents to live with their loss, or helped with their grief or feelings of finality.

Extrapolation of the findings to the neonatal population may be limited, as only 35% of the autopsies were in infants less than 3 months, and hospital and coronial cases were not differentiated; nevertheless, the study findings show the complexity of parental perceptions and seriously challenge the notion that an autopsy is psychologically supportive and a tool for the resolution of parental grief.

It is this type of nuanced finding that should give pause for everyone. The message to be taken from this study is that requesting consent from parents to perform an autopsy requires individualized assessment, sufficient detail (no parent considered the discussion too detailed), and the limitations of what an autopsy can offer, together with an appreciation of the potential impact the autopsy may invoke. It should be part of a bereavement support process with the promise of timely review of findings (absence of information and unanswered questions until the report is discussed create distress) be done in plain language and accompanied by monitoring of the parents' mourning pathway.

J. Hellman, MBBCh, FRCPC, MHSc

Categorizing neonatal deaths: a cross-cultural study in the United States, Canada, and The Netherlands
Verhagen AA, Janvier A, Leuthner SR, et al (Univ Med Ctr Groningen, The Netherlands)
J Pediatr 156:33-37, 2010

Objective.—To clarify the process of end-of-life decision-making in culturally different neonatal intensive care units (NICUs).

Study Design.—Review of medical files of newborns >22 weeks gestation who died in the delivery room (DR) or the NICU during 12 months in 4 NICUs (Chicago, Milwaukee, Montreal, and Groningen). We categorized deaths using a 2-by-2 matrix and determined whether mechanical ventilation was withdrawn/withheld and whether the child was dying despite ventilation or physiologically stable but extubated for neurological prognosis.

Results.—Most unstable patients in all units died in their parents' arms after mechanical ventilation was withdrawn. In Milwaukee, Montreal, and Groningen, 4% to 12% of patients died while receiving cardiopulmonary resuscitation. This proportion was higher in Chicago (31%). Elective extubation for quality-of-life reasons never occurred in Chicago and occurred in 19% to 35% of deaths in the other units. The proportion of DR deaths in Milwaukee, Montreal, and Groningen was 16% to 22%. No DR deaths occurred in Chicago.

Conclusions.—Death in the NICU occurred differently within and between countries. Distinctive end-of-life decisions can be categorized separately by using a model with uniform definitions of withholding/withdrawing mechanical ventilation correlated with the patient's physiological condition. Cross-cultural comparison of end-of-life practice is feasible and important when comparing NICU outcomes.

▶ Lack of explicit definitions and descriptions of practice in withdrawing life-sustaining medical treatment (LSMT) have limited the ability to know whether end-of-life (EOL) decisions in neonatal intensive care units are being made in infants whose death is impending or imminent or are being made in infants who might survive: so-called quality-of-life decisions. This retrospective study used a relatively simple 2-by-2 model regarding physiologic stability and degree of intervention to clarify this question and thereby highlight differences in the 4 units analyzed.

While the findings are to a degree reflective of the particular country's National Pediatric Societies' approach to the limits of viability guidelines, other differences cannot be accounted for by this, particularly in the 2 US units in which patterns of practice are fairly divergent. This raises the issue of unit culture—culture with a small c, namely, "the way we do things around here." What are the determinants of individual unit approaches to EOL decision making? Is it one leading proponent within that institution, a consensus of physicians and other health care professionals in the unit, the parent population and their homogeneity or heterogeneity? Is it the degree of tolerance of uncertainty, respect for parental views, manner of counseling, expectations of technology, religious/spiritual views of parents and the health care team, the use of assisted reproductive technique, or a myriad other reasons? Even though national guidelines may provide broad parameters and boundaries, it is still the culture of the particular unit that determines how these decisions are made. Further exploration of this complex issue would be intriguing.

J. Hellman, MBBCh, FRCPC, MHSc

Clinical Assessment of Extremely Premature Infants in the Delivery Room is a Poor Predictor of Survival
Manley BJ, Dawson JA, Kamlin COF, et al (Royal Women's Hosp, Melbourne, Victoria, Australia; et al)
Pediatrics 125:e559-e564, 2010

Background.—Some neonatologists state that at the delivery of extremely premature infants they rely on "how the baby looks" when deciding whether to initiate resuscitation. Previous studies have reported poor correlation between early clinical signs and prognosis.

Objective.—To determine if neonatologists can accurately predict survival to discharge of extremely premature infants on the basis of observations in the first minutes after birth.

Methods.—We showed videos of the resuscitation of 10 extremely premature infants (<26 weeks' gestation) to attending neonatologists and fellows from the 3 major perinatal centers in Melbourne, Australia. Antenatal information was available to the observers. A monitor visible in each video displayed the heart rate and oxygen saturation of the infant. Observers were asked to estimate the likelihood of survival to discharge for each infant at 3 time points: 20 seconds, 2 minutes, and 5 minutes after birth. The predictive ability of observers was expressed as the area (95% confidence interval [CI]) under the receiver-operating-characteristic curve.

Results.—Seventeen attending neonatologists and 17 neonatal fellows completed the study. Receiver-operating- characteristic curves were generated for the combined and individual groups. Observers' ability to predict survival was poor (combined results): 0.61 (95% CI: 0.54—0.67) at 20 seconds, 0.59 (95% CI: 0.52—0.64) at 2 minutes, and 0.61 (95% CI: 0.55—0.67) at 5 minutes. Level of experience did not affect the observers' accuracy of predicting survival.

Conclusion.—Neonatologists' reliance on initial appearance and early response to resuscitation in predicting survival for extremely premature infants is misplaced.

▶ As for a future life, every man must judge for himself between conflicting vague probabilities. Charles Robert Darwin (1809-1882).

Ethical decision making for premature infants has remained difficult since the dawn of neonatology. In the last few decades, with advancements such as improved ventilator capability, surfactant, nutrition, and antenatal steroids, these dilemmas now include extremely premature infants who in the best of circumstances face months in the intensive care unit and a high number of invasive procedures. For many parents and health care providers committed to doing what is best for the baby, it can be difficult to know if such care is truly in their best interests.

Ideally physicians meet with parents before delivery so that a trusting relationship can be established and a supportive environment created for the difficult decisions that must be made, often quickly and in the middle of the night.[1] A huge problem in these situations is the uncertainty that surrounds many decisions regarding resuscitation and treatment. Tools, such as the National Institute of Child Health and Human Development Outcomes Estimator [2] are helpful, but do not answer the most important question parents want answered: "what will happen to my baby?" Unable to answer this question, parents and physicians often agree to wait and "see how your baby looks" at delivery.

In this article, the authors use high-quality video recordings to determine the validity of this approach by determining whether neonatal fellows and attendings were able to accurately predict survival to discharge of 10 infants under 26 weeks' gestation in the first few minutes of life. The answer was a resounding NO. The overall ability of the 34 observers (17 fellows and 17 attendings) to predict survival was only slightly better than chance. Furthermore, the level of clinical experience did not affect accuracy. Additionally, during the first 5 minutes, attendings and fellows both changed their mind more than half the time about whether the baby would survive.

The results here are similar to studies performed by Meadow et al,[3] showing that predictions of death in the neonatal intensive care unit were often wrong.[1] It is difficult to be critical of the wait-and-see delivery approach. Without accurate ways to predict the future antenatally and the knowledge that often things are different than expected at delivery, along with chaotic circumstances that make it difficult to get truly informed consent, delaying a final decision until the clinician gets to evaluate the infant makes intrinsic sense. Unfortunately, the evidence does not back this approach, and clinicians and parents need to be aware of the severe limitations of early clinical evaluation. Ultimately the study is a reminder of the desperate need to improve our ability to provide individualized prognosis and treatment options.

J. M. Fanaroff, MD, JD

References

1. Griswold KJ, Fanaroff JM. An evidence-based overview of prenatal consultation with a focus on infants born at the limits of viability. *Pediatrics*. 2010;125: e931-e937.
2. Tyson JE, Parikh NA, Langer J, Green C, Higgins RD. National Institute of Child Health and Human Development Neonatal Research Network. Intensive care for extreme prematurity—moving beyond gestational age. *N Engl J Med*. 2008;358: 1672-1681.
3. Meadow W, Lagatta J, Andrews B, et al. Just, in time: ethical implications of serial predictions of death and morbidity for ventilated premature infants. *Pediatrics*. 2008;121:732-740.

Current empirical research in neonatal bioethics

Swinton CH, Lantos JD (The Univ of Chicago, IL; Univ of Missouri at Kansas City)
Acta Paediatr 99:1773-1781, 2010

Ethical dilemmas in neonatology can be analysed using both the theoretical tools of analytic philosophy and the empirical tools of clinical epidemiology and health services research. Both yield important insights into ways to think about the ethical issues that arise in clinical neonatology. In this paper, we review recent empirical research in neonatal bioethics. Studies published in the last 5 years shed light on issues that arise in prenatal consultation, prognostication, outcomes, quality-of-life and cost-effectiveness in neonatal intensive care. These studies show ways in which doctors vary in their decisions from country to country, hospital to hospital and for babies and children with different conditions but similar prognoses. Empirical research in bioethics can answer questions about what doctors and parents think and do. It does not answer questions about what they ought to do.

Conclusion.—Good ethics starts with good facts, even if good facts are not sufficient to get us to good ethics.

▶ Neonatology is a field rife with a number of complex ethical dilemmas. In this era of information overload, it is also increasingly difficult to keep abreast of the thousands of articles published each year in the field. Likened sometimes to "drinking from a fire hose," it is likely one of the major reasons you read this select. For this reason, it is wonderful that Drs Swinton and Lantos have written this article summarizing and discussing key research articles in neonatal bioethics.

Lantos, one of the leading pediatric ethicists in the country, and Swinton, a neonatal fellow studying clinical medical ethics, begin the article reminding us that empirical research tells us what is happening, but not necessarily what ought to be happening. Nevertheless, they note the value of such research for neonatologists and ethicists, stating that "[g]ood ethics starts with good facts, even if good facts are not sufficient to get us to good ethics."

The rest of the article then provides both a summary and critique of recent research in perinatal bioethics. The article is very well organized and covers many key subject areas in neonatal ethics: prenatal consultation, prognostication, outcomes, quality of life, and cost effectiveness. For each area, the authors review major recent studies and provide context and analysis. In many ways it has the feel of a Cochrane Review of neonatal ethics.

Throughout the article, there are humbling and thought-provoking facts as well as reminders of the importance of ethics in the daily lives of neonatologists. One survey finds that only 40% of doctors share decision-making responsibility with the parents, despite a heavy emphasis on shared decision making by the American Academy of Pediatrics and the Neonatal Resuscitation Program Guidelines.[1] Another comparison reminds us of the large variation in practice in this country and throughout the world, finding that 24% of infants die in the delivery room in the Netherlands compared with 0% in Chicago and 16% in Wisconsin.[2]

This variation in practice can even occur within an institution. The article discusses the importance of formal ethics teaching and reminds training programs to "be cognizant of the influence they have on the attitudes of their trainees with regard to ethical issues." In medicine, we are in a profession in which we are all lifelong learners and trainees, and while this article does not always tell us what we should do, it certainly provokes thought about what we are doing.

J. M. Fanaroff, MD, JD

References

1. Bastek TK, Richardson DK, Zupancic JA, Burns JP. Prenatal consultation practices at the border of viability: a regional survey. *Pediatrics.* 2005;116:407-413.

2. Verhagen AA, Janvier A, Leuthner SR, et al. Categorizing neonatal deaths: a cross-cultural study in the United States, Canada, and The Netherlands. *J Pediatr.* 2010; 156:33-37.

Current empirical research in neonatal bioethics

Swinton CH, Lantos JD (The Univ of Chicago, IL; Univ of Missouri at Kansas City)
Acta Paediatr 99:1773-1781, 2010

Ethical dilemmas in neonatology can be analysed using both the theoretical tools of analytic philosophy and the empirical tools of clinical epidemiology and health services research. Both yield important insights into ways to think about the ethical issues that arise in clinical neonatology. In this paper, we review recent empirical research in neonatal bioethics. Studies published in the last 5 years shed light on issues that arise in prenatal consultation, prognostication, outcomes, quality-of-life and cost-effectiveness in neonatal intensive care. These studies show ways in which doctors vary in their decisions from country to country, hospital to hospital and for babies and children with different conditions but similar prognoses. Empirical research in bioethics can answer questions about what doctors and parents think and do. It does not answer questions about what they ought to do.

Conclusion.—Good ethics starts with good facts, even if good facts are not sufficient to get us to good ethics.

▶ In their review of 5 years of empirical research in perinatal bioethics, Swinton and Lantos do a service for any neonatologist who has grappled with difficult ethical questions in the neonatal intensive care unit—in other words, all neonatologists. This article covers a wide range of complex and challenging problems that are commonly faced in the care of sick newborns, bringing to the foreground the productive and diverse work of empirical researchers whose efforts share the common goal of helping us find our way through the bioethical fog.

As the impetus to practice neonatal medicine in evidence-based fashion strengthens, so does the need to stay current on the growing body of knowledge that informs medical decision making. Amid a sea of clinical questions (intubate or try early continuous positive airway pressure? treat the patent ductus arteriosus or not?), keeping up with the literature can be a full-time job. While almost all of the studies reviewed here were initially published in high-impact journals, a busy neonatologist might miss out on the collective insight that can be gained from these empirical bioethics studies and continue to struggle in isolation with common ethical problems.

Swinton and Lantos review studies about decisions at the beginning and end of life, about counseling and prognostication, about quality of life, and how much money it takes to make all of this go. Each of these topics could fill a book, but rather than leaving us feeling completely overwhelmed by everything we don't know, the authors help us wrap our heads around these questions and remind us that working to find the answers is feasible and worthwhile. This article is also illustrative of the scope of the research tools available to tackle some of these problems; the studies cited in this article rely on survey methods, cost-benefit analysis, statistical models, and quality-of-life assessments, just to name a few. Neonatologists wishing to conduct their own empirical bioethics research might very well find inspiration and direction here.

What the authors don't share with us is how they identified the individual studies or the thematic framework they use to organize them. Is this comprehensive, or are there many other interesting empirical studies that didn't make the cut? Those who already have expertise in this field might have no problem placing this article in the larger landscape of neonatal bioethics literature, but for the dabblers among us, a little more context might be helpful. Nonetheless, even neonatologists with only passing interest in bioethics research are likely to find this review to be an informative current overview of what we have been learning about the process and outcomes of life-and-death decisions we make in the neonatal intensive care unit.

N. Laventhal, MD

Donation after cardiac death: the potential contribution of an infant organ donor population
Labrecque M, Parad R, Gupta M, et al (Children's Hosp Boston, MA)
J Pediatr 158:31-36, 2011

Objective.—To determine the percentage of deaths in level III neonatal intensive care unit (NICU) settings that theoretically would have been eligible for donation after cardiac death (DCD), as well as the percentage of these who would have been potential DCD candidates based on warm ischemic time.

Study Design.—We conducted a retrospective study of all deaths in 3 Harvard Program in Neonatology NICUs between 2005 and 2007. Eligible donors were identified based on criteria developed with our transplantation surgeons and our local organ procurement organization. Potential candidates for DCD were then identified based on an acceptable warm ischemic time.

Results.—Of the 192 deaths that occurred during the study period, 161 were excluded, leaving 31 theoretically eligible donors. Of these, 16 patients had a warm ischemic time of <1 hour and were potential candidates for DCD of 14 livers and 18 kidneys, and 14 patients had a warm ischemic time of <30 minutes and were potential candidates for DCD of 10 hearts.

Conclusions.—Eight percent of NICU mortalities were potential candidates for DCD. Based on the size of the potential donor pool, establishing an infant DCD protocol for level III NICUs should be considered.

▶ Deaths of infants on organ waiting lists are certainly a compelling reason to examine donation after cardiac death (DCD) as a potential route for organ donation. In DCD, organs are procured after cardiac arrest following the controlled withdrawal of life-sustaining assisted ventilation. The 3 Boston neonatal intensive care units (NICUs) retrospectively analyzed the deaths over a 3-year period to assess their eligibility for DCD. The authors' exclusionary criteria for which the infant would not be considered a donor were weight < 3 kg and age < 37 weeks; other exclusionary diagnostic criteria included active infection, malignancy, encephalopathy of unknown cause, brain death, and infants not requiring ventilation at the time of withdrawal of life-sustaining treatment. The remaining deaths were considered for liver, kidney, or heart donation, with a limit of up to 30 minutes from death for cardiac donation. They identified 31 theoretically eligible donors; this number was reduced to 16 potential donor candidates and 14 potentially eligible livers, 18 kidneys, and 10 hearts.

In addition to the controllable exclusionary criteria, many other factors come into play, particularly, parental consent rates. While we know that families often express a desire for something good to emerge from a tragic situation (in fact, 75% of conversations were initiated by parents), this does not translate into equivalent numbers, with a 40% chance of death not occurring within the 30-minute warm ischemia time limit, and other logistic realities that may preclude enactment of the process. These include the very real practical challenges of moving patients to a different location, the process and timing of the declaration of death, and the postdeclaration medical requirements, such as ventilation and heparinization. This is all in addition to the fact that DCD would require changes in current end-of-life practices, such as allowing families private time to hold their infant, to create memories, or to perform religious rituals. While transporting potential donors already within an institution from the NICU to a special preparation room is in itself difficult, the authors raise a significant issue in suggesting that because most potential donors die in the referral hospital, it might be worth considering moving these potential donors to a hospital with an independent infant DCD program specifically for this purpose. The practical and ethical issues raised by this suggestion are even more challenging.

While the criteria for organ eligibility that the authors cite may be contested by transplant personnel, both the discrepancy between the numbers of possible recipients and donors and parents' desire to derive something positive from a tragic situation stress the importance of understanding the potential role of an infant DCD program. This study raises this question for serious consideration. Moving from a conceptual framework to a practical, transparent, morally acceptable practice would need very thoughtful deliberation and careful planning among all stakeholders, including parents.

J. Hellman, MBBCh, FRCPC, MHSc

Ethically complex decisions in the neonatal intensive care unit: impact of the new French legislation on attitudes and practices of physicians and nurses

Garel M, Caeymaex L, Goffinet F, et al (INSERM U 953, Villejuif Cedex, France)
J Med Ethics 37:240-243, 2011

Objectives.—A statute enacted in 2005 modified the legislative framework of the rights of terminally ill persons in France. Ten years after the EURONIC study, which described the self-reported practices of neonatal caregivers towards ethical decision-making, a new study was conducted to assess the impact of the new law in neonatal intensive care units (NICU) and compare the results reported by EURONIC with current practices.

Setting and Design.—The study was carried out in the same two NICU as in the EURONIC qualitative study. A third centre was added to increase the sample size. From February to October 2007, 19 physicians and 17 nurses participated in semistructured interviews very similar to those for EURONIC. Content analysis identified the recurring themes emerging from the interviews.

Results.—Compared with the EURONIC results, the caregivers reported that they pay greater attention to the views of parents and provided respectful support to the neonates when life-sustaining treatment is withdrawn. Active termination of life has become exceptional. The possibility of withdrawal of treatment, the administration of sedatives to control pain even at the risk of hastening death, the emphasis on sparing parents the burden of decision, and the relative ignorance of the law were very similar to the EURONIC findings.

Conclusion.—Both the medical and the legal regulation of practices has allowed more dialogue with the parents and more humane care for dying newborns. A new European study is necessary to investigate the possible changes in practices and attitudes also in other countries.

▶ An earlier qualitative study, part of the EURONIC project comparing practice around ethical issues in European neonatal intensive care units (NICUs), had shown that in France, parents appeared to be the least directly involved in decision making about withholding and withdrawal of life-sustaining treatment. Thus, the impact of recent French legislation on the principle of patient autonomy and rights at the end of life was a worthy exploration via semistructured interviews of 19 French NICU physicians and 17 nurses. Overall, there did appear to be positive gains from the new legislation, either directly or indirectly, with more attention given to patients' end-of-life rights. There was an overall feeling of more honesty, more openness and transparency, increasing tendency of parents' presence during the dying process, and an increased rarity of drugs to actively end life.

An interesting finding from these interviews was that older physicians had a better knowledge of the law and expressed relief regarding the legislative changes, whereas younger physicians were more ambivalent, but acknowledged the necessity of the emotional work required in decision making with parents. They did not challenge the ethical principles underlying the new laws but appreciated the challenges of parental involvement in decision making and the need for training and, of course, experience.

A concern raised by the interviewees, one that cannot be resolved by law, is the inherent fear that by according respect for the principle of patient autonomy, physicians may potentially induce parental guilt for the responsibility for that decision. I am sure there is universal appreciation of this concern as we all struggle with how directive to be in each case, particularly in situations in which parents and physicians have divergent views on the best course to pursue. While knowledge of the national legislation certainly affects the process, the degree of certainty of diagnosis and prognosis, the openness and tolerance for uncertainty, the degree to which we inform parents of our own views and desire to share the burden of a decision, and the degree to which parents wish to be involved or demand to be the decision maker can only highlight that each case demands its own dynamic, interactive, deliberative negotiation.

J. Hellman, MBBCh, FRCPC, MHSc

Ethical and practical issues relating to the global use of therapeutic hypothermia for perinatal asphyxial encephalopathy
Wilkinson DJ, Thayyil S, Robertson NJ (Univ of Oxford, UK; Univ College London, UK)
Arch Dis Child Fetal Neonatal Ed 96:F75-F78, 2011

In intensive care settings in the developed world, therapeutic hypothermia is established as a therapy for term infants with moderate to severe neonatal encephalopathy due to perinatal asphyxia. Several preclinical, pilot and clinical trials conducted in such settings over the last decade have demonstrated that this therapy is safe and effective. The greatest burden of birth asphyxia falls, however, in low- and middle-income countries; it is still unclear whether therapeutic hypothermia is safe and effective in this context. In this paper, the issues around treatments that may be proven safe and effective in the developed world and the caution needed in translating these into different settings and populations are explored. It is argued that there are strong scientific and ethical reasons supporting the conduct of rigorous, randomised controlled trials of therapeutic hypothermia in middle-income settings. There also needs to be substantial and sustainable improvements in all facets of antenatal care and in the basic level of newborn resuscitation in low income countries. This will reduce the burden of disease and allow health workers to determine rapidly which infants are most eligible for potential neuroprotection.

▶ This article is a commentary that expresses concern over the implementation of therapeutic hypothermia following perinatal asphyxial encephalopathy in low- and middle-income countries. The authors address both population differences and practical and economic issues that might result in less successful outcomes than in the developed world.

Part of their caution depends upon how one interprets statistics. In a meta-analysis of randomized controlled trials (RCTs), the number needed to treat (NNT) for survival without neurological impairment is about 8, and there is a very wide margin of safety. In low- to middle-income countries, the incidence of postasphyxial encephalopathy is 10 to 20 times higher, and thus, differences between cooled and noncooled infants could be far greater, resulting in an even lower NNT in these settings.

Some of the population differences are real. There is no doubt a higher incidence of maternal malnutrition, intrauterine growth retardation, and less-sophisticated obstetrical and neonatal care; mothers with HIV and puerperal sepsis are more common, and multiple organ failure is more difficult to treat. The issue of infection is important, but even in the RCTs done to date, small study sizes have precluded stratification for the underlying cause of the encephalopathy, and virtually all studies have presumed that birth is time zero. Clearly, many enrolled babies were infected, and some sustained brain injury prior to the intrapartum period. Yet on balance, hypothermia still improved the outcomes of treated infants versus controls.

The authors are justifiably concerned about technological limitations and cost, but these should be solvable, even ice works.

Finally, the point is raised as to whether it would be ethical to undertake RCTs in low-resource settings. On one hand, babies assigned to standard care would be deprived of the established benefit of hypothermic neuroprotection. On the other hand, safety and feasibility issues could be addressed.

Stay tuned.

S. M. Donn, MD

6 Gastrointestinal Health and Nutrition

A Randomized, Double-Blind, Controlled Trial of the Effect of Prebiotic Oligosaccharides on Enteral Tolerance in Preterm Infants (ISRCTN77444690)
Modi N, Uthaya S, Fell J, et al (Imperial College London, UK)
Pediatr Res 68:440-445, 2010

Breast milk prebiotic oligosaccharides are believed to promote enteral tolerance. Many mothers delivering preterm are unable to provide sufficient milk. We conducted a multicenter, randomized, controlled trial comparing preterm formula containing 0.8 g/100 mL short-chain galacto-oligosaccharides/long-chain fructo-oligosaccharides in a 9:1 ratio and an otherwise identical formula, using formula only to augment insufficient maternal milk volume. Infants were randomized within 24 h of birth. The primary outcome (PO) was time to establish a total milk intake of 150 mL/kg/d PO and the principal secondary outcome (PSO) was proportion of time between birth and 28 d/discharge that a total milk intake of ≥150 mL/kg/d was tolerated. Other secondary outcomes included growth, fecal characteristics, gastrointestinal signs, necrotizing enterocolitis, and bloodstream infection. Outcomes were compared adjusted for prespecified covariates. We recruited 160 infants appropriately grown for GA <33 wk. There were no significant differences in PO or PSOs. After covariate adjustment, we showed significant benefit from trial formula in PSO with increasing infant immaturity (2.9% improved tolerance for a baby born at 28-wk gestation and 9.9% at 26-wk gestation; $p < 0.001$) but decreased or no benefit in babies > 31-wk gestation. Prebiotic supplementation appears safe and may benefit enteral tolerance in the most immature infants.

▶ It is easy to confuse prebiotics and probiotics. Probiotics are live microorganisms that, when administered in appropriate dose, confer health benefits on the host. The most commonly used probiotics are lactobacillus and bifidobacteria, but other species, including fungi, are used as probiotics. A meta-analysis Deshpande[1] included 15 trials and almost 3000 infants and demonstrated significant reductions in death or necrotizing enterocolitis (30%) without any significant side effects. Great benefits, no harm! However, probiotics have not been available in the United States for use in preterm infants because of problems in obtaining a standardized probiotic acceptable to the Food and Drug Administration.

Prebiotics typically comprise nondigestible carbohydrates. The most widely accepted prebiotics are the oligosaccharides inulin, fructo-oligosaccharides (FOS), galacto-oligosaccharides (GOS), and lactulose. FOS occur naturally in plants such as onion, chicory, garlic, asparagus, banana, and artichoke, among many others. Dietary FOS are not hydrolyzed by small intestinal glycosidases and reach the cecum structurally unchanged where they are metabolized by the intestinal microflora to form short-chain carboxylic acids, L-lactate, $CO(2)$, hydrogen, and other metabolites. As noted by Mihatsch,[2] prebiotic oligosaccharides reduce stool viscosity and accelerate gastrointestinal transport in preterm infants. They also appear to selectively stimulate the growth of lactobacilli in the gastrointestinal tract.

This well-conducted randomized trial from the team led by Modi supports the notion that prebiotics are beneficial for preterm infants. Feeding tolerance was improved most markedly for the least mature infants, but no benefits accrued beyond 31 weeks gestation. Also fewer babies in the prebiotic-treated group received total parenteral nutrition. The differences between the prebiotic treated group and those on standard feeds was no doubt dampened by the fact that both groups received a great deal of human milk, which contains large quantities of prebiotics. However, it would be unethical to withhold human milk from any infants. In a complementary study, Westerbeek[3] reported that enteral supplementation of a prebiotic mixture did not enhance the postnatal decrease in intestinal permeability in preterm infants in the first week of life. There are intriguing data accumulating to suggest that prebiotics, probiotics, and lactoferrin supplementation reduce mortality and serious morbidities, including sepsis and necrotizing enterocolitis. The randomized trials in preparation together with those in progress will help guide the clinician on the appropriate pathway to optimal nutrition.

A. A. Fanaroff, MD, FRCPE, FRCP&CH

References

1. Deshpande G, Rao S, Patole S, Bulsara M. Updated meta-analysis of probiotics for preventing necrotizing enterocolitis in preterm neonates. *Pediatrics.* 2010;125: 921-930.
2. Mihatsch WA, Hoegel J, Pohlandt F. Prebiotic oligosaccharides reduce stool viscosity and accelerate gastrointestinal transport in preterm infants. *Acta Paediatr.* 2006;95:843-848.
3. Westerbeek EA, van den Berg A, Lafeber HN, Fetter WP, van Elburg RM. The effect of enteral supplementation of a prebiotic mixture of non-human milk galacto-, fructo- and acidic oligosaccharides on intestinal permeability in preterm infants. *Br J Nutr.* 2011;105:268-274.

Dietary Intervention in Infancy and Later Signs of Beta-Cell Autoimmunity
Knip M, for the Finnish TRIGR Study Group (Univ of Helsinki and Helsinki Univ Central Hosp, Finland; et al)
N Engl J Med 363:1900-1908, 2010

Background.—Early exposure to complex dietary proteins may increase the risk of beta-cell auto-immunity and type 1 diabetes in children with genetic susceptibility. We tested the hypothesis that supplementing breast milk with highly hydrolyzed milk formula would decrease the cumulative incidence of diabetes-associated autoantibodies in such children.

Methods.—In this double-blind, randomized trial, we assigned 230 infants with HLA-conferred susceptibility to type 1 diabetes and at least one family member with type 1 diabetes to receive either a casein hydrolysate formula or a conventional, cow's-milk—based formula (control) whenever breast milk was not available during the first 6 to 8 months of life. Autoantibodies to insulin, glutamic acid decarboxylase (GAD), the insulinoma-associated 2 molecule (IA-2), and zinc transporter 8 were analyzed with the use of radiobinding assays, and islet-cell antibodies were analyzed with the use of immunofluorescence, during a median observation period of 10 years (mean, 7.5). The children were monitored for incident type 1 diabetes until they were 10 years of age.

Results.—The unadjusted hazard ratio for positivity for one or more autoantibodies in the casein hydrolysate group, as compared with the control group, was 0.54 (95% confidence interval [CI], 0.29 to 0.95), and the hazard ratio adjusted for an observed difference in the duration of exposure to the study formula was 0.51 (95% CI, 0.28 to 0.91). The unadjusted hazard ratio for positivity for two or more autoantibodies was 0.52 (95% CI, 0.21 to 1.17), and the adjusted hazard ratio was 0.47 (95% CI, 0.19 to 1.07). The rate of reported adverse events was similar in the two groups.

Conclusions.—Dietary intervention during infancy appears to have a long-lasting effect on markers of beta-cell autoimmunity—markers that may reflect an autoimmune process leading to type 1 diabetes. (Funded by the European Commission and others; ClinicalTrials.gov number, NCT00570102.)

▶ In this pilot study of the Trial to Reduce IDDM in the Genetically at Risk (TRIGR), nearly 500 newborn infants who had a first-degree relative with type 1 diabetes were randomized to receive a hydrolyzed protein formula or a regular nonhydrolyzed cow's milk—based formula whenever breast milk was not available. The children were followed until they were approximately 10 years of age for the development of diabetes-related antibodies and the development of overt diabetes. There were no differences in the development of diabetes between the 2 groups, but some significant differences were found in the development of autoantibody. Of interest is that those babies who were started on the hydrolyzed formula were started on the formula approximately 1.5 month later than the standard formula group ($P = .03$), suggesting a greater time of breast-feeding between birth and use of the intervention in the hydrolysate group. Could this be a confounding factor? Albeit very small numbers, the fact that there was no difference in onset of diabetes between the 2 groups is of interest, given that the autoantibodies were more prevalent in the control group compared with the hydrolysate group. It's possible that more time will be needed to determine if diabetes develops in more of the children who developed the antibodies. The ongoing and much larger TRIGR study conducted in 15 countries in 3 continents will provide more conclusive results. This study is intriguing, but a strong caveat should be made: protein hydrolysis destroys many potentially bioactive proteins present in milk. The amino acid content of the hydrolysate formula is far from ideal. Hydrolyzed formula should not be used more than necessary. It may be very helpful in those with allergies and, if additional studies show a decrease in type 1 diabetes, in those at very high genetic risk. It is likely that the report by Knip et al will stir exceptional interest in families with type 1 diabetes as well as many who do not have a familial risk. It is concerning that some people will preferentially begin to use the hydrolyzed formulas with their babies based on this report. This should be avoided because this study should be considered scientifically interesting and hypothesis generating but is not evidence to begin the widespread use of protein hydrolysate formulas without other specific indications. It is too premature to change feeding practices.

J. Neu, MD

Do Red Cell Transfusions Increase the Risk of Necrotizing Enterocolitis in Premature Infants?
Josephson CD, Wesolowski A, Bao G, et al (Emory Univ School of Medicine, Atlanta, GA; Longstreet Clinic, Gainesville, GA; Rollins School of Public Health, Atlanta, GA; et al)
J Pediatr 157:972-978, 2010

Objective.—To test the hypothesis that red blood cell (RBC) transfusions increase the risk of necrotizing enterocolitis (NEC) in premature infants, we investigated whether the risk of "transfusion-associated" NEC is higher in infants with lower hematocrits and advanced postnatal age.

Study Design.—Retrospective comparison of NEC patients and control patients born at <34 weeks gestation.

Results.—The frequency of RBC transfusions was similar in NEC patients (47/93, 51%) and control patients (52/91, 58%). Late-onset NEC (>4 weeks of age) was more frequently associated with a history of transfusion(s) than early-onset NEC (adjusted OR, 6.7; 95% CI, 1.5 to 31.2; $P = .02$). Compared with nontransfused patients, RBC-transfused patients were born at earlier gestational ages, had greater intensive care needs (including at the time of onset of NEC), and longer hospital stay. A history of RBC transfusions within 48-hours before NEC onset was noted in 38% of patients, most of whom were extremely low birth weight infants.

Conclusions.—In most patients, RBC transfusions were temporally unrelated to NEC and may be merely a marker of overall severity of illness. However, the relationship between RBC transfusions and NEC requires further evaluation in extremely low birth weight infants using a prospective cohort design.

▶ An association between red blood cell (RBC) transfusions and necrotizing enterocolitis (NEC) has now been reported by at least 4 different groups of investigators, but the nature of the relationship remains ambiguous. In this, the most recent of these reports, the authors use several statistical maneuvers to attempt to elucidate this question. This is the first of these reports to compare transfusion exposures in infants with NEC with those in infants without NEC. There was no difference in transfusion rates between infants with NEC and controls. Among infants with NEC who had received transfusions, the most recent transfusion was given more than 72 hours prior to the NEC episode in more than half and more than 1 week prior to the NEC episode in more than one-third, so there is not a compelling temporal relationship. Beyond suggesting that NEC and RBC transfusion may both be covariant with severity of illness and length of stay, the other analyses were largely unrevealing. While the authors conclude that additional studies are required, there is little evidence for a causal relationship in the data accrued to date. One wonders if the charm of this hypothesis lies more in our hope that there is an easy remedy for the scourge of NEC if only avoidance of transfusions could reduce or eliminate this disease. However, prospective trials comparing conservative and liberal transfusion criteria have not suggested an increased risk of NEC with more liberal use of RBC transfusions,[1-3] so it does not appear to be that simple. While these investigations may yet lead to some insight into the underlying biology of NEC, it is too soon to consider changing practice because of concerns about this association.

W. E. Benitz, MD

References

1. Bell EF, Strauss RG, Widness JA, et al. Randomized trial of liberal versus restrictive guidelines for red blood cell transfusion in preterm infants. *Pediatrics.* 2005; 115:1685-1691.
2. Chen H-L, Tseng H-I, Lu C-C, Yang S-N, Fan H-C, Yang R-C. Effect of blood transfusions on the outcome of very low body weight preterm infants under two different transfusion criteria. *Pediatr Neonatol.* 2009;50:110-116.
3. Kirpalani H, Whyte RK, Andersen C, et al. The Premature Infants in Need of Transfusion (PINT) study: a randomized, controlled trial of a restrictive (low) versus liberal (high) transfusion threshold for extremely low birth weight infants. *J Pediatr.* 2006;149:301-307.

Docosahexaenoic Acid and Amino Acid Contents in Pasteurized Donor Milk are Low for Preterm Infants
Valentine CJ, Morrow G, Fernandez S, et al (Ohio State Univ, Columbus; et al)
J Pediatr 157:906-910, 2010

Objective.—To evaluate whether pasteurized donor human milk meets the nutritional needs of preterm infants in terms of free fatty acid and amino acid contents.

Study Design.—Milk samples were prospectively collected from 39 donors to the Mothers' Milk Bank of Ohio. The fatty acid and amino acid compositions in donor milk samples were measured before and after pasteurization, and values were compared with previously published findings and preterm infant nutrition guidelines. The nutritional adequacy of donor milk for preterm infants was based on estimated daily intake of 150 mL/kg. Statistical significance was adjusted to account for multiple comparisons.

Results.—Pasteurization did not appreciably affect donor milk composition. Docosahexaenoic acid level (0.1 mol wt %), and concentrations of glycine, aspartate, valine, phenylalanine, proline, lysine, arginine, serine, and histidine in donor milk were all significantly lower than previously reported concentrations in milk.

Conclusions.—Donor milk is not substantially affected by pasteurization, but has low concentrations of docosahexaenoic acid and amino acids. Targeted nutritional supplementation of human donor milk for feeding preterm infants might be warranted (Fig 2).

▶ Studies showing benefits of human milk for premature infants have prompted significant shifts from formula to mother's milk in neonatal intensive care units. Often, the mother may not be able to provide her milk, and donor milk is commonly used in many neonatal intensive care units. As mentioned in this article, there seem to be benefits in the use of donor milk, but concern has been raised about altered composition and loss of bioactive components.

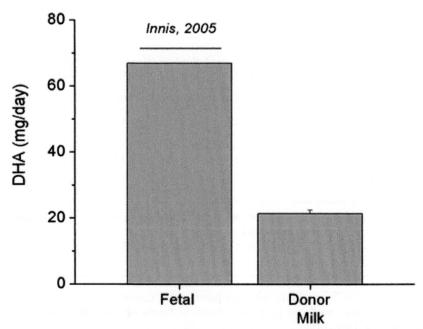

FIGURE 2.—DHA in human milk compared with fetal accretion levels. Total DHA consumption was calculated by the methods described by Innis[1] using 150 mL/day as the amount of a full enteral feed. The total DHA levels in donor human milk were substantially lower than fetal accretion levels. (Reprinted from Journal of Pediatrics, Valentine CJ, Morrow G, Fernandez S, et al. Docosahexaenoic acid and amino acid contents in pasteurized donor milk are low for preterm infants. *J Pediatr.* 2010;157:906-910. Copyright 2010 with permission from Elsevier.)

Docosahexaenoic acid (DHA) concentrations in human milk, formula, and numerous other food additives has been a focus of numerous studies in nutrition, especially as it pertains to infants, for more than a decade. Although still under debate, several studies suggest benefits in neurodevelopment and retinal function. In addition to the lipid composition, several other components of human milk have been under scrutiny. Among these are the free amino acids (FAA), which have been found to be higher in human colostrum but decreases through the transitional and mature milk stages. Despite this, FAA are higher in all human milks than in infant formulas.[1] The exact function of these free amino acids is only speculative.

The study by Valentine et al evaluated the effects of pasteurization on the composition of the fatty acids and free amino acids in donor breast milk and found very few differences before and after. Although not comprehensive, this adds to our knowledge that at least these components are not significantly altered by this process. However, the most interesting and disturbing finding in this study is the low quantity of DHA in donor milks. This by far does not reach the accretion rate of the fetus (Fig 2). In addition, many very low birth weight infants are provided little enteral feeding in their first several weeks after birth and receive their lipids intravenously, where there is no preformed DHA or some other nutritionally important very long chain polyunsaturated fatty acids. The continued use of human donor milk with these very low concentrations of DHA after a significant period of deprivation shortly after birth is likely to lead to deficits in DHA and other bioactively important very long chain polyunsaturated fatty acids. This is very disturbing in terms of its potential not only for neurodevelopmental delays and predisposition to retinal and other oxidative, and inflammatory damage but also intestinal inflammatory disease, such as necrotizing enterocolitis and lung inflammation, which contributes to bronchopulmonary dysplasia. This is an area that needs to be addressed in additional research and development of appropriate interventions.

J. Neu, MD

Reference

1. Chuang CK, Lin SP, Lee HC, et al. Free amino acids in full-term and pre-term human milk and infant formula. *J Pediatr Gastroenterol Nutr.* 2005;40:496-500.

Dynamics and Clinical Evolution of Bacterial Gut Microflora in Extremely Premature Patients

Jacquot A, Neveu D, Aujoulat F, et al (Hopital Arnaud de Villeneuve, Montpellier, France; Universite Montpellier, France; et al)
J Pediatr 158:390-396, 2011

Objective.—To determine baseline clinical characteristics that influence bacterial gut flora dynamics in very preterm infants and the relationship between gut flora dynamics and clinical evolution.

Study Design.—Prospective, monocentric study enrolling 29 consecutive very preterm infants. We collected data about growth, digestive tolerance, nutrition, and antibiotic use. Microflora in stool samples, collected between 3 and 56 days of life, was identified with direct molecular fingerprinting.

Results.—Median (interquartile range) body weight and gestational age at birth were 950 g (760-1060 g) and 27 weeks (27-29 weeks), respectively. The diversity score (number of operational taxonomic units) increased 0.45 units/week ($P < .0001$), with staphylococci as the major group. Bifidobacterium was poorly represented. Gestational age (≥ 28 weeks) and caesarean delivery independently correlated with better diversity scores during follow-up ($P < .05$). The 6-week diversity score inversely correlated with the duration of antibiotherapy ($P = .0184$) and parenteral feeding ($P = .013$). The microflora dynamics was associated with the digestive tolerance profile. Weight gain increased with increasing diversity score ($P = .0428$).

Conclusion.—Microflora diversity settled progressively in very preterm infants. Staphylococci were the major group, and few infants were colonized with Bifidobacterium spp. Measures that may improve microflora could have beneficial effects on digestive tolerance and growth.

▶ The intestinal microbiota is a complex ecosystem that has been shaped by millennia of evolution that usually exists in a symbiotic relationship with the host. In the last few years, emerging technologies derived largely from the Human Genome Project have been adapted to evaluate the intestinal microbiota; discoveries using these techniques have prompted initiatives, such as the Human Microbiome Roadmap, designed to evaluate the role of the intestinal microbiome in health and disease. In the term healthy infant, studies using non—culture-based techniques show that during early development, the microbiota undergoes changes based on diet, use of antibiotics, and C section versus vaginal mode of birth, among other perturbations.[1-7] Studies on preterm infants using new technologies are beginning to show how the microbes evolve over time and may shed light on necrotizing enterocolitis. In this study, fecal microbiota was analyzed in 29 consecutive extremely preterm infants between 3 and 56 days of life and analyzed using "fingerprinting" (gel separation, elution of bands from gels, and subsequent analysis of band sequences) correlated with clinical factors such as growth, digestive tolerance, nutrition, and antibiotic use to the major taxa present in the feces. As in a previous study in term healthy infants,[6] *Staphylococcus* species were by far the major group but Bifidobacterium poorly represented. The 6-week diversity score inversely correlated with the duration of antibiotic use and parenteral feeding. If one considers that diversity is likely to be related to a "healthy" microbial ecology, antibiotic use and lack of enteral feeding appeared to be significant contributory factors. The relative paucity of microbes other than *Staphylococcus* in babies who were feeding poorly (Fig 3) is of major significance since these are the most commonly represented genera with late-onset sepsis in the neonate. It is of interest but speculative that these are organisms

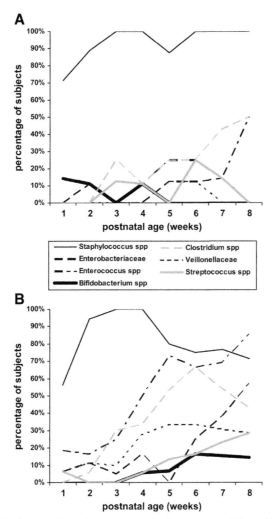

FIGURE 3.—Development of microflora, represented by the percentage of infants with species of each of the 6 main bacterial groups and with Bifidobacterium spp, **A**, in preterm infants with poor digestive tolerance (digestive score >2; n = 9) and **B**, infants with good digestive tolerance (n = 20). (Reprinted from Journal of Pediatrics, Jacquot A, Neveu D, Aujoulat F, et al. Dynamics and clinical evolution of bacterial gut microflora in extremely premature patients. *J Pediatr.* 2011;158:390-396. Copyright 2011 with permission from Elsevier.)

that may translocate through the intestinal barrier and cause bacteremia and subsequent sepsis.

J. Neu, MD

References

1. Dominguez-Bello MG, Costello EK, Contreras M, et al. Delivery mode shapes the acquisition and structure of the initial microbiota across multiple body habitats in newborns. *Proc Natl Acad Sci U S A.* 2010;107:11971-11975.

2. Biasucci G, Benenati B, Morelli L, Bessi E, Boehm G. Cesarean delivery may affect the early biodiversity of intestinal bacteria. *J Nutr.* 2008;138:1796S-1800S.
3. Grönlund MM, Lehtonen OP, Eerola E, Kero P. Fecal microflora in healthy infants born by different methods of delivery: permanent changes in intestinal flora after cesarean delivery. *J Pediatr Gastroenterol Nutr.* 1999;28:19-25.
4. Rushing J, Neu J. Cesarean versus vaginal delivery: long-term infant outcomes and the hygiene hypothesis. *Clin Perinatol.* 2011;38:321-331.
5. Palmer C, Bik EM, DiGiulio DB, Relman DA, Brown PO. Development of the human infant intestinal microbiota. *PLoS Biol.* 2007;5:e177.
6. Eggesbø M, Moen B, Peddada S, et al. Development of gut microbiota in infants not exposed to medical interventions. *APMIS.* 2011;119:17-35.
7. Koenig JE, Spor A, Scalfone N, et al. Succession of microbial consortia in the developing infant gut microbiome. *Proc Natl Acad Sci U S A.* 2011;108:4578-4585.

***Fucosyltransferase 2* Non-Secretor and Low Secretor Status Predicts Severe Outcomes in Premature Infants**
Morrow AL, Meinzen-Derr J, Huang P, et al (Cincinnati Children's Hosp Med Ctr, OH; et al)
J Pediatr 158:745-751, 2011

Objective.—To investigate secretor gene *fucosyltransferase 2* (FUT2) polymorphism and secretor phenotype in relation to outcomes of prematurity.

Study Design.—Study infants were ≤32 weeks gestational age. Secretor genotype was determined from salivary DNA. Secretor phenotype was measured with H antigen, the carbohydrate produced by secretor gene enzymes, in saliva samples collected on day 9 ± 5. The optimal predictive cutoff point in salivary H values was identified with Classification and Regression Tree analysis. Study outcomes were death, necrotizing enterocolitis (NEC, Bell's stage II/III), and confirmed sepsis.

Results.—There were 410 study infants, 26 deaths, 30 cases of NEC, and 96 cases of sepsis. Analyzed by genotype, 13% of 95 infants who were non-secretors, 5% of 203 infants who were heterozygotes, and 2% of 96 infants who were secretor dominant died ($P = .01$). Analyzed by phenotype, 15% of 135 infants with low secretor phenotype died, compared with 2% of 248 infants with high secretor phenotype (predictive value $= 76\%$, $P < .001$). Low secretor phenotype was associated ($P < .05$) with NEC, and non-secretor genotype was associated ($P = .05$) with gram negative sepsis. Secretor status remained significant after controlling for multiple clinical factors.

Conclusions.—Secretor genotype and phenotype may provide strong predictive biomarkers of adverse outcomes in premature infants (Fig 2).

▶ H antigens are indirect gene products consisting of fucose-containing oligosaccharide components of glycolipids or glycoproteins on cell surfaces or in mucinous secretions. These oligosaccharides are produced by 2 fucosyltransferases (FUT1 and FUT2) that link a fucose residue to a galactose. FUT1 is expressed in erythroid tissues and produces the immediate precursors of the

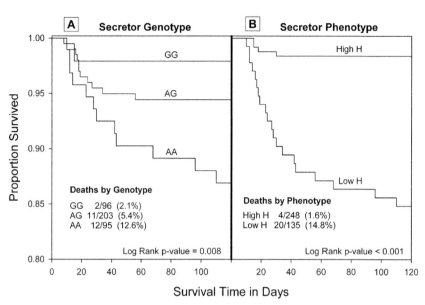

FIGURE 2.—Kaplan-Meier survival curves. A, Secretor genotype and B, secretor phenotype are each significantly associated with risk of death. Infants with the non-secretor genotype (AA) were at high risk of death, infants with the dominant secretor (GG) were at low risk of death, and the risk in infants who were heterozygotes (AG) was intermediate. Secretor phenotype was characterized as low salivary H (high risk of mortality) and high salivary H (low risk of mortality). (Reprinted from Journal of Pediatrics, Morrow AL, Meinzen-Derr J, Huang P, et al. *Fucosyltransferase 2* non-secretor and low secretor status predicts severe outcomes in premature infants. *J Pediatr*. 2011;158:745-751. Copyright (Year) with permission from Elsevier.)

ABO and Lewis blood-type antigens. FUT2 is expressed primarily in secretory epithelial cells; lack of FUT2 expression or activity results in mucins that lack the fucose-containing Se epitope. Individuals with those epitopes in their secretions are designated "secretors." Because of a common FUT2 gene polymorphism, about 20% of individuals lack these epitopes and are therefore "nonsecretors." The role of the Se epitopes is not fully understood, but several observations imply an important role in passive immunity. For example, nonsecretors appear to be resistant to norovirus infection but prone to development of Crohn disease.

This article documents a compelling relationship between FUT2 genotype or secretor phenotype and adverse outcomes for preterm infants. In a sample of infants with gestational age of 32 weeks or less, the risk of death was substantially greater among those with the nonsecretor genotype or phenotype (Fig 2). Although the risk for sepsis was not different between groups (odds ratio [OR] 1.03, 95% confidence interval [CI] 0.6—1.7), the odds of death from sepsis were greatly increased among infants with a nonsecretor phenotype (OR 17.9, 95% CI 2.4—789.0). Similarly, necrotizing enterocolitis (NEC) (OR 2.7, 95% CI 1.1—6.4), surgical NEC (OR 3.8, 95% CI 1.1—15.0), or death from NEC (OR 9.6, 95% CI 1.9-92.0) were much more frequent in nonsecretors. These fascinating results suggest an entirely new strategy for identifying infants at particular risk for these complications. Additional studies are anxiously awaited that confirm these data and explain how to develop novel tools for prediction and perhaps even prevention of NEC and sepsis in these vulnerable infants.

W. E. Benitz, MD

Human milk glycobiome and its impact on the infant gastrointestinal microbiota
Zivkovic AM, German JB, Lebrilla CB, et al (Univ of California, Davis)
Proc Natl Acad Sci U S A 108:4653-4658, 2011

Human milk contains an unexpected abundance and diversity of complex oligosaccharides apparently indigestible by the developing infant and instead targeted to its cognate gastrointestinal microbiota. Recent advances in mass spectrometry-based tools have provided a view of the oligosaccharide structures produced in milk across stages of lactation and among human mothers. One postulated function for these oligosaccharides is to enrich a specific "healthy" microbiota containing bifidobacteria, a genus commonly observed in the feces of breast-fed infants. Isolated culture studies indeed show selective growth of infant-borne bifidobacteria on milk oligosaccharides or core components therein. Parallel glycoprofiling documented that numerous *Bifidobacterium longum* subsp. *infantis* strains preferentially consume small mass oligosaccharides that are abundant early in the lactation cycle. Genome sequencing of numerous *B. longum* subsp. *infantis* strains shows a bias toward genes required to use mammalian-derived carbohydrates by comparison with adult-borne bifidobacteria. This intriguing strategy of mammalian lactation to selectively nourish genetically compatible bacteria in infants with a complex array of free oligosaccharides serves as a model of how to influence the human supraorganismal system, which includes the gastrointestinal microbiota.

▶ Breast-feeding has been clearly defined as providing the optimum nutrition for developing infants. As stated in this article, this optimization has occurred "over 200 million years of Darwinian evolution." Of the 3 components of human milk that are present in the highest concentration, oligosaccharides come in third place, with the first 2 places held by lactose and lipids. Human milk complex oligosaccharides are indigestible by the infant yet are consumed by microbial populations in the developing intestine. These oligosaccharides are related to the 4 human Lewis blood groups. The Lewis oligosaccharides, which coat red blood cells, are produced in the intestinal epithelium, where they are absorbed and transported into the plasma and adsorbed onto red blood cells. Of interest is that these blood groups are not present on the erythrocytes of newborns, but appear between 3 and 6 months and then begin to stabilize in concentration. Breast-feeding contributes large doses of Lewis structures. This raises the question of whether other cell surface components in immune system or other cells may also rely on their development from the ingestion of human milk oligosaccharides. In addition, these human milk oligosaccharides, which have similar structures as receptors found on intestinal epithelial and other cells, deflect pathogens from intestinal cell surfaces. In addition, these human milk oligosaccharides are thought to provide an environment that enriches the growth of beneficial microbiota, such as those belonging to the *Bifidobacterium* genus. When babies are weaned from their mother's milk, the microbiota abruptly changes and thus influences the human supraorganismal system. The implication of developing a better understanding of these interactions could reach far beyond simply adding these to formulas for babies who are not breast-fed. For example, could these potentially be used instead of antibiotics in the prophylaxis of infections?

J. Neu, MD

Ischemia-Reperfusion and Neonatal Intestinal Injury

Young CM, Kingma SDK, Neu J (Univ of Florida, Gainesville; Univ Med Ctr, Amsterdam, The Netherlands)
J Pediatr 158:e25-e28, 2011

We review research relating ischemia/reperfusion to injury in the neonatal intestine. Epidemiologic evidence suggests that the most common form of necrotizing enterocolitis is not triggered by a primary hypoxic-ischemic event. Its late occurrence, lack of preceding ischemic events, and evidence for microbial and inflammatory processes preclude a major role for primary hypoxic ischemia as the sentinel pathogenic event. However, term infants, especially those with congenital heart disease who have development of intestinal necrosis, and those preterm infants with spontaneous intestinal perforations, are more likely to have intestinal ischemia as a primary component of their disease pathogenesis.

▶ The concern that asphyxia or hypoxic-ischemic events may be causally associated with this necrotizing enterocolitis (NEC) is the underlying rationale for the common practice of withholding feedings from infants with low Apgar scores, stressful perinatal/neonatal events, or pharmacologic practices, such as providing indomethacin or other vasoactive agents that may relate to altered intestinal blood flow. This article challenges the dogma that has existed for more than 40 years that hypoxia-ischemia is the primary predisposing event that leads to the most common form of NEC seen in preterm infants. Although secondary microvascular ischemia is likely important, this is caused by more proximal factors, such as uncontrolled release of inflammatory and vasoactive mediators that have little or no relation to birth-related hypoxia ischemia and is not directly related to decreased mesenteric arterial flow as has been previously implicated to be causative of NEC. The latter predispose to ischemic intestinal injury, which probably should not even be named NEC or put in the same category as the disease that is most commonly seen in preterm infants. Examples of this would be babies who have left-sided cardiac failure or obstruction, and a better term for their disease would be cardiac-related intestinal ischemia. As discussed in the article, this revised concept has important implications in feeding infants by the enteral route. Should low Apgar scores be used as an indicator to not feed preterm infants for prolonged periods, as is common practice? This article provides fuel for challenging this concept.

J. Neu, MD

Mesentric oxygen saturations in premature twins with and without necrotizing enterocolitis
Zabaneh RN, Cleary JP, Lieber CA (Children's Hosp of Orange County, CA)
Pediatr Crit Care Med 2010 [Epub ahead of print]

Objective.—To report the use of near-infrared spectroscopic monitoring to recognize mesenteric oxygen desaturations in a preterm neonate with necrotizing enterocolitis as well as the demonstration of reassuring mesenteric tissue perfusion in a twin sibling with an uncomplicated course.

Design.—Case report.

Setting.—Neonatal intensive care unit in a tertiary care children's hospital.

Patients.—A 12-day-old growth-restricted preterm female twin with necrotizing enterocolitis and her twin who did not develop disease.

Interventions.—In the twin with symptoms of necrotizing enterocolitis, reduction in the mesenteric saturations was recorded in the injured bowel tissue as later confirmed during surgery. After resection of the ischemic bowel, mesenteric saturations returned to values comparable to those measured in the healthy twin. Reduced saturations were not observed in the asymptomatic twin.

Conclusions.—The use of optical oximetry to monitor mesenteric tissue saturation may provide a measure of bowel perfusion that could enhance clinical management in at-risk preterm neonates.

▶ Necrotizing enterocolitis (NEC) is the most common and fulminant gastrointestinal disease affecting neonates. This disease often has a rapid onset with few, if any, antecedent signs that can be used to reliably predict its occurrence. Its rapid onset and progression to death, as well as its severe morbidity when the infant survives, warrants the need for early noninvasive diagnostic tools. Optical oximetry based on near-infrared spectroscopy (NIRS) is being used increasingly as a useful noninvasive clinical tool for evaluating tissue oxygenation. NIRS correlates relative light absorption by oxy- and deoxyhemoglobin and displays saturation from smaller blood vessels (ie, arteriole, capillary, and venule) from which the level of tissue oxygenation can be estimated. Continuous monitoring of splanchnic or mesenteric tissue perfusion with NIRS might provide early signs of tissue hypoxia and injury leading to early diagnosis, prompt intervention, and potential prevention of NEC. Similarly, if normal mesenteric saturations reliably predicted a healthy bowel, interruptions in feedings and prolonged hyperalimentation might be avoided.

In this case report, Zabenah et al report the use of mesenteric NIRS monitoring in a 33-week premature neonate with NEC, the return of abdominal tissue perfusion after surgical intervention, and reassuring monitoring in a twin sibling with an uncomplicated clinical course. In their study, reduced mesenteric saturations were recorded over the injured bowel tissue as confirmed during surgery later. Several other studies have applied NIRS to the abdomen for investigating post-prandial changes, bowel ischemia, and NEC. Fortune et al[1] suggested the use of regional oxygen saturations as a way to detect the development of splanchnic ischemia. By comparing cerebral and splanchnic regional saturations, they were able to ascertain the presence of bowel ischemia by a reduction in cerebros-planchnic oxygenation ratio values. Stapleton et al[2] further described an associ-ation between mesenteric oxygen desaturation and the development of NEC in an infant with congenital heart disease. These studies highlight the potential application of NIRS in monitoring bowel disease progression and corroborating the diagnosis in high-risk neonates. However, further validation is necessary to determine applicability of the NIRS technology to studies involving NEC associ-ated with enteral feeding and feeding intolerance. Currently, NIRS is generally regarded to be a trend monitoring tool because of low resolution measurement that may resolve as technology evolves. A multisite measurement may provide more accurate information about regional tissue perfusion. Uncertainties still exist about the movement or geometrical changes of the intestines because of motility or distension from the intraluminal air. Pneumoperitoneum can also cause artifacts by pushing down the intestines, thus changing the optical path.

R. Sahni, MBBS

References

1. Fortune PM, Wagstaff M, Petros AJ. Cerebro-splanchnic oxygenation ratio (CSOR) using near infrared spectroscopy may be able to predict splanchnic ischaemia in neonates. *Intensive Care Med.* 2001;27:1401-1407.
2. Stapleton GE, Eble BK, Dickerson HA, Andropoulos DB, Chang AC. Mesenteric oxygen desaturation in an infant with congenital heart disease and necrotizing enterocolitis. *Tex Heart Inst J.* 2007;34:442-444.

Mucin dynamics and enteric pathogens

McGuckin MA, Lindén SK, Sutton P, et al (Mater Med Res Inst and The Univ of Queensland School of Medicine, South Brisbane, Australia; Gothenburg Univ, Sweden; Univ of Melbourne, Parkville, Victoria, Australia)
Nat Rev Microbiol 9:265-278, 2011

The extracellular secreted mucus and the cell surface glycocalyx prevent infection by the vast numbers of microorganisms that live in the healthy gut. Mucin glycoproteins are the major component of these barriers. In this Review, we describe the components of the secreted and cell surface mucosal barriers and the evidence that they form an effective barricade against potential pathogens. However, successful enteric pathogens have evolved strategies to circumvent these barriers. We discuss the interactions between enteric pathogens and mucins, and the mechanisms that these pathogens use to disrupt and avoid mucosal barriers. In addition, we

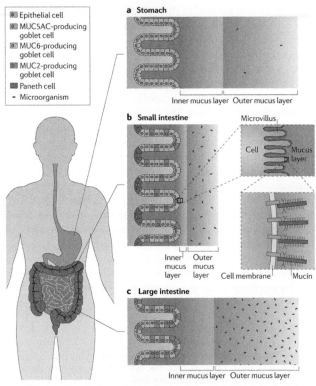

FIGURE 1.—The gastrointestinal mucosal barrier. The mucosa consists of a single layer of columnar epithelial cells covered by a layer of secreted mucus. The secreted mucus forms two layers, a thinner inner layer that is sterile and difficult to dislodge and an outer layer that is not sterile and is more easily removed. a| The outer layer of the stomach contains low numbers of transiting bacteria and measures ~120 μm in rats and mice, whereas the inner layer is sterile and measures ~100–150 μm. The mucus consists of mucin 5AC (MUC5AC) and MUC6 and is produced by mucus cells (stomach goblet cells). b| The mucus layer is thinner in the small intestine, consisting of an inner layer of ~15–30 μm and an outer layer of 100–400 μm; it is thickest in the ileum, where there are approximately 10^5–10^7 bacteria per gram of faeces in the lumen. Mucus in the small intestine (consisting of mainly MUC2) is produced by goblet cells and Paneth cells. c| Mucus in the large intestine (mainly MUC2) is predominantly produced by goblet cells and consists of a sterile inner layer of ~100 μm and a thick outer layer of ~700 μm. Numbers of bacteria are greater in the large intestine (10^{10}–10^{12} per gram) than in the small intestine owing to low numbers of bacteria in most food, bacterial killing by acid in the stomach, and the fast transit time and high concentration of bile acids in the small intestine, which limit bacterial growth. In the colon, the dwell time is longer, bile acid concentrations are low, endogenous mucus substrate is plentiful and Paneth cells and their secretions are sparse. Therefore, the environment in the colon (which is a fermentative organ analogous to the rumen) encourages a large, complex microbial consortium. Gastrointestinal epithelial cells, particularly those that do not produce mucus, are covered with microvilli containing a high density of transmembrane cell surface mucins. (Reprinted from McGuckin MA, Lindén SK, Sutton P, et al. Mucin dynamics and enteric pathogens. *Nat Rev Microbiol.* 2011;9:265-278, with permission from Macmillan Publishers Limited.)

describe dynamic alterations in the mucin barrier that are driven by host innate and adaptive immune responses to infection (Fig 1).

▶ This excellent review of mucin dynamics in the gastrointestinal tract presents a body of information that is very likely to play an important role in health and disease of preterm infants. Even though the neonate is not the focus of this article, it is not much of a stretch to extrapolate several of the principles presented to the importance of intestinal mucus in the developing preterm. The intestine, with its huge surface area, is lined by a mucus layer that can be very thick, as in the stomach and colon, or thin, such as in the small intestine (Fig 1). This provides a protective surface that separates luminal microorganisms from the intestinal epithelium and also prevents overly close interaction with intestinal receptors that may be involved with initiation of inflammatory responses. From a neonatal intensive care perspective, several entities, such as necrotizing enterocolitis, translocation of microbes (as in many cases of late-onset sepsis), and the systemic inflammatory response with its attendant consequences, come to mind in terms of protection by this barrier. This article clearly presents some of the conditions under which the mucus lining may be affected, including poor protein nutrition with attendant low threonine intake. This amino acid is important in the biosynthesis of mucin glycoproteins and may lead to diminished barrier function when not supplied adequately by either the enteral or parenteral routes. The interrelationship of mucin with commensal bacteria is of interest, where these resident microbes stimulate a baseline synthesis of the mucus, which in turn keeps pathogenic microorganisms at bay. It also serves as a medium for defensive proteins produced by Paneth cells that provide protection to the nearby stem cells and maintain turnover of intestinal epithelium. The fact that mucus also provides some of the same antigens seen in the Lewis blood group system, and when not present could predispose to infection or gut injury, also opens additional areas for future investigation.

J. Neu, MD

Necrotizing Enterocolitis
Neu J, Walker WA (Univ of Florida, Gainesville; Harvard Med School, Boston, MA)
N Engl J Med 364:255-264, 2011

Background.—Most very-low-birth-weight infants have intermittent gastrointestinal symptoms but do not have necrotizing enterocolitis. The mean prevalence of necrotizing enterocolitis in the United States and Canada is an estimated 7% in infants whose birth weight is 500 to 1500 g. Death occurs in 20% to 30% of cases, with higher rates in infants who need surgery. Although this disease is marked by feeding intolerance, abdominal distention, and bloody stools beginning 8 to 10 days after birth, the inflammatory process extends effects throughout the infant's system, affecting distant organs and raising the risk for neurodevelopmental delays. Abdominal radiography shows pneumatosis intestinalis, portal venous gas, or both. Dilated loops of bowel, little gas, and gas-filled loops of bowel remain in place on repeated examinations. In advanced cases, extraluminal air outside the bowel is seen. Within hours, symptoms can escalate from subtle signs to abdominal discoloration, intestinal perforation, and peritonitis, leading to systemic hypotension requiring intensive medical and/or surgical interventions. When short-bowel syndrome develops after necrotizing enterocolitis, the estimated cost of care over a 5-year period is nearly $1.5 million. The pathogenesis, differential diagnosis, treatments, and preventive strategies for this disorder were reviewed.

Pathogenesis.—Although the pathophysiology of necrotizing enterocolitis is poorly understood, observations strongly support a multifactorial cause. The principal combination suspected includes a genetic predisposition, intestinal immaturity, and unbalanced microvascular tone with abnormal microbial colonization in the intestine and a highly immunoreactive intestinal mucosa. Preterm infants are likely predisposed to an increased risk of intestinal injury because of their immature motility, digestion, absorption, immune defenses, barrier function, and circulatory regulation. After birth the normal human intestine is initially colonized by microbes and adapts to microbial stimulation by modifying the epithelial innate immune response. Fetal intestinal cells express lower levels of toll-like receptor 4 (TLR4) and a regulatory factor for transcription factor nuclear factor κB, which modulates inflammation. As a result, the enterocytes in preterm infants cannot handle the excessive stimulation. Increased interleukin-8 plus an excessive inflammatory response makes preterm infants more vulnerable to necrotizing enterocolitis. Inappropriate initial microbial colonization may contribute to the problem. Hypoxia-ischemia is an unlikely contributor to the disorder. The use of umbilical catheters and parenteral nutrition or elective transfusion of packed red cells appears to have no influence on necrotizing enterocolitis.

Differential Diagnosis.—The three common forms of neonatal intestinal injury are conditions seen in term infants, spontaneous intestinal perforations, and classic necrotizing enterocolitis. Necrotizing enterocolitis-n-like symptoms can occur in preterm, term, and late preterm infants, manifesting in older infants in the first week after birth and in association with problems such as maternal illicit drug use, intestinal anomalies, congenital heart disease, and perinatal stress on mesenteric blood flow. Spontaneous intestinal perforations in preterm infants occur in the first few days after birth, is not usually associated with enteral feeding, and involves minimal intestinal inflammation and necrosis. Indomethacin and glucocorticoid administration can be associated.

In classic necrotizing enterocolitis, the more premature the infant is, the later after birth the condition manifests. No universally reliable diagnostic criteria exist, but two staging systems exist. The Bell et al system identifies three stages: stage 1 shows highly nonspecific findings (feeding intolerance, mild abdominal distention, or both); stage 2 involves radiographic findings such as pneumatosis intestinalis; and stage 3 includes perforated viscus, perhaps associated with intestinal necrosis. The *Vermont Oxford Network Manual of Operations* identifies clinical signs as bilious gastric aspirate or emesis, abdominal distention, and occult gross blood in the stool without anal fissures and images showing pneumatosis intestinalis, hepatobiliary gas, and pneumoperitoneum. However, neither system adequately identifies when to treat surgically or indicates appropriate interventions early enough. A more reliable staging system is needed.

Treatment.—Medical intervention consists of abdominal decompression, bowel rest, broad-spectrum antibiotics, and intravenous hyperalimentation. Surgical interventions are needed if there is intestinal perforation or deteriorating clinical or biochemical status. Included are drain placement, exploratory laparotomy with resection of diseased bowel, and enterostomy with stoma creation. Advanced cases are managed with laparotomy and primary periotoneal drainage without laparotomy, but these approaches have questionable benefit. Once surgery is required, outcome is often poor.

Prevention.—The major preventive approaches are withholding enteral feedings, using enteral antibiotics, feeding the infant with maternal expressed breast milk, giving probiotic and/or prebiotic agents, and administering growth factors, anticytokine agents, and glucocorticoids. If feedings are completely withheld, prolonged parenteral nutrition, intestinal atrophy, increased permeability and inflammation, and late-onset sepsis can occur. Delaying feeding increases the severity of necrotizing entercoliitis should it occur. Exclusive use of human milk plus a human milk-n-derived fortifier is associated with a lower incidence of necrotizing entercolitis. Enteral aminoglycoside administration is often avoided to reduce risks of resistant microorganisms. The risk of necrotizing enterocolitis is increased with prolonged empirical use of intravenous antibiotics for preterm infants. Using probiotics can decrease the incidence of necrotizing enterocolitis but not the morbidity associated with it and may increase the risk of sepsis. Prebiotic agents, nutrients that enhance the growth of potentially beneficial microbes, include inulin, galactose, fructose, lactulose, and combinations of these. They enhance the proliferation of endogenous flora but the intestine must already be appropriately colonized, which is often not true in very-low-birth-weight preterm infants. Support is lacking for this approach and for the use of microbial components that modulate inflammation, such as those that affect TLR signaling.

Conclusions.—Prevention is the most likely avenue to obtain better results for infants at risk for necrotizing enterocolitis. Before effective strategies can be developed, clear, consistently used diagnostic criteria are needed. The development of highly sensitive specific biomarkers and new methods for detecting factors that predispose infants to necrotizing enterocolitis is needed. Research should focus on ways to enhance innate immunity using human milk and to avoid manipulations that can alter normal microbial ecology and diversity, such as the overuse of antibiotics.

▶ This review is an update on several aspects of necrotizing enterocolitis (NEC). One of the most important messages is that what we have been lumping into one disease is probably several different disease entities with different pathophysiologic mechanisms. For example, the intestinal necrosis seen in term infants with left-sided heart failure is different than the isolated ileal perforations seen in extremely low birth weight infants who have little intestinal necrosis. These are also different than those infants with the classic form of

NEC that is usually associated with inflammation and occurs more than 1 week after birth. Bell's criteria and their subsequent modifications, which have been the mainstay of NEC diagnosis, are discussed along with their limitations, especially stage 1 NEC, which is so poorly defined that it should be taken out of our diagnostic vocabulary. Some of the pathophysiology is also reviewed, with an emphasis placed on the need to better define the microbial ecology of the intestine in babies who develop NEC versus those who do not. The interaction with the intestinal microbes and intestinal cell surface innate receptors, such as toll-like receptor 4, are becoming a major focus of the pathophysiologic cascade involved in the pathogenesis of NEC. The need for better diagnostic and predictive biomarkers is discussed. A review of some of the newer preventative modalities, such as probiotics, is provided, with the suggestion that these are promising agents but that we also need to understand how they work, what they do, and have a clearer picture of both their short- and long-term effects before they become another misadventure in neonatal care.

J. Neu, MD

New Insights Into the Pathogenesis and Treatment of Necrotizing Enterocolitis: Toll-Like Receptors and Beyond
Afrazi A, Sodhi CP, Richardson W, et al (Univ of Pittsburgh School of Medicine, PA)
Pediatr Res 69:183-188, 2011

Necrotizing enterocolitis (NEC) is the leading cause of death from gastrointestinal disease in the preterm infant. The dismal results of current treatment for NEC highlight the urgent need for greater understanding of the pathogenesis of this disease, and the importance of discovering novel, molecular-specific therapies for it. Current dogma indicates that NEC development reflects an abnormal response by the premature infant to the microbial flora that colonizes the gastrointestinal tract, although the mechanisms that mediate these abnormal bacterial-enterocyte interactions and the reasons for the particularly increased susceptibility of the premature infant to the development of NEC remain incompletely explained. Recent evidence has shed light on an emerging role for the Toll-like receptors (TLRs) of the innate immune system as central players in the pathways that signal in response to enteric bacteria resulting in the development of NEC. We now review recent advances in the field of NEC and identify several exciting potential avenues for novel treatments by focusing on abnormal TLR4 signaling in the premature intestine in the pathogenesis of NEC. In so doing, we seek to offer new hope to the patients and their families who are affected by this devastating disorder.

▶ This review puts a spotlight on Toll-like receptor 4 (TLR4), one of at least 10 receptors found in various cell types, such as the intestinal epithelium, macrophages, antigen presenting cells, etc. The intestinal epithelium expresses TLR4, and this is a key proximal signaling molecule involved in the transduction of signals from microbes residing in the intestine and eventual transcription via nuclear factor kappa B movement into the nucleus and acting as a transcription factor for cytokine and chemokine production. The authors posit from their work and others that TLR4 is a signaling molecule that is crucial to the pathogenesis of necrotizing enterocolitis (NEC). Much of this work is based on studies in rodent models that involve major stressors, such as exposure to hypoxia, cold, formula rather than mothers' milk, etc, that cause an intestinal illness that many consider to be a model of NEC. In reality, most NEC that occurs in human preterm infants has little, if any, relationship to hypoxic episodes as induced in these animals and, unlike in the animal models, is not seen shortly after birth. Although the body of knowledge derived from these models likely represents intestinal injury associated with severe stress to the infant animal, I remain skeptical whether these are optimal for evaluating the pathogenesis of classic NEC.

Nevertheless, there is an emerging set of knowledge from human preterm infants, as described in this review, that the microbial milieu and the interaction of the innate immune system, including TLRs and other signaling molecules, play a role. TLR4 may be an important component in the pathogenesis, but there are several other signaling molecules, cell types other than the intestinal epithelial cell (which actually expresses TLR4 on the basolateral surface and needs to have an interepithelial opening for exposure to microbial ligands), that are likely to play a role. One of these (TLR9), as mentioned, may have important modulating effects. Simple preexposure to microbial ligands may induce counter-regulation to lipopolysaccharide and other ligands that can induce inflammation and actually promote intestinal healing and homeostasis.

Despite these caveats, the authors seem to be on the right track, and their work and others should provide a better understanding of the interaction between microbial components that interact with the immature intestine differently than the mature intestine, thereby providing a homeostatic mechanism that prevents disease.

J. Neu, MD

Non-Invasive Markers for Early Diagnosis and Determination of the Severity of Necrotizing Enterocolitis
Thuijls G, Derikx JPM, van Wijck K, et al (Nutrition and Toxicology Res Inst (NUTRIM), Maastricht, The Netherlands; et al)
Ann Surg 251:1174-1180, 2010

Objectives.—To improve diagnosis of necrotizing enterocolitis (NEC) by noninvasive markers representing gut wall integrity loss (I-FABP and claudin-3) and gut wall inflammation (calprotectin). Furthermore, the usefulness of I-FABP to predict NEC severity and to screen for NEC was evaluated.

Methods.—Urinary I-FABP and claudin-3 concentrations and fecal calprotectin concentrations were measured in 35 consecutive neonates suspected of NEC at the moment of NEC suspicion. To investigate I-FABP as screening tool for NEC, daily urinary levels were determined in 6 neonates who developed NEC out of 226 neonates included before clinical suspicion of NEC.

Results.—Of 35 neonates suspected of NEC, 14 developed NEC. Median I-FABP, claudin-3, and calprotectin levels were significantly higher in neonates with NEC than in neonates with other diagnoses. Cutoff values for I-FABP (2.20 pg/nmol creatinine), claudin-3 (800.8 INT), and calprotectin (286.2 μg/g feces) showed clinically relevant positive likelihood ratios (LRs) of 9.30, 3.74, 12.29, and negative LRs of 0.08, 0.36, 0.15, respectively. At suspicion of NEC, median urinary I-FABP levels of neonates with intestinal necrosis necessitating surgery or causing death were significantly higher than urinary I-FABP levels in conservatively treated neonates.

Of the 226 neonates included before clinical suspicion of NEC, 6 developed NEC. In 4 of these 6 neonates I-FABP levels were not above the cutoff level to diagnose NEC before clinical suspicion.

Conclusions.—Urinary I-FABP levels are not suitable as screening tool for NEC before clinical suspicion. However, urinary I-FABP and claudin-3 and fecal calprotectin are promising diagnostic markers for NEC. Furthermore, urinary I-FABP might also be used to predict disease severity.

▶ The current diagnostic criteria for necrotizing enterocolitis (NEC) are suboptimal at best. We currently have no specific and sensitive predictive or diagnostic biomarkers for this devastating disease. This article evaluates 3 new potential biomarkers (urinary intestinal fatty acid binding protein [I-FABP], claudin 3, and fecal calprotectin) and some already nonspecific markers for inflammatory processes, such as white blood cell and platelet counts. The theoretical advantage of the 3 new agents is that I-FABP is produced primarily by intestinal epithelium, and one would expect that damage to the intestinal epithelium would cause increased release of this into the bloodstream and subsequently in the urine. Likewise, claudin 3 (1 of about 20 claudin proteins) is found in interepithelial tight junctions and would also be expected to be released after intestinal epithelial injury. Calprotectin, found in neutrophils, might be expected to be found in the stool during intestinal inflammatory conditions. This study showed that C-reactive protein and platelet count to be no different in NEC cases and controls, but the white blood cell counts were lower in NEC. I-FABP, claudin 3, and calprotectin were sensitive and specific markers at the time of NEC diagnosis, with I-FABP appearing to have the best sensitivity and specificity. Unfortunately, the calprotectin from a practical standpoint is likely not to be a highly valuable indicator because babies do not provide stool at the will of the physician. Another concern is that the current gold standards used to diagnose NEC (eg, pneumatosis intestinalis) in these studies may actually not be a very good diagnostic tool to begin with. The fact that these 3 agents could not be used as predictive biomarkers comes of little surprise. They will only appear once the gut injury has already started. This should not blunt our enthusiasm for evaluating these and similar markers for use in diagnosis of NEC. Better tools are badly needed.

J. Neu, MD

Succession of microbial consortia in the developing infant gut microbiome
Koenig JE, Spor A, Scalfone N, et al (Cornell Univ, Ithaca, NY; et al)
Proc Natl Acad Sci U S A 108:4578-4585, 2011

The colonization process of the infant gut microbiome has been called chaotic, but this view could reflect insufficient documentation of the factors affecting the microbiome. We performed a 2.5-y case study of the assembly of the human infant gut microbiome, to relate life events to microbiome composition and function. Sixty fecal samples were collected from a healthy infant along with a diary of diet and health status. Analysis of >300,000 16S rRNA genes indicated that the phylogenetic diversity of the microbiome increased gradually over time and that changes in community composition conformed to a smooth temporal gradient. In contrast, major taxonomic groups showed abrupt shifts in abundance corresponding to changes in diet or health. Community assembly was nonrandom: we observed discrete steps of bacterial succession punctuated by life events. Furthermore, analysis of ≈ 500,000 DNA metagenomic reads from 12 fecal samples revealed that the earliest microbiome was enriched in genes facilitating lactate utilization, and that functional genes involved in plant polysaccharide metabolism were present before the introduction of solid food, priming the infant gut for an adult diet. However, ingestion of table foods caused a sustained increase in the abundance of Bacteroidetes, elevated fecal short chain fatty acid levels, enrichment of genes associated with carbohydrate utilization, vitamin biosynthesis, and xenobiotic degradation, and a more stable community composition, all of which are characteristic of the adult microbiome. This study revealed that seemingly chaotic shifts in the microbiome are associated with life events; however, additional experiments ought to be conducted to assess how different infants respond to similar life events.

▶ In this day of evidence-based medicine with blinded, multicenter trials and meta analyses involving hundreds and sometimes thousands of subjects, one would be surprised to see a study published in a very prestigious journal that involves only 1 subject. That is the case in this article, which in my opinion provides important and interesting information using novel technologies and raises the need to continue along this line of research. In this study, 1 baby was studied for 2.5 years after birth using 60 stool samples that were analyzed for nonculture-based microbial analysis using 16S pyrosequencing. Twelve of these samples were evaluated using a much broader analysis (called metagenomics) that involves studying the entire community of microbes usually focused on the entire microbial genome, which can in turn be used to probe existing databases for analysis of function. Several fascinating results were seen in this study. The first stools contained microbial DNA. Is it possible that this may have been of intrauterine origin? If so, it suggests that the fetus might be exposed to microbes before birth and that this may have some effect on the developing immune system via swallowing through the amniotic fluid. The pattern of microbial evolution over time was also of interest, with diversity increasing over time and microbes belonging to the phylum Firmicutes predominating in the first several months, then Proteobacteria, Bacteroidetes, and Actinobacteria taking over. The metagenomic studies were also of interest in that functional microbial genes associated with lactose-related activities were first detected, but with time, genes associated with other disaccharide and more complex carbohydrate metabolism were detected. Overall, this very detailed and extensive study in 1 baby offers an excellent start to more extensive population-based studies that will shed light on the microbiome that we have coexisted with since the beginning of our human species.

J. Neu, MD

Transfusion-Related Acute Gut Injury: Necrotizing Enterocolitis in Very Low Birth Weight Neonates after Packed Red Blood Cell Transfusion
Blau J, Calo JM, Dozor D, et al (Maria Fareri Children's Hosp at Westchester Med Ctr, Valhalla, NY)
J Pediatr 158:403-409, 2011

Objective.—This is a repeat cohort study in which we sought to determine whether an association of necrotizing enterocolitis (NEC) <48 hours of a packed red blood cells (PRBC) transfusion was a prior sampling artifact.

Study Design.—All very low birth weight neonates with NEC Stage ≥IIB admitted over an 18-month period were categorized for NEC: (1) <48 hours after a PRBC transfusion; (2) unrelated to the timing of PRBCs; and (3) never transfused.

Results.—Eight hundred eighty-three admissions over 18 months were reviewed; 256 were very low birth weight that resulted in 36 NEC cases and 25% were associated with PRBC (n = 9). PRBC-associated cases had lower birth weight, hematocrit, and rapid onset of signs (<5 hours). The timing of association of PRBC transfusion and NEC differed from random, showing a distribution that was not uniform over time ($\chi^2 = 170.7$, df = 40; $P < .000001$) consistent with the possibility of a causative relationship in certain cases of NEC. Current weight at onset of NEC did not differ; however, the more immature the neonate the later the onset of NEC creating a curious centering of occurrence at a median of 31 weeks postconceptual age.

Conclusions.—We conclude that PRBC-related NEC exists. Transfusion-related acute gut injury is an acronym we propose to characterize a severe neonatal gastrointestinal reaction proximal to a transfusion of PRBCs for anemia. The convergence at 31 weeks postconceptual age approximates the age of presentation of other O_2 delivery and neovascularization syndromes, suggesting a link to a generalized systemic maturational mechanism.

▶ This interesting report describes a subgroup of preterm infants with necrotizing enterocolitis (NEC) who developed the disease within hours after a packed red blood cell (PRBC) transfusion. Although only 25% of the infants with NEC at that center exhibited this temporal relationship, the timing is quite striking and appears to be statistically robust. (The Poisson probability of observing 9 of the 36 cases within a single 24-hour interval after transfusion is $< 10^{-9}$.) The authors therefore posit that instances of NEC following closely on red blood cell (RBC) transfusions may have a pathogenesis similar to that of transfusion-related acute lung injury and propose a new acronym for this putative syndrome: TRAGI, transfusion-related acute gut injury. In an accompanying editorial, Christensen[1] suggests 2 alternative explanations: ischemic bowel injury may be caused by the anemia that transfusion was intended to treat or effects of blood storage, such as depletion or red blood cell nitric oxide, may predispose to vasoconstriction and ischemic bowel injury. Diagnostic availability bias may provide another explanation: if the response to subtle early signs of NEC in anemic babies is PRBC transfusion because of ready availability of anemia as an explanatory diagnosis, then transfusion is likely to be soon followed by more overt signs of NEC. Whichever explanation is correct, this intriguing observation is already leading to new hypotheses that hold great promise for illuminating the pathogenesis, early diagnostic features, and/or potential preventive measures for NEC.

W. E. Benitz, MD

Reference

1. Christensen RD. Association between red blood cell transfusions and necrotizing enterocolitis. *J Pediatr.* 2011;158:349-350.

When to wean? How good is the evidence for six months' exclusive breastfeeding

Fewtrell M, Wilson DC, Booth I, et al (Univ College London Inst of Child Health, UK; Univ of Edinburgh, UK; Univ of Birmingham, UK)
BMJ 342:209-212, 2011

Background.—Early nutrition profoundly affects long-term health, including cognitive function, obesity, cardiovascular disease risk, cancer, and atopy. The World Health Organization (WHO) recommended in 2001 that infants be exclusively breast fed for 6 months. However, many Western countries, including 65% of the European member states and the United States, chose not to comply fully with this guideline, but in 2003 the United Kingdom chose to follow it. The evidence supporting this stance was not well characterized earlier but has been reassessed because of new data and a recent expert review completed for the European Food Safety Authority (EFSA) that recommends adding complementary foods to infants' diets between ages 4 and 6 months.

Evidence Supporting WHO's Recommendation.—The evidence for breast feeding itself is extensive, but that specific to 6 months' exclusive breast feeding is less impressive. The WHO recommendation is primarily based on a systematic review of infant and maternal health effects after 6 months versus 3 or 4 months of exclusive breast feeding. Seven of the 16 eligible studies reviewed were from developing nations, and all but two were observational. The conclusions supported 6 months' exclusive breast feeding to reduce infection and the risk of gastroenteritis in developed nations. No compelling evidence indicated a need to change from the then-current recommendation that solids be introduced between ages 4 and 6 months.

New Evidence.—Four observational studies in developed nations found that 6 months of exclusive breast feeding lowers the risk of pneumonia and recurrent otitis media, reduces the risk of hospital admission for infant infections, lowers the incidence of gastroenteritis, and helped prevent chest infection. However, the introduction of infant formula, not solid foods, predicted increased hospital admissions. In addition, whether exclusive breast feeding for 6 months reliably supports adequate growth is a concern. The WHO found only limited data in support of exclusive breast feeding for 6 months. In addition, it is likely that parents whose child signals hunger with exclusive breast feeding will begin to introduce weaning foods earlier. Many mothers who exclusively breast fed cannot support an infant's energy requirements for 6 months. In the United States, iron requirements are not met with exclusive breast feeding, with infants developing anemia and low serum ferritin levels, which can have irreversible long-term adverse effects on motor, mental, and social development. Improved iron status in pregnancy, delayed umbilical cord clamping, and supplements for infants at risk may help avoid adverse effects. Many developing nations also have increasing rates of food allergy even though potentially allergenic foods, such as cows' milk, eggs, fish, gluten, peanuts, and seeds, are not given to infants early. Conversely, some countries where peanuts are used as weaning foods have low incidences of peanut allergy. Some evidence shows immune tolerance develops with repeated exposure in a critical early time window and perhaps in the context of other dietary factors, including breast feeding. For example, evidence suggests that gluten can be introduced at age 3 to 6 months, while waiting until after age 6 months has an increased risk of wheat allergy at age 4 years. Longer term effects of exclusive breast feeding are not known for blood pressure, cognition, atopy, and dental caries but are suggested for fatness or overweight.

Conclusions.—In resource-poor countries with high morbidity and mortality from infections exclusive breast feeding for 6 months has a clearly positive effect. In Western nations, exclusive breast feeding for 6 months is linked to less infection. Areas of concern associated with this longer period of breast feeding include higher rates of iron deficiency anemia, food allergies, and celiac disease, along with the accompanying long-term complications of these conditions. It is advised that, before making global public health recommendations, there should be an evidence-based approach to appraising the available scientific data, a synthesis balancing the risks and benefits of the proposed change, and an auditing mechanism developed to detect adverse population effects of the implemented change. Based on the current evidence for the EFSA's member nations, complementary foods can be safely introduced between ages 4 to 6 months. Exclusive breast feeding may not always provide sufficient nutrition for optimal growth and development. When breast milk is no longer adequate nutrition will vary with the infant's size, activity, growth rate, and gender as well as the quality and volume of the breast milk supply. A hungry infant is most likely a mechanism whereby the timing of weaning can be individualized for the specific mother-infant pair.

▶ This review provides an important critique on a practice that has received support by the World Health Organization (WHO) since 2001 and become public policy in many countries, that is, exclusive breast milk feeding for at least 6 months. It is of interest that a majority of countries have adopted this policy, with the exception of the United States and a few European Union countries. The WHO recommendation was based largely on one systematic review[1] of the maternal and infant health effects on infants of breast-feeding for 6 months versus 3 to 4 months. This review included 16 eligible studies, of which only 2 were randomized trials. The review suggested that exclusive breast-feeding for 6 months resulted in no apparent growth deficits or allergies but longer time to return to menses in the mothers. There was a suggestion of not only reduced infection but also iron deficiency. The American Academy of Pediatrics (AAP) Committee on Nutrition suggested that in developed countries, complementary foods may be introduced at 4 to 6 months despite a difference of opinion from the AAP Committee on Breastfeeding, which recommended exclusive breast-feeding for 6 months.[2]

In a concurrent systematic review,[3] 33 studies were analyzed and no compelling evidence was found to change the pre-2001 recommendations (breast-feed and introduce solid foods between 4 and 6 months). Newer evidence is emerging that the practice of exclusive breast-feeding for 6 months may not be the best practice for all infants. Some mothers may not be able to provide adequate quantities of milk for their rapidly growing infant. Studies are showing that US infants exclusively breast-fed for 6 months in comparison to continuing breast-feeding but introducing complementary foods 4 to 5 months are more likely to develop anemia and low serum ferritin. This is of major concern given the relationship of early iron deficiency to irreversible mental and motor deficits. Furthermore, a critical period appears to exist for development of food allergies with the delayed exposure to potentially allergenic foods, including cow's milk, eggs, fish, gluten, and peanuts. The lack of early introduction of bitter tastes has also been associated with unwillingness to eat vegetables when these individuals mature.[4] Whether introduction of solids between 4 and 6 months results in obesity in adulthood still needs to be determined. Because the evidence to support advantages of exclusive breast-feeding for 6 months has been shown to be weak and since there may be significant detrimental effects, the European Food Safety Authority has concluded that for infants across the European Union, complementary foods may be introduced safely between 4 and 6 months.

This review provides a strong lesson that broad policy decisions based on systematic reviews, especially those based on observational studies rather than strong randomized clinical trials, may cause harm. Not all infants and their mothers are the same, and such sweeping public policies should be based on very solid evidence and prerequisites prior to adoption as described in this review.

J. Neu, MD

References

1. Kramer MS, Kakuma R. Optimal duration of exclusive breastfeeding. *Cochrane Database Syst Rev.* 2002;(1). CD003517.
2. Kleinman, RE. *Pediatric Nutrition Handbook from the American Academy of Pediatrics.* 5th ed. American Academy of Pediatrics; 2004. 108.
3. Lanigan JA, Bishop J, Kimber AC, Morgan J. Systematic review concerning the age of introduction of complementary foods to the healthy full-term infant. *Eur J Clin Nutr.* 2001;55:309-320.
4. Prescott SL, Smith P, Tang M, et al. The importance of early complementary feeding in the development of oral tolerance: concerns and controversies. *Pediatr Allergy Immunol.* 2008;19:375-380.

Fucosyltransferase 2 Non-Secretor and Low Secretor Status Predicts Severe Outcomes in Premature Infants
Morrow AL, Meinzen-Derr J, Huang P, et al (Cincinnati Children's Hosp Med Ctr, OH; et al)
J Pediatr 158:745-751, 2011

Objective.—To investigate secretor gene fucosyltransferase 2 (FUT2) polymorphism and secretor phenotype in relation to outcomes of prematurity.

Study Design.—Study infants were $\leq$32 weeks gestational age. Secretor genotype was determined from salivary DNA. Secretor phenotype was measured with H antigen, the carbohydrate produced by secretor gene enzymes, in saliva samples collected on day 9 ± 5. The optimal predictive cutoff point in salivary H values was identified with Classification and Regression Tree analysis. Study outcomes were death, necrotizing enterocolitis (NEC, Bell's stage II/III), and confirmed sepsis.

Results.—There were 410 study infants, 26 deaths, 30 cases of NEC, and 96 cases of sepsis. Analyzed by genotype, 13% of 95 infants who were non-secretors, 5% of 203 infants who were heterozygotes, and 2% of 96 infants who were secretor dominant died ($P = .01$). Analyzed by phenotype, 15% of 135 infants with low secretor phenotype died, compared with 2% of 248 infants with high secretor phenotype (predictive value = 76%, $P < .001$). Low secretor phenotype was associated ($P < .05$) with NEC, and non-secretor genotype was associated ($P = .05$) with gram negative sepsis. Secretor status remained significant after controlling for multiple clinical factors.

Conclusions.—Secretor genotype and phenotype may provide strong predictive biomarkers of adverse outcomes in premature infants.

▶ Several clinical scoring systems with varying acronyms (eg, CRIB, SNAP) have been developed to predict neonatal morbidity and mortality and these have been compared, but none seem to offer a striking advantage over birth weight in a very low birth weight ventilated group.[1] The development of readily accessible biomarkers that would provide the clinician with a better grading system for degree of illness and potential to develop necrotizing enterocolitis and sepsis would be very helpful in anticipatory guidance. This study evaluated the secretor gene *fucosyltranferase 2* (*FUT2*) collected from saliva. The H antigen plays important roles in mucosal maturation and immunity. H antigen is expressed on mucosal surfaces and in saliva and other secretions. Polymorphisms in the secretor gene (*FUT2*) produce variable expression of H antigen. This study evaluated the associations between the secretor gene polymorphism and outcomes of prematurity. They found that the secretor H antigen normally increases in the saliva of premature infants in the first postnatal weeks. At 2 weeks, the nonsecretor genotype and low expression of the secretor H antigen in infants' saliva samples were predictive of an increased incidence of death and necrotizing enterocolitis. Differences in salivary H distribution between death and survivor groups were not caused by confounding by gestational age, birth weight, and controlling for multiple other clinical factors. It begs the question of why the H antigen was found to be low in the individuals with the greatest risk of illness. One caveat is that the H antigen secretor status was measured by immunoassay at a time when many of these infants are either at the peak of their illness associated with prematurity or just overcoming some of the major respiratory problems and whether nutritional status in the sicker infants may have been the cause of the lower levels. Nevertheless, this is a potentially valuable finding and deserves additional investigation so that it might be implemented for practical use in these infants.

J. Neu, MD

Reference

1. Fleisher BE, Murthy L, Lee S, Constantinou JC, Benitz WE, Stevenson DK. Neonatal severity of illness scoring systems: a comparison. *Clin Pediatr (Phila).* 1997;36:223-227.

7 Genetics and Teratology

Assessment of the ductus venosus, tricuspid blood flow and the nasal bone in second-trimester screening for trisomy 21
Stressig R, Kozlowski P, Froehlich S, et al (Praenatal.de - Praenatal Medicine and Genetics, Duesseldorf/Cologne, Germany; et al)
Ultrasound Obstet Gynecol 37:444-449, 2011

Objective.—To examine the prevalence of reversed a-wave in the ductus venosus, tricuspid regurgitation and absent nasal bone, in a second-trimester population undergoing amniocentesis, after exclusion of major fetal defects and to estimate the performance in screening for trisomy 21 based on maternal age and these markers in a general population.

Methods.—This was a retrospective study involving pregnancies undergoing amniocentesis due to increased risk for trisomy 21, mainly because of advanced maternal age. Before the invasive procedure, an ultrasound examination was carried out to exclude major fetal defects and to examine the ductus venosus, tricuspid blood flow and the presence of the fetal nasal bone. Modeling techniques were used based on 20 000 euploid pregnancies and 20 000 pregnancies with trisomy 21 to assess the screening performance in a general population.

Results.—The study population consisted of 3613 euploid pregnancies and 35 cases with trisomy 21. In the euploid group, reversed flow in the ductus venosus, tricuspid regurgitation and an absent nasal bone was observed in 1.7%, 1.5% and 0.1% of cases, respectively. In the trisomic group, these markers were found in 14.3%, 11.4% and 14.3% of cases, respectively. For a 5% false-positive rate, the detection rate in screening for trisomy 21, based on maternal age and either ductus venosus, tricuspid blood flow or nasal bone would be 33.8%, 32.4% or 31.4%, respectively. Screening by maternal age alone would detect 29.0% of the fetuses with trisomy 21. Receiver–operating characteristics curve analysis showed a slight but significant improvement in screening performance for trisomy 21 based on the inclusion of these markers.

Conclusion.—Second-trimester ultrasound screening for trisomy 21 based on maternal age with additional assessment of the ductus venosus, tricuspid blood flow and the fetal nasal bone in otherwise normal-appearing fetuses is only marginally better than is screening by maternal age alone.

▶ We have become accustomed to the modern era of sophisticated technology for evaluation of karyotype and individual chromosomes; such technology includes fluorescence, in situ hybridization, and microarray chips. I thought a look backward might be sobering. Although Down syndrome was described in 1866 by physician John Langdon Down, it took almost 100 years for the cause of the disorder to be identified as a chromosome 21 trisomy by Jerome Lejeune in 1959. Only 3 years before, it was determined that the actual number of human chromosomes was 46. This exciting new discovery led to identifying the cause of numerous syndromes, including Down syndrome (trisomy 21), the most common chromosome disorder.[1] The condition has been recognized with increased frequency in utero, and all pregnant women should be offered screening for trisomy 21. If the screen is positive, she should have rapid access to appropriate counseling by trained staff.

Beth A Pletcher[2] noted in 1998, "Just as maternal serum screening has become more sensitive with the addition of multiple biochemical markers, it is likely that only by combining screening for several ultrasound markers as well as maternal age and maternal serum results will the utility of ultrasound in the diagnosis of trisomy 21 and other aneuploidies be realized. Until such time as the correct identification of affected fetuses (sensitivity) approaches that of serum screening and maternal age, it is unlikely that ultrasound will replace amniocentesis as a diagnostic test." Her words hold true today.

In the report from Stressig and colleagues in Tubingen, Germany, if there are no major defects identified in the fetus but there is reversed flow in the ductus venosus or tricuspid regurgitation, the risk of trisomy 21 is approximately 5% to 10%. However, if the nasal bone is not visible, the risk is about 50%. Nonetheless, second-trimester screening by maternal age and these markers is only marginally better than screening by maternal age alone.

In the combined data from two large first-trimester screening studies at 11 to 13 weeks of gestation, involving approximately 39 000 euploid fetuses and 261 fetuses with trisomy 21, an abnormal nasal bone (abnormally small or absent) is seen in almost 60% of trisomy 21 but only 1.6% of the euploid cases.[3]

Kozlowski[4] noted that an absent nasal bone was observed in only approximately 30% of the fetuses with trisomy 21 and in 0.1% of the euploid fetuses.

In evaluating the nasal bone, Sressig magnified the image so that only the head with a midsagittal view of the fetal profile was shown on the screen. The nasal bone was classified as abnormal if it was not present and as normal if it was present. Hypoplastic nasal bones were not considered separately but were classified as normal. Tricuspid regurgitation is considered to be a transient and physiological finding in the second half of pregnancy and in postnatal life, but at 11 to 13 weeks of gestation, tricuspid regurgitation is observed in about half of fetuses with trisomy 21 and in only 1% of the euploid fetuses. Because fetuses with congenital heart disease were excluded from Sressig's study, the prevalence of Tricuspid incompetence was identified in only 14.3% in his series.

Reversed flow in the ductus venosus has been reported in two thirds of fetuses with trisomy 21 and 3% of Euploid fetuses. Perhaps it is disappointing that the ultrasound findings only marginally assisted in the diagnosis of trisomy 21. Maternal age remains a prominent if not the dominant risk factor, and the combination of biochemical markers with ultrasound including nuchal thickness, evaluation of the nasal bone, and presence of cardiac and gastrointestinal malformations all help to make the diagnosis of trisomy 21, which can of course be confirmed by amniocentesis or chorionic villus analysis.

A. A. Fanaroff, MD, FRCPE, FRCP&CH

References

1. Warkany J. Etiology of mongolism. *J Pediatr.* 1960;56:412-419.
2. Pletcher J. Ultrasound findings in Trisomy 21. May 1998. http://njms.umdnj.edu/genesweb2/topics/ob_gyn/prenatal_ultrasound.html.
3. Kagan KO, Cicero S, Staboulidou I, Wright D, Nicolaides KH. Fetal nasal bone in screening for trisomies 21, 18 and 13 and Turner syndrome at 11-13 weeks of gestation. *Ultrasound Obstet Gynecol.* 2009;33:259-264.
4. Kozlowski P, Knippel AJ, Froehlich S, Stressig R. Additional performance of nasal bone in first trimester screening. *Ultraschall Med.* 2006;27:336-339.

Associations Between Maternal Fever and Influenza and Congenital Heart Defects
Oster ME, Riehle-Colarusso T, Alverson CJ, et al (Emory Univ, Atlanta, GA; Ctrs for Disease Control and Prevention, Atlanta, GA)
J Pediatr 158:990-995, 2011

Objective.—To examine associations between maternal reports of prenatal fever or influenza and congenital heart defects (CHDs), and to evaluate whether those associations varied with antipyretic use.

Study Design.—We analyzed case infants with CHD (n = 2361) and control infants without CHD (n = 3435) from the Baltimore-Washington Infant Study (1981-1989). Participating mothers were asked whether they experienced a "fever of 101°F or higher," had "influenza (flu)," or used an antipyretic agent (ie, acetaminophen, salicylate, or nonsteroidal anti-inflammatory drug) during the period extending from 3 months before pregnancy through the end of the third month of pregnancy. We used logistic regression to compute ORs and 95% CIs while controlling for potential confounders.

Results.—There were significant associations between fever and influenza and specific CHDs, namely right-sided obstructive defects (fever: OR, 2.04; 95% CI, 1.27 to 3.27; influenza: OR, 1.75; 95% CI, 1.16 to 2.62) and atrioventricular septal defects in infants with Down syndrome (fever: OR, 1.92; 95% CI, 1.10 to 3.38; influenza: OR, 1.66; 95% CI, 1.04 to 2.63). Maternal antipyretic use in the setting of fever or influenza tended to decrease these associations.

Conclusions.—Prenatal maternal fever or influenza may be associated with right-sided obstructive lesions in all infants and with atrioventricular septal defects in infants with Down syndrome. The use of antipyretics might attenuate such associations.

▶ It has always appeared odd to me that there is so much information regarding the effects of rubella and cytomegalovirus on the fetus, yet so little is known regarding the most common virus, influenza. This article addresses that gap in our knowledge and fills in some of the details. The strength of the study is that it is a large population-based study; however, maternal recall rather than viral studies or patient records are used to document the presence of an influenzalike illness in the periconceptual period. Furthermore, the mother's memory is needed to establish the presence or absence of fever and the medications used to treat the febrile illness. In contrast to other publications on influenza during pregnancy, a clear relationship is established between maternal reports of fever or influenza during the 3 months before and after conception and a significantly increased risk of having an offspring with a right-sided obstructive heart defect, especially tricuspid atresia and pulmonary atresia with intact ventricular septum. In addition, for the first time, the authors document that if mothers reported fever or influenza during the aforementioned time period, there was a significantly increased risk for atrioventricular septal defects (AVSD) in infants with Down syndrome, perhaps representing a gene environment interaction.

The use of antipyretic agents tended to attenuate the associations between fever or influenza and congenital heart disease (CHD). However, because fever and influenza tended to occur together, the authors were unable to separate the independent effects of these 2 variables. These findings confirm those from previous studies of CHD that demonstrated an association between fever or influenza and right-sided obstructive heart defects, particularly tricuspid atresia.[1] There was no association between maternal fever and cono-truncal defects, atrial septal defects, perimembranous ventricular septal defects, AVSD without Down syndrome, total anomalous pulmonary venous return, or left-sided obstructive defects. The association of fever and influenza with AVSD in patients with Down syndrome has not been reported previously, mainly because previous studies excluded subjects with Down syndrome from their analyses. It remains unclear why AVSD in patients with Down syndrome may be associated with fever and influenza but AVSD in patients without Down syndrome is not.

The take-home message is that future prospective studies documenting influenza, fever, and its treatment are needed to validate these findings of increased right-sided lesions following febrile illnesses or influenza in the periconceptual period. However, based on this study, prompt relief of fever and prevention of influenza in the periconceptual period is warranted.

A. A. Fanaroff, MD, FRCPE, FRCP&CH

Reference

1. Cleves MA, Malik S, Yang S, Carter TC, Hobbs CA. Maternal urinary tract infections and selected cardiovascular malformations. *Birth Defects Res A Clin Mol Teratol*. 2008;82:464-473.

Genetic Factors in Isolated and Syndromic Esophageal Atresia

Geneviève D, de Pontual L, Amiel J, et al (Université Montpellier 1, France; Université Paris-Descartes, France)
J Pediatr Gastroenterol Nutr 52:S6-S8, 2011

Esophageal atresia (EA) and tracheoesophageal fistulae (TEF) are frequent congenital malformations (1/3500 births) characterized by a discontinuity of the lumen of the esophagus.

EA/TEF is anatomically divided into 5 subtypes based on the location and type of anastomosis between trachea and esophagus. To our best knowledge, no differences in developmental origin could be identified for each of the 5 subtypes, and no correlation has been established between subtypes of EA and specific genetic disorders. EA is clinically divided into 2 different forms: isolated EA (IEA, 50%) and syndromic EA (SEA, 50%).

Epidemiological studies do not support the existence of strong genetic factors in IEA. In IEA, recurrence risk is estimated to 1%, and twin concordance rate is low (2.5%). However, in SEA, first-degree relatives are more likely to present malformations of the VACTERL spectrum. In addition, identification of several disease genes involved in SEA, mouse models, and chromosomal anomalies argues in favor of genetic factors in EA (Table 1).

▶ This article is a brief summary of factors associated with esophageal atresia/ tracheoesophageal fistula (EA/TEF), splitting it into 2 major categories: isolated and syndromic. Each of these constitutes about 50% of the total. The 5 subtypes of EA/TEF based on location and type of anastomosis between the trachea and esophagus do not appear to exhibit differences in developmental origin, and there does not appear to be a correlation between subtypes and specific genetic disorders. The isolated form of EA/TEF shows little relationship to genetic factors: twin concordance is low as is recurrence risk. With the syndromic forms of EA/TEF, first-degree relatives are more likely to present VACTERL spectrum malformations. There are now several disease genes that have been found to be involved with syndromic EA/TEF. Environmental factors have also been associated with a small number of babies who present with this anomaly. A summary of the etiologies of syndromic EA/TEF is provided in Table 1. Of interest is the emerging data on chromosome 13, 16, 17, and 22 deletions. Epigenetic alterations are also being suspected in at lease one of the subsets involving histone acetylation of BAXP1 in oculo-auriculo-vertebral

TABLE 1.—Principal Genetic Syndromes with Esophageal Atresia

Environmental Agents	Chromosomal Anomalies	Malformative Associations	(Gene/MIM)	Polymalformative Genetic Disorders	(Gene/MIM)
Fetal alcohol syndrome	Trisomy 21	VATER/VACTERL association	ZIC3? FOX cluster? (214800)	Feingold syndrome	(MYCN/164280)
Maternal phenylketonuria	Trisomy 13	OAVS spectrum	(Epigenetic anomaly? BPAX1/164210)	Charge syndrome	(CHD7/214800)
Maternal diabetes	Trisomy 18	MURCS	(601076)	AEG syndrome	(SOX2/206900)
Fetal carbimazole syndrome	Del 22q11.2			Fanconi anemia	(FANCA to M/227645)
Adriamycine (animal models)	Del 17q21.3-q23			G syndrome	(MID-1/30000)
	Del 16q24.1			Mitochondrial DNA mutations	
				Bartsocas-Papas/lethal popliteal pterygium syndrome	(263650)
				Fryns syndrome	(229850)

syndrome (a rare cause of EA/TEF). It's exciting to see the emergence of new technologies being applied to a better understanding of this condition.

J. Neu, MD

Maternal nutrition and gastroschisis: findings from the National Birth Defects Prevention Study
Feldkamp ML, Carmichael SL, Shaw GM, et al (Univ of Utah, Salt Lake City; Stanford Univ School of Medicine, Palo Alto, CA; et al)
Am J Obstet Gynecol 204:404.e1-404.e10, 2011

Objective.—Gastroschisis is increasing in many countries, especially among young women. Because young women may have inadequate nutrition, we assessed the relationship between individual nutrients and the risk for gastroschisis.

Study Design.—We analyzed data from the National Birth Defects Prevention Study, a population-based case-control study. Cases were ascertained from 10 birth defect surveillance systems. Controls were randomly selected from birth certificates or hospital records. Nutrient intake was estimated for the year prior to conception from maternal interviews based on a 58-item food frequency questionnaire and cereal consumption reported. A total of 694 cases and 6157 controls were available for analysis.

Results.—Reported intake of individual nutrients did not substantially affect the risk for gastroschisis. Stratification by maternal age, preconception body mass index, folic acid–containing supplements, or energy intake (kilocalories) did not alter risk estimates.

Conclusion.—This study does not support an increased risk for gastroschisis with decreasing tertiles of individual nutrients.

▶ The prevalence of gastroschisis appears to be increasing according to several studies.[1-3] In fact, the gastroschisis prevalence has increased 10-fold over the past 3 decades in Utah.[2] Maternal factors that appear to be associated with gastroschisis include a lower maternal age and maternal smoking. This study used data from the National Birth Defects Prevention study where 694 cases and 6154 controls were available for analysis. Because of the association with younger mothers, it was hypothesized that these younger mothers might have poorer nutrition than older mothers. Using dietary recall methods (not a very sensitive technique), it was found that maternal macronutrient and micronutrient intake did not affect the odds of gastroschisis. Again, in this study, a fascinating finding was an odds ratio of 7.1 if the mother was younger than 20 years and 0.3 if the mother was older than 30 years. Since there is no known genetic predisposition, this still suggests environmental influences related to age. For the most part, this study appears to have ruled out the likelihood that the different dietary habits of younger women are a likely causative factor for the development of gastroschisis. Nevertheless, the relationship between age and the development of the disease is so strong that additional investigation along the line of causative pathogenesis in relation to maternal age remains in order.

J. Neu, MD

References

1. Chabra S, Gleason CA, Seidel K, Williams MA. Rising prevalence of gastroschisis in Washington State. *J Toxicol Environ Health A.* 2011;74:336-345.
2. Hougland KT, Hanna AM, Meyers R, Null D. Increasing prevalence of gastroschisis in Utah. *J Pediatr Surg.* 2005;40:535-540.
3. Vu LT, Nobuhara KK, Laurent C, Shaw GM. Increasing prevalence of gastroschisis: population-based study in California. *J Pediatr.* 2008;152:807-811.

8 Hematology and Bilirubin

Bilirubin Binding Contributes to the Increase in Total Bilirubin Concentration in Newborns with Jaundice
Ahlfors CE, Parker AE (Stanford Univ, CA; California Pacific Med Ctr, San Francisco)
Pediatrics 126:e639-e643, 2010

Objective.—This study tests the hypothesis that the hourly rate of increase in plasma bilirubin concentration (ΔB_T) would increase significantly with increasing binding avidity.

Methods.—The plasma total bilirubin concentration (B_T), unbound bilirubin concentration, and albumin concentration values for healthy newborns with jaundice (≤ 100 hours of age, ≥ 35 weeks of gestation, and ≥ 2.5 kg at birth) were obtained from medical records. ΔB_T (in milligrams per deciliter per hour) was calculated as the slope of B_T versus age (in hours). Binding avidity was quantified as the product of the albumin concentration and its bilirubin binding constant (K). Linear correlation was used to test the hypothesis that ΔB_T would increase significantly with $K \cdot$albumin concentration.

Results.—The ranges of B_T, unbound bilirubin concentration, albumin concentration, and K values for the 21 patients studied were 7.6 to 28.5 mg/dL, 0.53 to 2.52 μg/dL, 2.9 to 4.6 g/dL, and 38 to 163 L/μmol, respectively. ΔB_T correlated significantly with $K \cdot$albumin concentration ($r^2 = 0.23$; $P = .026$).

Conclusions.—Plasma bilirubin binding avidity contributes significantly to ΔB_T. This component of ΔB_T is associated with a lower risk of bilirubin neurotoxicity, and studies aimed at incorporating plasma bilirubin binding avidity measurements into the algorithms used for management of newborn jaundice seem warranted.

▶ In this brief report, Ahlfors and Parker use decades of intimate familiarity with the problem of hyperbilirubinemia and bilirubin neurotoxicity to leverage a small amount of new data into a very important conclusion. Based on observations in only 21 patients, they demonstrate a weak ($r^2 = 0.23$) but statistically significant ($P = .026$) direct correlation between plasma bilirubin binding avidity and the estimated rate of rise in total serum bilirubin levels (B_T). The rate of rise in B_T, long used to estimate risk for development of severe hyperbilirubinemia and presumably bilirubin encephalopathy, may therefore have a negative correlation with the latter. In effect, more avid binding of bilirubin by albumin would reduce the risk of kernicterus through redistribution of bilirubin from the extravascular to the intravascular compartments. The authors reach this important conclusion: "Prospective studies measuring Δ BT, peak BT, plasma bilirubin binding, and carbon monoxide production in newborn populations are needed to develop appropriate laboratory algorithms for screening for and managing transient neonatal jaundice."

Whether these are the most important measurements or the focus should shift to development of rapid inexpensive methods for identification of genetic polymorphisms with strong associations with severe hyperbilirubinemia and bilirubin neurotoxicity (eg, glucose-6-phosphate dehydrogenase and uridine 5'-diphospho-glucuronosyltransferase) is debatable, but the point that we lack reliable tools for identification of infants at risk for kernicterus should not be.

W. E. Benitz, MD

Excessively high bilirubin and exchange transfusion in very low birth weight infants
Kuint J, Maayan-Metzger A, Boyko V, et al (Tel Aviv Univ, Israel)
Acta Paediatr 100:506-510, 2011

Aim.—To evaluate the performance of exchange transfusion in very low birth weight (VLBW) infants with excessively high serum bilirubin levels.

Methods.—A population-based observational study using data collected by the Israel National VLBW Infant Database. The study sample comprised 13 499 infants. Two definitions of excessively high-peak bilirubin levels that might be considered as threshold levels for performance of exchange transfusion were used. First, a bilirubin level of ≥15 mg/dL for all infants (PSB-15), and second, incremental bilirubin levels ranging from 12 to 17 mg/dL according to gestational age (PSB-GA).

Results.—Four hundreds sixty-eight (3.5%) and 1035 infants (7.7%) infants in the PSB-15 and in the PSB-GA groups respectively had peak serum bilirubin levels above thresholds for exchange transfusion. Exchange transfusions were performed in 66 (14.1%) of these infants in the PSB-15 group and 91 (8.8%) in the PSB-GA group. Using logistic regression analysis, peak serum bilirubin was found as an independent factor for performing exchange transfusion.

Conclusion.—Exchange transfusion was performed in only 9–14% of VLBW infants with excessively high bilirubin levels. We speculate that this may be a result of an absence of definitive guidelines or the possible belief that the risks of exchange transfusion outweigh the potential risk of bilirubin-induced neurological injuries.

▶ The authors performed a population-based observational study to compare the total serum bilirubin (TSB) levels at which exchange transfusions were performed in very low birth weight (VLBW) infants compared with published guidelines. There is nothing wrong with this exercise if the intention is to demonstrate the existing variation in practice. But the implication that the observed practice variations are examples of inappropriate care must be questioned. It is well known that the data on which existing guidelines are based are extremely limited and that, in practice, there are wide variations with regard to the use of exchange transfusions in these infants.[1-3] Estimating the risk that various TSB levels pose for brain damage in this population is difficult, if not impossible, and although the American Academy of Pediatrics produced guidelines for the management of hyperbilirubinemia in infants < 35 weeks' gestation in 1994 and 2004,[4,5] they have yet to come up with a guideline for the management of VLBW or extremely low birth weight (ELBW) infants. This provides some sense of how difficult it is to achieve agreement among experts on when and how these infants should be treated.

In the large, recently published Neonatal Network study,[6] the protocol called for an exchange transfusion if the TSB level exceeded the threshold value after 8 hours of intensive phototherapy. The TSB threshold was > 13 mg/dL for infants with 501 to 750 g birth weight and > 15 mg/dL for those with 751 to 1000 g birth weight. Such levels would be considered excessive by Kuint et al, yet were agreed to by academic neonatologists at 16 Neonatal Research Network centers in the United States. The veiled implication that some 9% to 14% of VLBW infants in Israel are being managed inappropriately produced a vigorous rebuttal by 2 senior Israeli neonatologists.[7]

The ultimate decision to be made in a VLBW infant whose bilirubin level continues to rise in spite of intensive phototherapy is when the risk of bilirubin-induced neurological damage exceeds the risk of exchange transfusion. At present, the answer to that question is unknown, but it should soon become moot because exchange transfusions in these infants are becoming increasingly rare.[6,8,9] In the Neonatal Network study, only 5 of 1974 (0.25%) ELBW infants required an exchange transfusion.[6]

M. J. Maisels, MB, BCh, DSc

References

1. Maisels MJ, Watchko JF. Treatment of jaundice in low birthweight infants. *Arch Dis Child Fetal Neonatal Ed.* 2003;88:F459-F463.
2. Hansen TWR. Therapeutic approaches to neonatal jaundice: an international survey. *Clin Pediatr (Phila).* 1996;35:309-316.
3. Rennie JM, Sehgal A, De A, Kendall GS, Cole TJ. Range of UK practice regarding thresholds for phototherapy and exchange transfusion in neonatal hyperbilirubinaemia. *Arch Dis Child Fetal Neonatal Ed.* 2009;94:F323-F327.
4. American Academy of Pediatrics Subcommittee on Hyperbilirubinemia. Management of hyperbilirubinemia in the newborn infant 35 or more weeks of gestation. *Pediatrics.* 2004;114:297-316.
5. Practice parameter: management of hyperbilirubinemia in the healthy term newborn. American Academy of Pediatrics. Provisional Committee for Quality Improvement and Subcommittee on Hyperbilirubinemia. *Pediatrics.* 1994;94: 558-562.
6. Morris BH, Oh W, Tyson JE, et al. Aggressive vs. conservative phototherapy for infants with extremely low birth weight. *N Engl J Med.* 2008;359:1885-1896.

7. Kuint J, Maayan-Metzger A, Boyko V, et al. Excessively high bilirubin and exchange transfusion in very low birth weight infants. *Acta Paediatr.* 2011;100:506-510.
8. O'Shea TM, Dillard RG, Klinepeter KL, Goldstein DJ. Serum bilirubin levels, intracranial hemorrhage, and the risk of developmental problems in very low birth weight infants. *Pediatrics.* 1992;90:888-892.
9. Maisels MJ. Phototherapy—traditional and nontraditional. *J Perinatol.* 2001;21: S93-S97.

Excessively high bilirubin and exchange transfusion in very low birth weight infants

Kuint J, Maayan-Metzger A, Boyko V, et al (Tel Aviv Univ, Israel)
Acta Paediatr 100:506-510, 2011

Aim.—To evaluate the performance of exchange transfusion in very low birth weight (VLBW) infants with excessively high serum bilirubin levels.

Methods.—A population-based observational study using data collected by the Israel National VLBW Infant Database. The study sample comprised 13 499 infants. Two definitions of excessively high-peak bilirubin levels that might be considered as threshold levels for performance of exchange transfusion were used. First, a bilirubin level of ≥15 mg/dL for all infants (PSB-15), and second, incremental bilirubin levels ranging from 12 to 17 mg/dL according to gestational age (PSB-GA).

Results.—Four hundreds sixty-eight (3.5%) and 1035 infants (7.7%) infants in the PSB-15 and in the PSB-GA groups respectively had peak serum bilirubin levels above thresholds for exchange transfusion. Exchange transfusions were performed in 66 (14.1%) of these infants in the PSB-15 group and 91 (8.8%) in the PSB-GA group. Using logistic regression analysis, peak serum bilirubin was found as an independent factor for performing exchange transfusion.

Conclusion.—Exchange transfusion was performed in only 9–14% of VLBW infants with excessively high bilirubin levels. We speculate that this may be a result of an absence of definitive guidelines or the possible belief that the risks of exchange transfusion outweigh the potential risk of bilirubin-induced neurological injuries.

▶ From an Israeli database, 13 499 infants were evaluated for bilirubin levels and use of exchange transfusions. Using criteria of bilirubin levels of greater than or equal to 15 mg/dL or incremental ranges from 12 to 17 mg/dL according to gestational age, 3.5% and 7.7% of infants had peak serum bilirubin concentrations above "thresholds" for exchange transfusion. Exchange transfusions were performed in 14.1% and 8.8% of these groups, respectively. The authors related this to guidelines from several textbooks and suggest that the number of exchange transfusions according to written textbook guidelines is low and that this could present a hazard to these neonates. However, there are no data on follow-up of these babies. How many of these infants might actually have developed bilirubin-induced encephalopathy? How good is the evidence from the textbooks and the studies on which the recommendations are based in preterm infants? Are exchange transfusions (especially now when so few are being done) really benign? Do these studies take into account the real-time scenarios: for example, when a bilirubin concentration result is obtained and comes back "high" but responds nicely to phototherapy, hydration, and other common measures? The latter is a common scenario and may have been a very reasonable approach in a large number of these infants. In summary, I only partially agree with the implication that many of the clinicians are underperforming exchange transfusions, but do agree that better evidence-based guidelines, including algorithms of when to transfuse if other measures such as phototherapy and hydration fail, would be useful.

J. Neu, MD

Interpreting Conjugated Bilirubin Levels in Newborns
Davis AR, Rosenthal P, Escobar GJ, et al (California Pacific Med Ctr, San Francisco; Univ of California, San Francisco; Northern California Kaiser Permanente, San Francisco, CA)
J Pediatr 158:562-565, 2011

Objective.—To examine the clinical significance of elevated conjugated bilirubin (CB) levels in newborns.

Study Design.—This retrospective study evaluated a birth cohort of 271 186 full-term newborns born within a Northern California hospital network from 1995 to 2004. All CB and direct bilirubin (DB) levels were available in a database and were correlated with the patients' inpatient and outpatient *International Classification of Diseases, 9th Revision* diagnoses.

Results.—The 99th percentile for CB is 0.5 mg/dL, and the 99th percentile for DB is 2.1 mg/dL. CB levels between 0.5 and 1.9 mg/dL can be associated with infection, but most often remain unexplained. Liver and biliary disease become increasingly likely as CB levels increase; for CB ≥5 mg/dL, 47% of newborns have biliary disease and 43% have liver disease.

Conclusions.—CB and DB levels are not interchangeable. In newborns with CB levels ≥0.5 mg/dL and <2 mg/dL, infection must be ruled out, and the newborn should be observed. In newborns with levels ≥2 mg/dL, a more in-depth assessment of the hepatobiliary system is indicated.

▶ In this study, the investigators used the large database available in the Northern California Kaiser Permanente Medical Care Program to evaluate the difference between the measurement of conjugated bilirubin (CB), as measured by the Vitros instrument, and direct bilirubin (DB), using the diazo method. They then looked at the association of different disease states with elevations of CB and DB.

Although frequently used interchangeably in the literature, CB and DB are not the same. CB is the product of the conjugation of unconjugated bilirubin with glucuronic acid and, when measured with the Vitros technique,[1] only CB is measured. The measurement of DB includes the measurement of delta bilirubin—the component of conjugated bilirubin that is covalently bound to albumin—but in the neonate, delta bilirubin is generally present in negligible amounts and does not affect DB measurement. What does affect the measurement of DB, however, is the total serum bilirubin (TSB) level. With increasing TSB levels, DB measurements become spuriously elevated. This occurs because some of the unconjugated bilirubin also reacts with the diazo reagent, without the addition of the accelerant normally required for the measurement of indirect reacting (unconjugated) bilirubin. As a result, DB measurements tend to overestimate the concentrations of CB.

The differences between the maximum CB and DB found in the first 2 weeks of life in the populations studied were striking: 81.2% of infants had a CB of ≤0.1 mg/dL, whereas only 0.16% had a DB of that level; 99.7% of CB measurements were ≤2.0 mg/dL compared with 98.6% of DB. We measured TSB and DB values in our nursery in 610 infants prior to discharge from the well-baby nursery.[2] In our population, the 95th percentile for DB was 1.0 mg/dL and for the 99th percentile, DB was 1.3 mg/dL. There was a significant correlation between TSB and DB ($r = 0.22$, $P = .003$), confirming the effect of increasing TSB levels on DB.

The Vitros technique is now widely used and has a small coefficient of variation (CV) at low CB levels (CV 6.5% at a CB of 1.4 mg/dL).[1] Nevertheless, unlike with TSB levels, I am unaware of any data comparing interlaboratory CB levels with the Vitros technique, so we do not know the CV between different laboratories as we do for the TSB.[3]

It is clear from the study of Davis et al that CB and DB measurements cannot be used interchangeably and this is particularly the case with levels < 2 mg/dL. On the other hand, 96% of infants whose CB levels were between 0.5 and 1.9 mg/dL had no diagnosis associated with this finding. Although 2% with CB 0.5 to 1.9 mg/dL were diagnosed with severe bacterial infection, one would expect such infants to look sick in addition to having a slightly elevated CB. When the CB was < 2 mg/dL, the risk of severe bacterial infection, gastrointestinal abnormality, or liver disease increased significantly and there was a direct relationship between increasing CB levels and the likelihood of a significant pathological diagnosis being made.

What this study shows, and our experience confirms, is that although slightly elevated levels of DB or CB are not rare in the neonatal period, the vast majority of such elevated levels are not associated with any significant disease state. When faced with a slightly elevated DB in an otherwise well-looking infant, our practice is to repeat the value in a week. In most infants, the DB will return to normal. In those in whom this does not occur, we need to consider the diagnoses listed by Davis et al and do the appropriate investigations. For those institutions that use the Vitros technique, infants with CB levels between 0.5 and 2.0 mg/dL should be evaluated for the possibility of severe bacterial infection. For levels < 2 mg/dL, additional investigations are needed.

Normative data for CB and DB are hard to find, and these investigators have performed a valuable service by telling us when we need to worry and when we can wait.

M. J. Maisels, MB, BCh, DSc

References

1. Wu TW, Dappen GM, Spayd RW, Sundberg MW, Powers DM. The Ektachem clinical chemistry slide for simultaneous determination of unconjugated and sugar-conjugated bilirubin. *Clin Chem.* 1984;30:1304-1309.
2. Maisels MJ, Kring EA. Should we measure direct bilirubin (DB) levels on all infants of the nursery? E-PAS. 618441.6. 2007.
3. Lo SF, Jendrzejczak BA, Doumas BT; College of American Pathologists. Laboratory performance in neonatal bilirubin testing using commutable specimens: a progress report on a College of American Pathologists study. *Arch Pathol Lab Med.* 2008;132:1781-1785.

Intravenous Immunoglobulin in Neonates With Rhesus Hemolytic Disease: A Randomized Controlled Trial

Smits-Wintjens VEHJ, Walther FJ, Rath MEA, et al (Leiden Univ Med Ctr, Netherlands; et al)
Pediatrics 127:680-686, 2011

Background.—Despite limited data, international guidelines recommend the use of intravenous immunoglobulin (IVIg) in neonates with rhesus hemolytic disease.

Objective.—We tested whether prophylactic use of IVIg reduces the need for exchange transfusions in neonates with rhesus hemolytic disease.

Design and Setting.—We performed a randomized, double-blind, placebo-controlled trial in neonates with rhesus hemolytic disease. After stratification for treatment with intrauterine transfusion, neonates were randomly assigned for IVIg (0.75 g/kg) or placebo (5% glucose). The primary outcome was the rate of exchange transfusions. Secondary outcomes were duration of phototherapy, maximum bilirubin levels, and the need of top-up red-cell transfusions.

Results.—Eighty infants were included in the study, 53 of whom (66%) were treated with intrauterine transfusion(s). There was no difference in the rate of exchange transfusions between the IVIg and placebo groups (7 of 41 [17%] vs 6 of 39 [15%]; $P = .99$) and in the number of exchange transfusions per patient (median [range]: 0 [0–2] vs 0 [0–2]; $P = .90$) or in duration of phototherapy (4.7 [1.8] vs 5.1 [2.1] days; $P = .34$), maximum bilirubin levels (14.8 [4.7] vs 14.1 [4.9] mg/dL; $P = .52$), and proportion of neonates who required top-up red-cell transfusions (34 of 41 [83%] vs 34 of 39 [87%]; $P = .76$).

Conclusions.—Prophylactic IVIg does not reduce the need for exchange transfusion or the rates of other adverse neonatal outcomes. Our findings do not support the use of IVIg in neonates with rhesus hemolytic disease.

► On the basis of randomized or quasi-randomized controlled trials as well as observational studies in the 1990s,[1-4] many neonatologists have been using intravenous immunoglobulin (IVIG) in the management of neonatal hemolytic disease for a decade or more. Thus, the results of this study will come as a surprise.

As noted by the investigators, a review by the Cochrane Collaboration of the 3 previously published randomized controlled trials that met the criteria for inclusion concluded that none of these studies was of high quality and that "further well designed studies are needed before routine use of intravenous immunoglobulin can be recommended for the treatment of isoimmune haemolytic jaundice."[5] When one examines these data carefully, it is true that these studies did not meet the highest standards of randomized controlled trials.[5] Nevertheless, the effect size was dramatic. In the groups who received IVIG plus phototherapy, only 14 of 96 (15%) infants required an exchange transfusion compared with 48 of 93 (52%) of those who received phototherapy alone, a relative risk (RR) of 0.28, 95% confidence interval (CI) 0.17 to 0.47, $P < .00001$.[1-3,5] However, these studies were not explicit in describing how they used phototherapy; they did not use placebos, and they were not adequately blinded. Some studies included infants with Rh disease as well as ABO incompatibility,[2,6,7] which is known to cause less severe hemolysis than Rh disease, and this could be one reason IVIG might not work as well in Rh disease as it does in ABO isoimmunization. Hammerman et al[7] investigated this question by measuring corrected carboxyhemoglobin (COHbc) levels in neonates with ABO isoimmunization. These infants received IVIG if, despite phototherapy, the serum bilirubin level reached 13 mg/dL by age 24 hours or 16 mg/dL after 24 hours. They classified their infants according to the response to IVIG as "responders" or "nonresponders." The responders were those in whom the total serum bilirubin (TSB) levels either remained stable or decreased following IVIG administration, and the nonresponders were those whose TSBs increased by 2 mg/dL within 24 hours after IVIG administration. Four of 5 nonresponders required exchange transfusions, but 0 of 18 of the responders did ($P < .001$). The hemoglobin levels were lower and the COHbc levels higher in the nonresponders, indicating that they were suffering from more severe hemolytic disease. This suggests that the severity of hemolysis is a determining element in the response of these infants to IVIG.

In their systematic review of randomized and quasi-randomized control trials of IVIG and phototherapy compared with phototherapy alone in neonates with both Rh and/or ABO incompatibility, Gottstein and Cooke concluded that high-dose IVIG reduced the risk of exchange transfusion by 72% (RR = 0.28, 95% CI 0.17-0.47).[8] Based on these observations, the number needed to treat with IVIG to prevent 1 exchange transfusion was only 2.7 (95% CI 2.0-3.8).

The incidence of complications related to high-dose IVIG has been low but includes pyrogenic reactions, volume overload, and hypoglycemia. In the studies reviewed,[1-4] none of these side effects were observed in any of the infants. A recent Spanish study suggested that there was an association between the use of IVIG and necrotizing enterocolitis (NEC).[9] In this retrospective analysis, 167 infants received IVIG for the treatment of Rh or ABO hemolytic disease and 10 (6%) developed NEC. The gestational age of these infants was 37 to 39 weeks, not a group that is normally associated with NEC. In this population, NEC is most likely the result of intestinal hypoxia-ischemia as a result of thrombosis rather than infection. Deep vein thrombosis has been associated with the use of IVIG in adults.[10] In a letter in response to this,

Hansen[11] noted that they had used IVIG in almost 200 infants over a period of 10 years at their institution in Oslo and had not had a single case of NEC. He questioned whether the IVIG preparation used in the study might be responsible for this complication.

Most recently, Huizing et al[12] conducted a review of their experience with IVIG in 176 infants with both Rh and ABO incompatibility over 2 time periods: 1993 to 1998 and 1999 to 2003. Before using IVIG, 49% of these infants were exchanged vs 12% following the use of IVIG (odds ratio 0.11, 95% CI 0.046-0.26).

What should we do with this information? The historical data and several randomized and quasi-randomized trials, plus observational studies, support the benefits of IVIG in preventing the need for exchange transfusion in infants who have not responded adequately to phototherapy. One of the intangibles in all of these studies is how phototherapy was used, something that could affect the outcomes. The observations of Hammerman et al[7] are also intriguing and suggest that perhaps it is the infants with severe hemolysis who are less likely to respond to IVIG. If this is the case, however, one would expect that infants with less severe hemolysis should respond to phototherapy and be less likely to need an exchange transfusion. In the Western world, severe Rh disease is now uncommon. With effective use of phototherapy and the prevention of Rh disease, exchange transfusions have become a rarity in most neonatal intensive care units. Eventually, the need for IVIG use should become equally rare.

M. J. Maisels, MB, BCh, DSc

References

1. Rübo J, Albrecht K, Lasch P, et al. High-dose intravenous immune globulin therapy for hyperbilirubinemia caused by Rh hemolytic disease. *J Pediatr.* 1992;121:93-97.
2. Alpay F, Sarici S, Okutan V, Erdem G, Ozcan O, Gökçay E. High-dose intravenous immunoglobulin therapy in neonatal immune haemolytic jaundice. *Acta Paediatr.* 1999;88:216-219.
3. Dağoğlu T, Ovali F, Samanci N, Bengisu E. High-dose intravenous immunoglobulin therapy for rhesus haemolytic disease. *J Int Med Res.* 1995;23:264-271.
4. Voto LS, Sexer H, Ferreiro G, et al. Neonatal administration of high-dose intravenous immunoglobulin in rhesus hemolytic disease. *J Perinat Med.* 1995;23:443-451.
5. Alcock GS, Liley H. Immunoglobulin infusion for isoimmune haemolytic jaundice in neonates. *Cochrane Database Syst Rev.* 2002;(3). CD003313.
6. Miqdad AM, Abdelbasit OB, Shaheed MM, Seidahmed MZ, Abomelha AM, Arcala OP. Intravenous immunoglobulin G (IVIG) therapy for significant hyperbilirubinemia in ABO hemolytic disease of the newborn. *J Matern Fetal Neonatal Med.* 2004;16:163-166.
7. Hammerman C, Kaplan M, Vreman HJ, Stevenson DK. Intravenous immune globulin in neonatal ABO isoimmunization: factors associated with clinical efficacy. *Biol Neonate.* 1996;70:69-74.
8. Gottstein R, Cooke R. Systematic review of intravenous immunoglobulin in haemolytic disease of the newborn. *Arch Dis Child Fetal Neonatal Ed.* 2003;88:F6-F10.
9. Figueras-Aloy J, Rodríguez-Miguélez JM, Iriondo-Sanz M, Salvia-Roiges MD, Botet-Mussons F, Carbonell-Estrany X. Intravenous immunoglobulin and necrotizing enterocolitis in newborns with hemolytic disease. *Pediatrics.* 2010;125:139-144.

10. Go RS, Call TG. Deep venous thrombosis of the arm after intravenous immunoglobulin infusion: case report and literature review of intravenous immunoglobulin-related thrombotic complications. *Mayo Clin Proc.* 2000;75:83-85.
11. Hansen TWR. Necrotizing enterocolitis and IVIG. *Pediatrics.* 2010, www.pediatrics.org. 2010.
12. Huizing KMN, Røislien J, Hansen TWR. Intravenous immune globulin reduces the need for exchange transfusions in rhesus and AB0 incompatibility. *Acta Paediatr.* 2008;97:1362-1365.

Intravenous Immunoglobulin in Neonates With Rhesus Hemolytic Disease: A Randomized Controlled Trial

Smits-Wintjens VEHJ, Walther FJ, Rath MEA, et al (Leiden Univ Med Ctr, Netherlands; et al)
Pediatrics 127:680-686, 2011

Background.—Despite limited data, international guidelines recommend the use of intravenous immunoglobulin (IVIg) in neonates with rhesus hemolytic disease.

Objective.—We tested whether prophylactic use of IVIg reduces the need for exchange transfusions in neonates with rhesus hemolytic disease.

Design and Setting.—We performed a randomized, double-blind, placebo-controlled trial in neonates with rhesus hemolytic disease. After stratification for treatment with intrauterine transfusion, neonates were randomly assigned for IVIg (0.75 g/kg) or placebo (5% glucose). The primary outcome was the rate of exchange transfusions. Secondary outcomes were duration of phototherapy, maximum bilirubin levels, and the need of top-up red-cell transfusions.

Results.—Eighty infants were included in the study, 53 of whom (66%) were treated with intrauterine transfusion(s). There was no difference in the rate of exchange transfusions between the IVIg and placebo groups (7 of 41 [17%] vs 6 of 39 [15%]; $P = .99$) and in the number of exchange transfusions per patient (median [range]: 0 [0−2] vs 0 [0−2]; $P = .90$) or in duration of phototherapy (4.7 [1.8] vs 5.1 [2.1] days; $P = .34$), maximum bilirubin levels (14.8 [4.7] vs 14.1 [4.9] mg/dL; $P = .52$), and proportion of neonates who required top-up red-cell transfusions (34 of 41 [83%] vs 34 of 39 [87%]; $P = .76$).

Conclusions.—Prophylactic IVIg does not reduce the need for exchange transfusion or the rates of other adverse neonatal outcomes. Our findings do not support the use of IVIg in neonates with rhesus hemolytic disease.

▶ Administration of intravenous immunoglobulin (IVIG) for prevention of exchange transfusion in infants with rhesus (Rh) isoimmunization has long been considered an efficacious practice. The American Academy of Pediatrics (AAP) recommends the use of IVIG for neonates with isoimmune hemolytic disease and a total serum bilirubin within 2 to 3 mg/dL of the exchange threshold, despite the lack of studies that demonstrate efficacy in the context of current prenatal intrauterine transfusion and intensive phototherapy practices.

This double-blind, randomized controlled trial of 80 infants with Rh isoimmunization found that with early white light phototherapy (12—20 µw/cm²/nm, started immediately after birth), there was no significant difference in the number of neonates requiring exchange transfusions (17% in the IVIG group vs 15% in the control group) or the number of exchange transfusions performed per neonate. These conclusions extended to subgroup analyses performed on the infants with a history of prenatal intrauterine transfusions, as well as those without. Notably, the study was powered based on an expected exchange transfusion rate of 30% in the control group, almost double what was found, and 6% in the treatment group. Although it therefore remains possible that a significant difference was not detected because of insufficient statistical power, the very similar rates of exchange transfusion make that unlikely. The lower than expected prevalence of exchange transfusion is likely a result of aggressive early phototherapy, although the type of light was not as intense, nor of the blue-green spectrum that is currently recommended by the AAP. Overall, however, the investigators should be applauded for a well-designed trial that is reflective of the current prenatal and postnatal interventions. These results rightly call into question a long-held empiric practice. Practitioners should be circumspect about the efficacy of IVIG in neonates with Rh isoimmunization in light of this relevant, high-quality evidence.

A. K. Rajani, MD

Postponing or eliminating red blood cell transfusions of very low birth weight neonates by obtaining all baseline laboratory blood tests from otherwise discarded fetal blood in the placenta
Christensen RD, Lambert DK, Baer VL, et al (Intermountain Healthcare, Salt Lake City, UT; McKay-Dee Hosp Ctr, Ogden, UT; Univ of Utah School of Medicine, Salt Lake City; et al)
Transfusion 51:253-258, 2011

Background.—Safely reducing the proportion of very low birth weight neonates (<1500 g) that receive a red blood cell (RBC) transfusion would be an advance in transfusion practice.

Study Design and Methods.—We performed a prospective, single-centered, case-control, feasibility analysis, preparatory to designing a definitive trial. Specifically, we sought to determine whether we could obtain all baseline neonatal intensive care unit blood tests from the placenta, after placental delivery, thereby initially drawing no blood from the neonate.

Results.—Ten cases where all baseline blood tests were drawn from the placenta, and 10 controls where all tests were drawn from the neonate, were closely matched for birth weight, gestational age, sex, and race. Early cord clamping was used for all 20. Over the first 18 hours the hemoglobin increased in nine cases versus two controls (p = 0.005). During the first 72 hours one case versus five controls qualified for and received an RBC transfusion. In the first week the cases received four transfusions and the controls received 16 (p = 0.02). None of the cases had an intraventricular hemorrhage (IVH) but four of the controls had a Grade 1 and two had a Grade 3 (p = 0.01).

Conclusion.—We speculate that this method is feasible and generally postpones the first RBC transfusion until beyond the period of peak vulnerability to IVH.

▶ The frequency of intraventricular hemorrhage (IVH) has remained static for more than a decade, particularly among extremely preterm infants. This pilot study adds to the emerging body of evidence suggesting that a contributing factor may be an inadequate circulating blood volume at birth or shortly thereafter. None of the babies who had their initial baseline tests done with blood obtained from the placenta had an IVH compared with 40% who had baseline tests done on blood drawn through an umbilical line after admission to the newborn intensive care unit. As noted by the authors, the amount of blood withdrawn for these initial tests can equal 10% of the calculated blood volume for extremely low birth weight infants. The deficit can be as high as 20%, at least temporarily, if the sample is drawn through an umbilical catheter, because excess blood is withdrawn to clear the catheter of intravenous fluid.

Another clinical practice that is associated with depletion of circulating blood volume is early cord clamping. In a recently published meta-analysis,[1] the benefit of delayed cord clamping in preterm infants consisted of better blood pressure and less need for inotropic support during the first 24 hours after birth. Other benefits included reduced number of blood transfusions ($P = .0004$); despite that fact, no significant difference was found in hematocrit in the first 24 hours. There was no significant difference in infant deaths; however, a significant difference in the incidence of IVH was reported ($P = .002$).

Could it be that a large proportion of IVH is iatrogenic? Randomized clinical trials of delayed cord clamping, or the use of placental blood for initial baseline tests, or a combination of both practices might answer this question. However, there may be insufficient equipoise regarding delayed cord clamping since the American College of Obstetricians and Gynecologists Committee on Obstetric Practice is in the process of developing a technical bulletin encouraging delayed cord clamping for preterm infants.

L. A. Papile, MD

Reference

1. Rabe H, Reynolds G, Diaz-Rossello J. A systematic review and meta-analysis of a brief delay in clamping the umbilical cord of preterm infants. *Neonatology.* 2008;93:138-144.

9 Infectious Disease and Immunology

A Pilot Study to Determine the Safety and Feasibility of Oropharyngeal Administration of Own Mother's Colostrum to Extremely Low-Birth-Weight Infants
Rodriguez NA, Meier PP, Groer MW, et al (NorthShore Univ HealthSystem, Chicago, IL; Rush Univ College of Nursing, Chicago, IL; Univ of South Florida, Tampa, FL)
Adv Neonatal Care 10:206-212, 2010

Own mother's colostrum is rich in cytokines and other immune agents that may stimulate oropharyngeal-associated lymphoid tissue if administered oropharyngeally to extremely low-birth-weight (ELBW) infants during the first days of life when enteral feeding is contraindicated. However, the safety and feasibility of the oropharyngeal route for the administration of colostrum have not been determined.

Purpose.—To determine the safety of oropharyngeal administration of own mother's colostrum to ELBW infants in first days of life. A secondary purpose was to investigate the feasibility of (1) delivering this intervention to ELBW infants in the first days of life and (2) measuring concentrations of secretory immunoglobulin A and lactoferrin in tracheal aspirate secretions and urine of these infants.

Subjects.—Five ELBW infants (mean birth weight and gestational age = 657 g and 25.5 weeks, respectively).

Design.—Quasi-experimental, 1 group, pretest-posttest design.

Methods.—Subjects received 0.2 mL of own mother's colostrum administered oropharyngeally every 2 hours for 48 consecutive hours, beginning at 48 hours of life. Concentrations of secretory immunoglobulin A and lactoferrin were measured in tracheal aspirates and urine of each subject at baseline, at the completion of the intervention and again 2 weeks later.

Results.—All infants completed the entire treatment protocol, each receiving 24 treatments. A total of 15 urine specimens were collected and 14 were sufficient in volume for analysis. A total of 15 tracheal aspirates were collected, but only 7 specimens (47%) were sufficient in volume for analysis. There was wide variation in concentrations of secretory immunoglobulin A and lactoferrin in urine and tracheal aspirates among the 5 infants; however, several results were outside the limits of assay detection. All infants began to suck on the endotracheal tube during the administration of colostrum drops. Oxygen saturation measures remained stable or increased slightly during each of the treatment sessions. There were no episodes of apnea, bradycardia, hypotension, or other adverse effects associated with the administration of colostrum.

Conclusions.—Oropharyngeal administration of own mother's colostrum is easy, inexpensive, and well-tolerated by even the smallest and sickest ELBW infants. Future research should continue to examine the optimal procedure for measuring the direct immune effects of this therapy, as well as the clinical outcomes such as infections, particularly ventilator-associated pneumonia.

▶ Over the past several years, there has been increasing attention paid to decreasing the frequency of nosocomial infection, especially among extremely low birth weight (ELBW) infants. The main focus for preventing nosocomial infection has been reducing the exposure of these immunologically compromised infants to potential pathogens. As previously suggested by the authors, a complementary strategy might be to give colostrum, a biologic fluid that is rich in protective immune factors, via the oropharyngeal route, a strategy that has been shown to be effective for the delivery of immunotherapy in adults unable to tolerate parenteral administration.

In the previous pilot study, the authors evaluated the safety and feasibility of administering own mother's colostrum to ELBW infants shortly after birth. ELBW infants were eligible for enrollment in the study as long as they were not receiving vasopressor medications more than 10 mcg/kg/min. A total of 4.8 mL of colostrum was needed to complete the study protocol; however, treatment was initiated when a minimum of 2.4 mL of colostrum was available. Colostrum was delivered using a needle-less tuberculin syringe. Approximately 0.1 mL of colostrum was delivered to the right and left buccal mucosa with the tip directed posteriorly toward the oropharynx every 2 hours for 48 hours. Vital signs were monitored throughout the treatment protocol. Concentrations of lactoferrin and secretory immunoglobulin A in tracheal aspirates and urine were used as markers of immune response.

There were no adverse effects associated with the administration of colostrum. An observation of interest was that even the sickest infants were noted to suck on the endotracheal tube when receiving colostrum, an activity that was interpreted by mothers as their infants tasting the colostrum.

The data regarding immune response are inconclusive, in part because there are no reference values for immune markers in ELBW infants in the first few days after birth. As a surrogate, it would have been helpful if the authors had reported the frequency of nosocomial infection in the study group. Nonetheless, the pilot study showed that giving colostrum early is easy, inexpensive, and well tolerated by acutely ill ELBW infants.

L. A. Papile, MD

Antibiotic weight-watching: slimming down on antibiotic use in a NICU
Liem TY, van den Hoogen A, Rademaker CMA, et al (Univ Med Centre Utrecht, The Netherlands)
Acta Paediatr 99:1900-1902, 2010

Background.—Units such as the neonatal intensive care unit (NICU) use antibiotics extensively and face the accompanying challenge of avoiding antibiotic-resistant infections. In NICU patients the symptoms of infection are aspecific, immune defenses are immature, and multitudes of risk factors for infection accompany the invasive treatment procedures often needed for preterm infants. It is difficult to rule out infection in these infants, so the use of antimicrobial agents is widespread. Multidrug-resistant infections can have a major impact on morbidity, mortality, and healthcare costs, so it is important to develop a policy of restricted and appropriate antibiotic use. Multidisciplinary infectious disease teams (IDTs) have been established to help cope with the problem of overtreatment.

Methods.—The evaluation process followed in the authors' NICU included daily discussions with the IDT concerning all cases of infection and policies for antibiotic treatment. These are incorporated into the routine care regimen. The IDT consists of a pediatric infectious disease specialist, a medical microbiologist, and neonatologists interested in neonatal infectious disease. Participants in the discussions include the IDT, neonatologists, fellows, and registrars. All cases of suspected or proven infection are reviewed systematically to monitor the accuracy of the antimicrobial therapy being used and determine how long it should be continued.

Results.—The antibiotic use in the authors' institution was evaluated from 1990 to the present, revealing that 85% to 90% of all infants admitted to the NICU received antibiotic treatment for suspected infection or risk factors, with few treated for proven sepsis. Total antimicrobial use was expressed as mean days of therapy (DOT). It declined significantly, from 9.0 to 5.8, even though a high proportion of the infants received antimicrobial treatment. The clinical and demographic characteristics of infants admitted to the NICU showed no significant change. The greatest change was a decline in the mean DOT of antimicrobials (specifically, amoxicillin-clavulanic acid and gentamicin) used for suspected early-onset sepsis and risk for infection after birth, but a decline was also noted for the use of first-generation cephalosporins (specifically, cefazolin). Vancomycin use showed no specific trend, but its DOT was only 0.1 to 1 days. No increased incidence of infection or higher mortality resulted; in fact, the mortality declined from 17% to 9%. No evidence of increasing antibiotic resistance of the four most often identified causative microorganisms was found. Because the DOT for sepsis treatment is dictated by protocol to be 7 to 14 days, the decrease in duration of treatment was the result of fewer days of treatment for cases of suspected but unproven infection and risk factor prophylaxis.

Conclusions.—It remains challenging to identify infants with infections and restrict further the use of antimicrobial therapy to avoid resistant

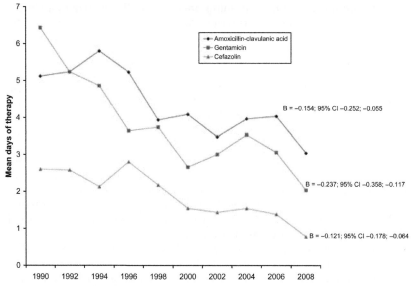

FIGURE 2.—Duration of treatment with the most frequently used antimicrobial agents in the neonatal intensive care units, expressed as mean number of days of treatment for each admitted infant (1990–2008). (Reprinted from Liem TY, van den Hoogen A, Rademaker CMA, et al. Antibiotic weight-watching: slimming down on antibiotic use in a NICU. *Acta Paediatr.* 2010;99:1900-1902. Reprinted with permission of John Wiley & Sons, Inc.)

disease strains. The current best practice is to stop giving antibiotics in cases where infection can be ruled out. The multidisciplinary IDT can help in forming guidelines and making decisions in this area (Fig 2).

▶ This short communication underlines what many neonatologists already know but find a difficult challenge to surmount: our overuse of antibiotics in the neonatal intensive care unit (NICU). This study shows no change in the percentage of babies treated with antibiotics in an NICU in Utrecht since the early 1990s. The percentage treated was 85% to 90%, but with only a 15% to 18% incidence of infection. However, after the institution of antibiotic stewardship with an infectious disease team that met weekly to review cases of all patients with suspected or proven infection and discuss duration of treatment, the duration of treatment with amoxicillin-clavulanic acid and gentamicin dropped by approximately 50% (Fig 2).

In the United States, ampicillin and gentamicin are by far the most commonly used drugs in the NICU, with a 2- to 3-fold increase in the use of iron and multivitamins.[1] The use of antibiotics shortly after birth in most very low birth weight infants is based on several factors, very few of which have a strong scientific foundation that prove a need. These include the presumption that premature labor is caused by infection, the difficulty of discerning respiratory distress syndrome caused by surfactant deficiency from bacterial pneumonia, and the immaturity of the neonatal immune system. The emergence of resistant microorganisms is certainly a concern, as raised in this article, but more recently, other concerns, such as altering the microbial ecology of the gastrointestinal tract and thereby increasing the likelihood of necrotizing enterocolitis[2,3] are also being recognized.

The antibiotic stewardship approach as mentioned in this article appeared to be successful in decreasing the length of time babies remained on antibiotics (without increasing morbidity or mortality), but did not have an effect on the percentage of babies treated. A similar approach involves simply not routinely treating on a knee jerk and carefully evaluating risk factors before beginning or continuing treatment. As stated in the article, better diagnostic factors are needed that could be used at the bedside. This is certainly attainable with some of the "omic" technologies.

A question that we need to ask and answer is whether we have lost all equipoise to do a prospective randomized study that involves one group that is given antibiotics using our usual approach versus not giving routine antibiotics in the first several days after birth in very low birthweight infants. If not, such a study would require courage and a very careful design, but it should be done.

J. Neu, MD

References

1. Clark RH, Bloom BT, Spitzer AR, Gerstmann DR. Reported medication use in the neonatal intensive care unit: data from a large national data set. *Pediatrics*. 2006; 117:1979-1987.
2. Wang Y, Hoenig JD, Malin KJ, et al. 16S rRNA gene-based analysis of fecal microbiota from preterm infants with and without necrotizing enterocolitis. *ISME J*. 2009;3:944-954.
3. Cotten CM, Taylor S, Stoll B, et al. NICHD Neonatal Research Network. Prolonged duration of initial empirical antibiotic treatment is associated with increased rates of necrotizing enterocolitis and death for extremely low birth weight infants. *Pediatrics*. 2009;123:58-66.

Clinical signs and CRP values associated with blood culture results in neonates evaluated for suspected sepsis

Ohlin A, Björkqvist M, Montgomery SM, et al (Örebro Univ Hosp, Sweden; Örebro Univ, Sweden)
Acta Paediatr 99:1635-1640, 2010

Aim.—To identify which clinical signs at presentation are most predictive of sepsis subsequently confirmed by blood culture and to investigate whether the predictive power of the clinical signs varies by gestational age.

Methods.—Among 401 newborn infants <28 days of age with suspected sepsis, nine signs of sepsis and C-reactive protein (CRP) values were prospectively recorded. Logistic regression assessed the association of these signs and laboratory values with a subsequently confirmed diagnosis of sepsis by positive blood culture. The analysis was stratified by gestational age with mutual simultaneous adjustment for the signs and sex.

Results.—Five of the nine clinical signs (feeding intolerance, distended abdomen, blood pressure, bradycardia and apnoea), along with CRP were statistically significantly associated with a positive blood culture. After simultaneous adjustment for all of the signs, apnoea, hypotension and CRP were independently predictive of positive blood culture. When the material was stratified by gestational age, differences in the association with positive blood culture were found for bradycardia, tachypnea and irritability/seizures.

Conclusion.—In this selected population of infants with suspected sepsis, apnoea and hypotension are independently predictive of a confirmed diagnosis, while bradycardia is more predictive among preterm infants and tachypnea among term infants.

▶ This report from a single regional neonatal intensive care unit (NICU) updates and adds to the extensive literature relating clinical signs of illness in newborn infants to the probability of culture-proven bacteremia. Multivariate analysis of prospectively collected data from infants in the NICU demonstrated significant associations between bacteremia and apnea, hypotension, and an initial serum C-reactive protein (CRP) level >10 mg/L. Bradycardia, feeding intolerance, or distended abdomen correlated with sepsis only in univariate analyses; tachypnea, increased oxygen requirement, irritability or seizures, and patent ductus arteriosus were not predictive of sepsis. Bradycardia appeared to be a sign of sepsis in preterm but not in full-term infants, and tachypnea seemed to be a weak sign for sepsis in full-term infants, but was clearly not useful among preterm infants. The implications of this report are limited by commingling cases of early and late-onset sepsis, which appear to be distinct entities in this population (as in previous reports), since only 10% of the infants evaluated at <48 hours of age were bacteremic, but 43% of older infants were bacteremic. The authors correctly emphasize that the reported odds ratios for each clinical finding are strongly dependent on the nature of the reference group: in this instance, infants with at least one of the selected clinical signs, several of which turned out not to be predictive of sepsis. It is essential to recognize that elimination of those signs as potential predictors of sepsis would skew the odds ratios for other findings. This phenomenon may account for the apparent high sensitivity (93%) of the initial CRP level in this report, which exceeds that in most prior studies, in which the criteria for evaluation may have been much less constrained. Collectively, these observations suggest that pattern recognition algorithms for detection of neonatal infections by computerized expert systems will likely need to be stratified by both gestational and postnatal age. The search for an effective diagnostic tool for neonatal sepsis is not over.

W. E. Benitz, MD

Congenital and neonatal varicella: impact of the national varicella vaccination programme in Australia
Khandaker G, Marshall H, Peadon E, et al (Children's Hosp at Westmead and Univ of Sydney, New South Wales, Australia; Women's and Children's Hosp and Univ of Adelaide, South Australia, Australia; Univ of Sydney, New South Wales, Australia; et al)
Arch Dis Child 96:453-456, 2011

Objective.—Routine varicella zoster vaccination for children aged 18 months began in Australia from November 2005. The aim of this study was to compare the current incidence and outcomes of congenital and neonatal varicella in Australia with similarly collected data from 1995 to 1997.

Methods.—Active national prospective surveillance was carried out for congenital and neonatal varicella using the Australian Paediatric Surveillance Unit (APSU) for 3.5 years from June 2006. Around 1300 clinicians reported monthly according to predefined case criteria.

Results.—During the study period the mean monthly return rate of APSU report cards was 93.7%. Two cases of congenital varicella (0.19 per 100 000 live births per annum) and 16 cases of neonatal varicella (2.0 per 100 000 live births per annum) were identified. During 2008 and 2009 no cases of congenital varicella were reported; neonatal varicella rates declined to 0.7 per 100 000 live births per annum, a significant trend (p=0.005) and a reduction of over 85% compared with rates during 1995–1997 (the prevaccination era) and the first year of the current surveillance study. Eleven of 16 neonatal cases followed prenatal maternal infection; seven of the 11 infections were acquired from children, four of whom were living in the same household. Ten (62.5%) infants with neonatal varicella were admitted to hospital, one of whom developed varicella pneumonitis requiring ventilatory support, but none died. Only one infecting contact had been vaccinated.

Conclusions.—There has been an apparent reduction of congenital varicella and a significant reduction of neonatal varicella in Australia following the introduction of universal varicella vaccination in 2005.

▶ Neonatologists spend a lot of time discussing the so-called TORCH syndrome but pay little attention to congenital and neonatal varicella because it is so rare. The rewards of universal immunization are highlighted in this report from Khandaker et al. The congenital varicella syndrome (CVS) was first reported in 1947.[1] In 1994, Enders et al[2] added a considerable number of cases to the sparse literature on the topic. They studied 1373 women who had varicella and 366 who had herpes zoster during the first 36 weeks of gestation. They speculated that the incidence of CVS per 100 000 births could be estimated from the incidence of varicella in pregnancy and the risk of CVS according to the gestational stage observed in their joint prospective study in Germany and the United Kingdom between 1980 and 1993. From UK surveillance data, they estimated that the incidence of varicella in pregnancy is 3 per

1000, giving an incidence of CVS of approximately 1.6 per 100 000 births in England and Wales. They further speculated that a vaccine would significantly decrease the burden of disease. This has indeed come to pass.

In the report from Australia, Khandaker et al report that the incidence of CVS was 0.8/100 000 births prior to the introduction of the vaccine and 0.19 after the introduction of the vaccine, a very satisfactory reduction. For their purposes, CVS was defined as any termination, stillbirth, newborn infant, or child up to the age of 2 years with definite or suspected CVS, with or without defects, who met at least 1 of the following criteria:

1 Cicatricial skin lesions in a dermatomal distribution and/or poxlike skin scars and/or limb hypoplasia
2 Development of herpes zoster in the first year of life

Cases that did not come to a pediatrician's attention (eg, those ending in therapeutic abortion) are not routinely reported and could not be included in this study. Neonatal varicella was defined as any infant with neonatal varicella based on history, clinical findings, or laboratory findings (eg, culture, polymerase chain reaction, immunoglobulin M, or immunofluorescence positive or seroconversion) in the first month of life but without features of CVS. Also, the estimated incidence of neonatal varicella, 2.05 per 100 000 live births per year, was significantly lower ($P = .00002$) during this study period compared with the incidence reported in 1995 to 1997 of 5.8 per 100 000 live births per year prior to universal immunization.

Remember that in addition to the skin and limb abnormalities, the brain and eye may be targeted in CVS. Brain anomalies include cortical atrophy, ventriculomegaly, microcephaly, and involvement of the autonomic nervous system resulting in bowel and bladder dysfunction. The eye pathology ranges from cataracts to microphthalmia, chorioretinitis, and optic atrophy.

In summary, congenital and neonatal varicella infections are associated with significant morbidity and mortality. Universal varicella vaccination is associated with reductions in the incidence of both congenital and neonatal varicella. Vigilant clinicians using antivirals and zoster immune globulin can prevent the serious morbidity associated with neonatal varicella.

A. A. Fanaroff, MD, FRCPE, FRCP&CH

References

1. Laforet EG, Lynch CL Jr. Multiple congenital defects following maternal varicella: report of a case. *N Engl J Med.* 1947;236:534-537.
2. Enders G, Miller E, Cradock-Watson J, Bolley I, Ridehalgh M. Consequences of varicella and herpes zoster in pregnancy: prospective study of 1739 cases. *Lancet.* 1994;343:1548-1551.

Early Onset Neonatal Sepsis: The Burden of Group B Streptococcal and E. coli Disease Continues

Stoll BJ, for the Eunice Kennedy Shriver National Institute of Child Health and Human Development Neonatal Research Network (Emory Univ School of Medicine, Atlanta, GA; et al)
Pediatrics 127:817-826, 2011

Background.—Guidelines for prevention of group B streptococcal (GBS) infection have successfully reduced early onset (EO) GBS disease. Study results suggest that *Escherichia coli* is an important EO pathogen.

Objective.—To determine EO infection rates, pathogens, morbidity, and mortality in a national network of neonatal centers.

Methods.—Infants with EO infection were identified by prospective surveillance at Eunice Kennedy Shriver National Institute of Child Health and Human Development Neonatal Network centers. Infection was defined by positive culture results for blood and cerebrospinal fluid obtained from infants aged ≤72 hours plus treatment with antibiotic therapy for ≥5 days. Mother and infant characteristics, treatments, and outcomes were studied. Numbers of cases and total live births (LBs) were used to calculate incidence.

Results.—Among 396 586 LBs (2006–2009), 389 infants developed EO infection (0.98 cases per 1000 LBs). Infection rates increased with decreasing birth weight. GBS (43%, 0.41 per 1000 LBs) and *E coli* (29%, 0.28 per 1000 LBs) were most frequently isolated. Most infants with GBS were term (73%); 81% with *E coli* were preterm. Mothers of 67% of infected term and 58% of infected preterm infants were screened for GBS, and results were positive for 25% of those mothers. Only 76% of mothers with GBS colonization received intrapartum chemoprophylaxis. Although 77% of infected infants required intensive care, 20% of term infants were treated in the normal newborn nursery. Sixteen percent of infected infants died, most commonly with *E coli* infection (33%).

Conclusion.—In the era of intrapartum chemoprophylaxis to reduce GBS, rates of EO infection have declined but reflect a continued burden of disease. GBS remains the most frequent pathogen in term infants, and *E coli* the most significant pathogen in preterm infants. Missed opportunities for GBS prevention continue. Prevention of *E coli* sepsis, especially among preterm infants, remains a challenge.

▶ This update on the characteristics of early-onset neonatal sepsis is a reminder that this problem has not been eliminated. Although these data from a consortium of university-based neonatal intensive care units (NICUs) may not be representative of neonatal infections across the full range of obstetrical and neonatal services, the trends and challenges identified by this survey are generally applicable. The most common causes of sepsis remain *Escherichia coli* in preterm infants and group B streptococcus (GBS) in term infants, despite significant success in reducing rates of the latter disease. The authors' conclusion that recommendation of ampicillin and gentamicin as the first-line choice for empiric antimicrobial therapy remains appropriate is reassuring, but the observation that 78% of the isolated *E coli* strains were resistant to ampicillin is a reason for concern. Ampicillin resistance was not correlated with exposure to intrapartum antibiotics, but the relationship to prolonged antepartum antibiotic exposure reported by others[1] was not explored. Fortunately, 97% of the *E coli* strains remain sensitive to gentamicin; however, *E coli* caused 40% of the cases of early-onset meningitis, which may not be optimally treated by gentamicin monotherapy, indicating the importance of both diagnostic lumbar puncture and timely adjustments in antibiotic coverage. Of the 160 infants with GBS sepsis, 61 (38%) were born to women who had received intrapartum antibiotics, demonstrating the imperfect efficacy of that intervention; 41 (26%) were born to women with negative antepartum screening cultures or cesarean delivery, who did not qualify for and did not receive intrapartum prophylaxis, reflecting incomplete ascertainment of at-risk infants by the current algorithm. Noncompliance with the Centers for Disease Control and Prevention guidelines (failure to provide intrapartum prophylaxis despite maternal GBS bacteriuria, colonization, intrapartum risk factor with unknown colonization, or preterm birth without a screening culture within 5 weeks) was confirmed in 30 (19%) and possible in 28 (17%) of the GBS cases, suggesting the potential for an additional 35% reduction in GBS attack rates through more comprehensive implementation of prophylaxis strategies. No similar opportunity for prevention of *E coli* infections is apparent. As these authors point out, however, "strategies to reduce the unacceptably high rates of preterm birth in the United States are more likely to reduce deaths associated with early onset infections, as well as deaths related to other complications of prematurity."

W. E. Benitz, MD

Reference

1. Terrone DA, Rinehart BK, Einstein MH, Britt LB, Martin JN Jr, Perry KG. Neonatal sepsis and death caused by resistant Escherichia coli: Possible consequences of extended maternal ampicillin administration. *Am J Obstet Gynecol.* 1999;180:1345-1348.

Effect of vitamin supplements on HIV shedding in breast milk
Villamor E, Koulinska IN, Aboud S, et al (Univ of Michigan School of Public Health, Ann Arbor; Harvard School of Public Health, Boston, MA; Muhimbili Univ of Health and Allied Sciences, Dar es Salaam, Tanzania)
Am J Clin Nutr 92:881-886, 2010

Background.—Supplementation in lactating HIV-1—infected women with preformed vitamin A and β-carotene (VA/BC) increases the risk of mother-to-child transmission of HIV through breastfeeding. Identifying a biological mechanism to explain this unexpected finding would lend support to a causal effect.

Objective.—The aim of the study was to evaluate the effect of VA/BC or multivitamin (B complex, vitamin C, and vitamin E) supplementation of

HIV-infected women on HIV shedding in breast milk during the first 2 y postpartum.

Design.—We quantified viral (cell-free) and proviral (cell-associated) HIV loads in breast-milk samples collected ≤15 d after delivery and every 3 mo thereafter from 594 Tanzanian HIV-1—infected women who participated in a randomized trial. Women received 1 of the following 4 daily oral regimens in a 2 × 2 factorial fashion during pregnancy and throughout the first 2 y postpartum: multivitamin, VA/BC, multivitamin including VA/BC, or placebo.

Results.—The proportion of breast-milk samples with detectable viral load was significantly higher in women who received VA/BC (51.3%) than in women who were not assigned to VA/BC (44.8%; $P = 0.02$). The effect was apparent ≥6 mo postpartum (relative risk: 1.34; 95% CI: 1.04, 1.73). No associations with proviral load were observed. The multivitamin had no effects. In observational analyses, β-carotene but not retinol breast-milk concentrations were significantly associated with an increased viral load in milk.

Conclusions.—VA/BC supplementation in lactating women increases the HIV load in breast milk. This finding contributes to explaining the adverse effect of VA/BC on mother-to-child transmission. β-Carotene appears to have an effect on breast-milk viral load, independent of pre-formed vitamin A. This trial was registered at clinicaltrials.gov as NCT00197756.

▶ The surprising results of this study of 720 women infected with human immu-nodeficiency virus (HIV) in Tanzania suggest that vitamin A and β-carotene, but not multivitamin, supplementation to lactating mothers increases HIV shedding in the breast milk, thereby increasing viral load in the infants. The effect of the vitamin A/β-carotene on the breast milk viral load was apparent at or after 6 months postpartum, resulting in a 34% increase in the risk of HIV shedding in milk after 6 months. The mechanisms of this are unclear, but the results are compelling in light of previous studies. Whether the retinoic acid has an effect on mammary epithelium (as seen in studies of keratinocytes where the vitamin caused a decrease in the intracellular junction protein claudin-1[1]), which may in turn lead to increased shedding of virus, remains speculative. This finding should underline the need for caution in providing these vitamins to HIV-infected mothers.

J. Neu, MD

Reference

1. Hatakeyama S, Ishida K, Takeda Y. Changes in cell characteristics due to retinoic acid; specifically, a decrease in the expression of claudin-1 and increase in claudin-4 within tight junctions in stratified oral keratinocytes. *J Periodontal Res.* 2010;45:207-215.

Inter-Alpha Inhibitor Protein Level in Neonates Predicts Necrotizing Enterocolitis

Chaaban H, Shin M, Sirya E, et al (Women & Infants Hosp, Providence, RI; ProThera Biologics, East Providence, RI; et al)
J Pediatr 157:757-761, 2010

Objectives.—To compare inter-alpha inhibitor protein (IaIp) levels in neonates with proven necrotizing enterocolitis (NEC) and neonates with other, nonspecific abdominal disorders.

Study Design.—This was a prospective observational study of neonates in the neonatal intensive care unit. NEC was diagnosed according to Bell's staging criteria. The neonates in the control group had a nonspecific abdominal disorder, but no radiographic evidence of NEC and no disease progression. All neonates with radiographically confirmed NEC were included. Plasma IaIp levels were quantitated by enzyme-linked immunosorbent assay.

Results.—Seventeen neonates had confirmed NEC, and 34 neonates had nonspecific abdominal disorders that improved rapidly. Gestational age, postnatal age, weight, sex, maternal obstetric variables, rupture of membranes, and mode of delivery did not differ between the two groups. Mean IaIp level was significantly lower in the NEC group compared with the control group (137 ± 38 mg/L; 95% confidence interval [CI], 118-157 mg/L vs 258 ± 53 mg/L; 95% CI, 238-277 mg/L; $P < .0001$).

Conclusions.—The finding of significantly lower IaIp levels in neonates with NEC suggests that IaIp might be a useful, sensitive biomarker, allowing initiation of appropriate therapy and reducing antibiotic overuse in neonates with suspected but unproven NEC. Administration of IaIp may significantly reduce the severity of systemic inflammation and associated tissue injury.

▶ Necrotizing enterocolitis (NEC) remains a complex and poorly understood neonatal disease with an unacceptably high incidence of morbidity and mortality. Recent studies suggest that an altered intestinal microbiome coupled with an unbalanced proinflammatory response in a high-risk premature infant may lead to the final common pathway of intestinal necrosis. Although probiotic prophylaxis may reduce the risk for disease, identifying a predictive marker would significantly improve clinical decision making and may reduce NEC-related morbidity and mortality.

This study identifies a new predictive marker, inter-alpha inhibitor protein (IaIp), which may have a clinically useful profile with strong positive and negative predictive values. In this cohort of 17 NEC patients and 34 controls with abdominal symptoms/signs and no radiographic evidence of NEC, there was essentially no overlap between plasma IaIp levels at the time of diagnosis. These data suggest that the plasma IaIp level alone could predict NEC with near certainty, a most impressive result. Previous reports evaluating potential predictive markers of NEC are far less reliable or consistent, although some might have clinical use, including C-reactive protein, hydrogen breath test, interleukin-8, platelet activating factor, and most recently, complement 5a, cytosolic beta-glucosidase, serum amyloid A, and salivary H secretor phenotype 1 to 4. In these studies, most markers were measured at the time of NEC diagnosis, and unfortunately, patients will benefit only if a marker is discovered that predicts NEC before a diagnosis is made. As such, additional studies characterizing plasma Ialp in a larger patient population and at time points that precede the clinical diagnosis of NEC are needed before this approach becomes clinically useful.

The impact of Ialp may be significantly greater than that of a reliable predictive marker for NEC; Ialp may be useful in the treatment of this dreaded disease. It has been shown that serine proteases initiate a cell death pathway in epithelial cells, and this mechanism may contribute to the pathogenesis of NEC 5. If so, low Ialp levels due to consumption or immaturity would lead to prolonged serine protease exposure and may contribute to increased epithelial cell death. It seems plausible that exogenous Ialp could reduce serine protease effects, and in animals, Ialp treatment has been shown to reduce the risk of death in a neonatal sepsis model 6. Additional studies are needed to explore the possible role of Ialp in the diagnosis and treatment of neonatal NEC, but this preliminary report highlights the exciting potential of this understudied molecule.

M. S. Caplan, MD

Maternal Influenza Vaccination and Effect on Influenza Virus Infection in Young Infants
Eick AA, Uyeki TM, Klimov A, et al (Johns Hopkins Bloomberg School of Public Health, Baltimore, MD; Natl Ctr for Immunization and Respiratory Diseases, Atlanta, GA)
Arch Pediatr Adolesc Med 165:104-111, 2011

Objective.—To assess the effect of seasonal influenza vaccination during pregnancy on laboratory-confirmed influenza in infants to 6 months of age.

Design.—Nonrandomized, prospective, observational cohort study.

Setting.—Navajo and White Mountain Apache Indian reservations, including 6 hospitals on the Navajo reservation and 1 on the White Mountain Apache reservation.

Participants.—A total of 1169 mother-infant pairs with mothers who delivered an infant during 1 of 3 influenza seasons.

Main Exposure.—Maternal seasonal influenza vaccination.

Main Outcome Measures.—In infants, laboratory-confirmed influenza, influenzalike illness (ILI), ILI hospitalization, and influenza hemagglutinin inhibition antibody titers.

Results.—A total of 1160 mother-infant pairs had serum collected and were included in the analysis. Among infants, 193 (17%) had an ILI hospitalization, 412 (36%) had only an ILI outpatient visit, and 555 (48%) had no ILI episodes. The ILI incidence rate was 7.2 and 6.7 per 1000 person-days for infants born to unvaccinated and vaccinated women, respectively. There was a 41% reduction in the risk of laboratory-confirmed influenza virus infection (relative risk, 0.59; 95% confidence interval, 0.37-0.93) and a 39% reduction in the risk of ILI hospitalization (relative risk, 0.61; 95% confidence interval, 0.45-0.84) for infants born to influenza-vaccinated women compared with infants born to unvaccinated mothers. Infants born to influenza-vaccinated women had significantly higher hemagglutinin inhibition antibody titers at birth and at 2 to 3 months of age than infants of unvaccinated mothers for all 8 influenza virus strains investigated.

Conclusions.—Maternal influenza vaccination was significantly associated with reduced risk of influenza virus infection and hospitalization for an ILI up to 6 months of age and increased influenza antibody titers in infants through 2 to 3 months of age.

▶ During the H1N1 influenza epidemic of 2009, immunization of pregnant women was advocated primarily because of the remarkable vulnerability of pregnant women to development of very severe infection with that viral strain. Many of us encouraged women to get vaccinated by noting the additional potential for immunoprotection of their newborn infants. This report confirms that this secondary benefit is not merely hypothetical. Reporting data gathered during the 3 influenza seasons from the fall of 2002 through the summer of 2005, these authors document protective antibody titers in infants born to recipients of the annual influenza vaccine, from birth through at least 2 to 3 months of age. Antibody titers decline to those of unimmunized infants by 6 months of age. Nonetheless, there were substantial reductions in laboratory-confirmed influenza infections and in hospital admissions for influenza-like illnesses in the first 6 months after birth, the period of greatest risk of severe influenza illness. Passive immunity afforded by maternal immunization, although incomplete, provides critical protection of infants from influenza infection during this crucial interval, until the infants become eligible for influenza vaccination themselves at 6 months of age. Notably, rates of influenza-like illness for infants born to unimmunized and immunized mothers were virtually identical, highlighting the necessity for specific diagnoses in these follow-up studies. Sometimes it really is possible to get 2 for the price of 1, and once again, we are indebted to our obstetrical colleagues for making it happen.

W. E. Benitz, MD

Nosocomial Infection Reduction in VLBW Infants With a Statewide Quality-Improvement Model
Wirtschafter DD, Powers RJ, Pettit JS, et al (David D. Wirtschafter, MD, Inc, San Jose, CA; Good Samaritan Hosp, San Jose, CA; Kaiser Permanente Med Ctr, Modesto, CA; et al)
Pediatrics 127:419-426, 2011

Objective.—To evaluate the effectiveness of the California Perinatal Quality Care Collaborative quality-improvement model using a toolkit supplemented by workshops and Web casts in decreasing nosocomial infections in very low birth weight infants.

Design.—This was a retrospective cohort study of continuous California Perinatal Quality Care Collaborative members' data during the years 2002–2006. The primary dependent variable was nosocomial infection, defined as a late bacterial or coagulase-negative staphylococcal infection diagnosed after the age of 3 days by positive blood/cerebro-spinal fluid culture(s) and clinical criteria. The primary independent variable of interest was voluntary attendance at the tool-kit's introductory event, a direct indicator that at least 1 member of an NICU team had been personally exposed to the toolkit's features rather than being only notified of its availability. The intervention's effects were assessed using a multivariable logistic regression model that risk adjusted for selected demographic and clinical factors.

Results.—During the study period, 7733 eligible very low birth weight infants were born in 27 quality-improvement participant hospitals and 4512 very low birth weight infants were born in 27 non–quality-improvement participant hospitals. For the entire cohort, the rate of nosocomial infection decreased from 16.9% in 2002 to 14.5% in 2006. For infants admitted to NICUs participating in at least 1 quality-improvement event, there was an associated decreased risk of nosocomial infection (odds ratio: 0.81 [95% confidence interval: 0.68–0.96]) compared with those admitted to nonparticipating hospitals.

Conclusions.—The structured intervention approach to quality improvement in the NICU setting, using a toolkit along with attendance at a workshop and/or Web cast, is an effective means by which to improve care outcomes.

▶ Nosocomial infections occur worldwide and affect both developed and resource-poor countries. Infections acquired in health care settings are among the major causes of death and increased morbidity among hospitalized patients. Neonatal hospital-acquired infections add to the functional disability and emotional stress of the family and may also lead to neurocognitive impairment. Nosocomial infections are also one of the leading causes of death. The economic costs are considerable, with the increased length of stay contributing most to the costs.

Efficient progress in decreasing neonatal nosocomial infection rates can be achieved when statewide quality-improvement collaboratives using structured interventions (toolkits) are augmented with brief interactions that introduce, orient, and motivate potential users. Central line—associated bloodstream infections (CLABSIs) have come to be recognized as preventable adverse events that result from lapses in technique at multiple levels of care. CLABSIs have been significantly reduced with the use of central-line bundles. (A bundle is a protocol put in place to ensure that a procedure is performed using the latest evidence-based techniques.) To further reduce these lines and other nosocomial infections requires not only an understanding of the scientific data and technology but the ability to get buy-in to the program from all the personnel and families and the creation of a multidisciplinary team within the intensive care unit. Continued staff education, awareness of practice changes, strict adherence to the elements of the bundle, and close monitoring and reporting to all of the staff of the rates of infection all become essential components of the bundle implementation. Self-study modules with pretests and posttests, the use of pictorials and other informational tools, prohibition of line invasion, and meticulous care of the hub all support a culture of zero tolerance for infection.[1] After all, that is our goal: zero line infections and zero ventilator-associated pneumonias. It is not rocket science, but good teamwork and adherence to policy that gets the job done. Continuing educational reinforcement and positive feedback to the staff are also essential elements of this process.

A. A. Fanaroff, MD, FRCPE, FRCP&CH

Reference

1. Zack J. Zeroing in on zero tolerance for central line-associated bacteremia. *Am J Infect Control*. 2008;36:S176.e1-S176.e2.

Ohio Statewide Quality-Improvement Collaborative to Reduce Late-Onset Sepsis in Preterm Infants
Kaplan HC, for the Ohio Perinatal Quality Collaborative (Cincinnati Children's Hosp Med Ctr, OH; et al)
Pediatrics 127:427-435, 2011

Objective.—We aimed to reduce late-onset bacterial infections in infants born at 22 to 29 weeks' gestation by using collaborative quality-improvement methods to implement evidence-based catheter care. We hypothesized that these methods would result in a 50% reduction in nosocomial infection.

Patients and Methods.—We conducted an interrupted time-series study among 24 Ohio NICUs. The intervention began in September 2008 and continued through December 2009. Sites used the Institute for Healthcare Improvement Breakthrough Series quality-improvement model to facilitate implementation of evidence-based catheter care. Data were collected monthly for all catheter insertions and for at least 10 observations of indwelling catheter care. NICUs also submitted monthly data on catheter-days, patient-days, and episodes of infection. Data were analyzed by using statistical process control methods.

Results.—During the intervention, NICUs submitted information on 1916 infants. Of the 242 infections reported, 69% were catheter associated. Compliance with catheter-insertion components was >90% by April 2009. Compliance with components of evidence-based indwelling catheter care reached 80.4% by December 2009. There was a significant reduction in the proportion of infants with at least 1 late-onset infection from a baseline of 18.2% to 14.3%.

Conclusions.—There was a 20% reduction in the incidence of late-onset infection after the intervention, but the magnitude was less than hypothesized, perhaps because compliance with components of evidence-based care of indwelling catheters remained <90%. Because nearly one-third of infections were not catheter associated, improvement may require attention to other aspects of care such as skin integrity and nutrition.

▶ Reducing health care—associated or nosocomial infection in preterm infants remains a major challenge. Late-onset infections cause significant morbidity and mortality in preterm infants. These low birth weight, immature infants with multiorgan system failure are vulnerable to infection because of their immature and impaired host defense system, poor skin integrity, and prolonged exposure to invasive vascular access devices. Quality improvement interventions focused on catheter care have reduced nosocomial infections in adult and pediatric patients but have yet to be proven effective in preterm neonates.

Kaplan et al show that application of evidence-based venous catheter care as part of a state-based quality improvement collaborative in Ohio can reduce infections in preterm neonates. "They highlight the important role of reliability principles in evidence implementation." The authors were disappointed that the compliance was less than 90%, but this offers the opportunity to do even better in the future as centers become more familiar with and apply the evidence in a uniform manner. Also, at least one-third of the infections were unrelated to the catheters.

Dr Jill Baley's commentary covers three communications, all related to nosocomial infections, that appeared in the journal *Pediatrics* in March 2011.

As neonatologists, we have to accept and even embrace a rapid rate of change in both our knowledge base and in technology. It comes with the territory. However, for unclear reasons, we seem to have accepted that our babies will get infections, and lots of them. That also seems to come with the territory. After all, our babies are small. They have immature immune systems. They undergo many invasive procedures. Their immature skin does not provide much of a barrier to microbial invasion. We have noted what the risk factors are for infections and have tried to develop better screening tools for prediction of which infant will need care and antibiotics. We have paid close attention to which antibiotics provide the best coverage and how to minimize the development of resistance. Likewise, we have improved our supportive care for infants in septic shock and respiratory failure. Our efforts at preventing infections, though, seem to have focused on interventions: intravenous immunoglobin infusions did little to help. Prophylactic fluconazole remains controversial. Oral gentamicin failed to prevent necrotizing enterocolitis. So we continue to believe that our babies will get infections, and lots of them. At least that has been our assumption until recently. Now these 3 collaborative efforts in California, Ohio, and New York have demonstrated that paying attention to the most basic and straightforward methods of care can do what all our interventions have failed to accomplish to date. All 3 collaborative groups focused on central line—related infections in babies. The populations varied a bit: from all neonates to very low birth weight neonates to 22- to 29-weeks'-gestation neonates. The interventions, though, were remarkably similar: the need to have a standardized procedure, maintaining a checklist of the steps in the procedure, remembering sterility, making certain that all items necessary to complete the placement of the line are present before starting the procedure, and providing routine care of the dressings and tubing. These simple methods, which we learned in medical school, can make a difference, if there is adherence to their practice. What a humbling experience! Our interventions have been of less value than simply putting together a bundle of straightforward best practices. Undoubtedly, that is also why having a high patient neonatal intensive care unit volume makes a large difference. A large volume necessitates a standardized method to placement and maintenance of central lines. Kudos to basic practices.

A. A. Fanaroff, MD, FRCPE, FRCP&CH
J. E. Baley, MD

Randomised controlled trial of prophylactic fluconazole versus nystatin for the prevention of fungal colonisation and invasive fungal infection in very low birth weight infants
Aydemir C, Oguz SS, Dizdar EA, et al (Zekai Tahir Burak Maternity Hosp, Ankara, Turkey)
Arch Dis Child Fetal Neonatal Ed 96:F164-F168, 2011

Background.—Invasive fungal infections are a major cause of morbidity and mortality in preterm infants. The authors conducted the first prospective, randomised controlled trial of nystatin compared with fluconazole for the prevention of fungal colonisation and invasive fungal infection in very low birth weight (VLBW) neonates.

Methods.—During a 12-month period, all VLBW neonates were assigned randomly to receive nystatin (1 ml suspension, 100 000 U/ml, every 8 h), fluconazole (3 mg/kg body weight, every third day) or placebo from birth until day 30 of life (day 45 for neonates weighing <1000 g at birth). The authors performed weekly surveillance cultures and systemic fungal susceptibility testing.

Results.—During the study period, 278 infants (fluconazole group, n = 93; nystatin group, n = 94; control group, n = 91) weighing <1500 g at birth were admitted. There were no differences in birth weight, gestation, gender or risk factors for fungal infection among the groups. Fungal colonisation occurred in 11.7% of the nystatin group and 10.8% of the fluconazole group, as compared with 42.9% of the control group. The incidence of invasive fungal infection was 4.3% in the nystatin group and 3.2% in the fluconazole group, as compared with 16.5% in the control group. There were no differences in fungal colonisation and invasive fungal infection between the nystatin and fluconazole groups.

Conclusions.—Prophylactic nystatin and fluconazole reduce the incidence of colonisation and invasive fungal infection in VLBW neonates.

The authors believe that nystatin is an alternative to fluconazole, because nystatin is safe, inexpensive, well tolerated and effective.

▶ There is consensus that invasive fungal infection is an important cause of mortality and morbidity in very low birth weight (VLBW), extremely preterm infants. Some specific risk factors include prolonged use of parenteral nutrition with central lines and extended exposure to broad-spectrum antibiotics, histamine type 2 receptor blockers, and postnatal steroids. Prevention of fungal colonization and infection is more effective than treatment of an established infection. An ever-expanding literature has addressed the value of early empirical and prophylactic treatment. There is A-1 evidence supporting antifungal prophylaxis with fluconazole. The literature supports targeting infants who weigh less than 1000 g and/or those who are at 27 weeks of gestation or less, because this group has high infection-related mortality and neurodevelopmental impairment.[1-3] Antifungal prophylaxis nearly eliminates infection-related mortality. Concern exists about the impact that widespread use of prophylaxis may have on the emergence of antifungal resistance, but to date these fears have been unfounded. To resolve the clinical uncertainty about the effect of prophylactic oral/topical nonabsorbed antifungals to reduce mucocutaneous colonization and so limit the risk of invasive fungal infection in this population, Austin et al[4] completed a Cochrane review. Although there was evidence of a reduction in risk of invasive fungal infection in infants treated with nystatin, the data needed to be interpreted with caution, as the trials had methodological weaknesses, including quasi-randomization, lack of allocation concealment, lack of blinding of intervention and outcomes assessment, and high rates of invasive fungal infection in the control groups. The investigators called for further prospective randomized trials with long-term follow-up. Kaufman and Manzoni[3] noted that "Fluconazole is more efficacious than nystatin prophylaxis in infants weighing less than 1000 g, is less expense, requires less frequent dosing (twice weekly intravenous [IV] dosing), and can be given when infants are not feeding." Reed et al[5] commented that "Although fluconazole prophylaxis appears to reduce the rates of colonization and invasive fungal infections, no trial in this review was able to demonstrate a significant difference in long-term morbidity or mortality."

Aydemir et al have responded to the call by Austin et al for randomized controlled trials (RCTs). They have performed the first prospective RCT comparing nystatin with fluconazole for the prevention of fungal colonization and invasive fungal infection in VLBW infants. This study demonstrated that nystatin prophylaxis is similar in efficacy to fluconazole prophylaxis in VLBW infants with no signs of adverse effects or harm. There is still a need for more data before practitioners will switch from fluconazole to nystatin. In the meantime, encouraging data are emerging on the use of probiotics, prebiotics, and lactoferrin to reduce nosocomial infections, including fungal infections.[6,7]

A. A. Fanaroff, MD, FRCPE, FRCP&CH

References

1. Manzoni P, Jacqz-Aigrain E, Rizzollo S, et al. Antifungal prophylaxis in neonates. *Early Hum Dev.* 2011;87:S59-S60.

2. Wilkerson J, McPherson C, Donze A. Fluconazole to prevent systemic fungal infections in infants: reviewing the evidence. *Neonatal Netw.* 2010;29(5):323-333.
3. Kaufman DA, Manzoni P. Strategies to prevent invasive candidal infection in extremely preterm infants. *Clin Perinatol.* 2010;37:611-628.
4. Austin N, Darlow BA, McGuire W. Prophylactic oral/topical non-absorbed antifungal agents to prevent invasive fungal infection in very low birth weight infants. *Cochrane Database Syst Rev.* 2009;(4). CD003478.
5. Reed BN, Caudle KE, Rogers PD. Fluconazole prophylaxis in high-risk neonates. *Ann Pharmacother.* 2010;44:178-184.
6. Manzoni P, Rinaldi M, Cattani, et al. Italian Task Force for the Study and Prevention of Neonatal Fungal Infections, Italian Society of Neonatology. Bovine lactoferrin supplementation for prevention of late-onset sepsis in very low-birth-weight neonates: a randomized trial. *JAMA.* 2009;302:1421-1428.
7. Venkatesh MP, Abrams SA. Oral lactoferrin for the prevention of sepsis and necrotizing enterocolitis in preterm infants. *Cochrane Database Syst Rev.* 2010;(5). CD007137.

Randomised controlled trial of prophylactic fluconazole versus nystatin for the prevention of fungal colonisation and invasive fungal infection in very low birth weight infants

Aydemir C, Oguz SS, Dizdar EA, et al (Zekai Tahir Burak Maternity Hosp, Ankara, Turkey)
Arch Dis Child Fetal Neonatal Ed 96:F164-F168, 2011

Background.—Invasive fungal infections are a major cause of morbidity and mortality in preterm infants. The authors conducted the first prospective, randomised controlled trial of nystatin compared with fluconazole for the prevention of fungal colonisation and invasive fungal infection in very low birth weight (VLBW) neonates.

Methods.—During a 12-month period, all VLBW neonates were assigned randomly to receive nystatin (1 ml suspension, 100 000 U/ml, every 8 h), fluconazole (3 mg/kg body weight, every third day) or placebo from birth until day 30 of life (day 45 for neonates weighing <1000 g at birth). The authors performed weekly surveillance cultures and systemic fungal susceptibility testing.

Results.—During the study period, 278 infants (fluconazole group, n=93; nystatin group, n=94; control group, n=91) weighing <1500 g at birth were admitted. There were no differences in birth weight, gestation, gender or risk factors for fungal infection among the groups. Fungal colonisation occurred in 11.7% of the nystatin group and 10.8% of the fluconazole group, as compared with 42.9% of the control group. The incidence of invasive fungal infection was 4.3% in the nystatin group and 3.2% in the fluconazole group, as compared with 16.5% in the control group. There were no differences in fungal colonisation and invasive fungal infection between the nystatin and fluconazole groups.

Conclusions.—Prophylactic nystatin and fluconazole reduce the incidence of colonisation and invasive fungal infection in VLBW neonates.

The authors believe that nystatin is an alternative to fluconazole, because nystatin is safe, inexpensive, well tolerated and effective.

▶ Invasive fungal infections in newborn infants are associated with significant short- and long-term morbidity.[1] Prevention measures have focused on generic infection control practices and avoidance of modifiable neonatal intensive care unit—related risk factors.[2] Chemoprophylaxis with a systemically absorbed antifungal agent such as fluconazole achieves fungicidal concentrations but raises concern for emergence of antifungal resistance. Prophylaxis with an oral/topical nonabsorbed antifungal agent has been proposed as a potentially cheap and easy alternative.

This study is the first prospective randomized controlled trial comparing nystatin with fluconazole for prevention of fungal colonization and invasive fungal infection. However, there are multiple methodological issues that limit the generalizability of the study findings. Eligible infants were randomly allocated by computer-generated randomization into 3 groups in a 1:1:1 ratio, but caregivers were not blinded to study status. Differences in frequency of drug/placebo administration and route of administration were readily apparent, which may lead to surveillance and ascertainment bias secondary to adjustments in thresholds for investigation and diagnosis of suspected invasive disease. Despite a statistical reduction in colonization and invasive infection in both intervention groups compared with the control group, high baseline rates in the control group (42.9% colonization and 16.5% infection) were observed, which the authors attributed to the injudicious and long-term administration of antibiotics as well as the usage of total parenteral nutrition and invasive procedures. Neither intervention had any effect on the association between colonization and subsequent progression to invasive infection. Overall mortality and mortality associated with invasive disease were similar in all 3 groups. Power and sample size calculations were not addressed by the authors beyond the acknowledgement that the study was not powered to examine differences in mortality. There was also no selection of natively resistant *Candida* species documented; however, detection of clinically significant shifts in *Candida* species or emergence of acquired resistance mutations likely requires a longer surveillance than the 12-month study period. Lastly, the authors did not examine long-term outcomes, such as disability-free survival. Given these limitations, the study's summary findings are insufficient to warrant routine antifungal chemoprophylaxis.

J. S. Lee, MD, MPH

References

1. Austin N, Darlow BA, McGuire W. Prophylactic oral/topical non-absorbed antifungal agents to prevent invasive fungal infection in very low birth weight infants. *Cochrane Database Syst Rev.* 2009;(4). CD003478.
2. Manzoni P, Stolfi I, Pugni L, et al. A multicenter, randomized trial of prophylactic fluconazole in preterm neonates. *N Engl J Med.* 2007;356:2483-2495.

Real-Time PCR Assay Provides Reliable Assessment of Intrapartum Carriage of Group B *Streptococcus*

Alfa MJ, Sepehri S, De Gagne P, et al (Univ of Manitoba, Winnipeg, Canada)
J Clin Microbiol 48:3095-3099, 2010

The objective of this study was to determine the reliability of the real-time PCR assay for determining the group B *Streptococcus* (GBS) status of women in labor. In this prospective study we compared the results of culture and PCR testing of vaginal and rectal samples collected by nursing staff when women were in labor. Patients' charts were also reviewed to obtain relevant information about pregnancy risk factors. Our results demonstrated a sensitivity, specificity, positive predictive value (PPV), and negative predictive value (NPV) of 90.5%, 96.1%, 86.4%, and 97.4%, respectively, for rapid PCR. Of the 196 women evaluated, 29 (14.8%) presented with unknown GBS status, 11 (37.9%) of whom received unnecessary intrapartum antibiotics. The rapid real-time PCR test was robust and was able to reliably detect the presence of GBS in women in labor within 1 h of specimen submission to the laboratory. We recommend that the rapid PCR test be targeted to women who present in labor with unknown GBS status. In cases where the laboratory does not offer 24-h availability of testing, sample collection followed by PCR testing the next morning is still valuable and provides reliable results 24 to 48 h faster than culture and will aid appropriate decision-making regarding continuing or stopping antibiotics for neonates of women with unknown GBS status.

▶ The devil is in the details. This report adds another series to a growing body of literature documenting correlation between conventional culture and molecular methods for detection of group B streptococcal (GBS) colonization. Rapid polymerase chain reaction (PCR) appears to be comparable to conventional laboratory methods. Because PCR can be performed quickly (in less than 1 hour) after presentation for delivery, it offers an alternative to risk factor–based prophylaxis strategies for women whose GBS colonization status is unknown. However, the logical foundations of this approach bear scrutiny. As these authors document, rapid PCR on rectovaginal specimens is a reasonable predictor of rectovaginal GBS colonization as ascertained by enhanced broth culture methods. Rectovaginal cultures performed at 35 to 37 weeks' gestation are good predictors of vaginal GBS colonization at delivery. Vaginal colonization is the relevant determinant of risk since 98% of infants with early-onset GBS sepsis are born to women with that finding. Although collection of both vaginal and rectal specimens for antepartum screening is a necessity for ascertainment of risk for vaginal colonization at birth, one-third of women with rectovaginal colonization do not have vaginal colonization. Consequently, intrapartum prophylaxis is provided to many women who do not have vaginal colonization and whose infants are at little risk. A rapid PCR method for identification of women with vaginal colonization would permit a more selective approach with little or no reduction in prophylaxis efficacy. Unfortunately, available data suggest that the sensitivity of commercially available rapid PCR may be substantially lower for vaginal specimens, possibly reflecting smaller bacterial inocula. A rapid PCR method with sensitivity sufficient to reliably identify women with vaginal colonization would therefore be ideal. Until one is developed, currently available commercial assays (such as that used in this report) on rectovaginal specimens may be a useful complement to, or even a replacement for, antepartum screening cultures. Rapid bedside testing would obviate the logistical challenge of ensuring availability of antepartum screening at the time and place of delivery, eliminate the problem of missed antepartum screening, and permit extension of the screening-based strategy to women who present in labor before scheduled screening at 35 weeks' gestation. The major barrier to adopting such a strategy is the observation that about 20% of women in this study delivered within 4 hours of presentation. More detailed information about the potential impact of an hour's delay in initiation of prophylaxis in this group is needed.

W. E. Benitz, MD

Statewide NICU Central-Line-Associated Bloodstream Infection Rates Decline After Bundles and Checklists
Schulman J, the New York State Regional Perinatal Care Centers (Weill Cornell Med College, NY; et al)
Pediatrics 127:436-444, 2011

Objective.—In 2008, all 18 regional referral NICUs in New York state adopted central-line insertion and maintenance bundles and agreed to use checklists to monitor maintenance-bundle adherence and report checklist use. We sought to confirm whether adopting standardized bundles and using central-line maintenance checklists reduced central-line-associated bloodstream infections (CLABSI).

Methods.—This was a prospective cohort study that enrolled all neonates with a central line who were hospitalized in any of 18 NICUs. Each NICU reported CLABSI and central-line utilization data and checklist use. We used χ^2 to compare CLABSI rates in the preintervention (January to December 2007) versus the postintervention (March to December 2009) periods and Poisson regression to model adjusted CLABSI rates.

Results.—Each study period included more than 55 000 central-line days and more than 200 000 patient-days. CLABSI rates decreased 67% statewide (risk ratio: 0.33 [95% confidence interval: 0.27−0.41]; $P < .0005$); after adjusting for the altered central-line−associated bloodstream infection definition in 2008, by 40% (risk ratio: 0.60 [95% confidence interval: 0.48−0.75]; $P < .0005$). A total of 13 of 18 NICUs reported using maintenance checklists for 10% to 100% of central-line days. The checklist-use rate was associated with the CLABSI rate (coefficient: −0.57, $P = .04$). A total of 10 of 18 NICUs were independent CLABSI rate predictors, ranging from 1 site with greatly reduced risk (incidence

TABLE 1.—Central-Line Insertion and Maintenance Bundle Elements

Insertion Bundle	Maintenance Bundle
a) Establish a central line kit or cart to consolidate all items necessary for the procedure	a) Perform hand hygiene with hospital approved alcohol-based product or antiseptic-containing soap before and after accessing a catheter or before and after changing the dressing
b) Perform hand hygiene with hospital-approved alcohol-based product or antiseptic-containing soap before and after palpating insertion sites and before and after inserting the central line	b) Evaluate the catheter insertion site daily for signs of infection and to assess dressing integrity
c) Use maximal barrier precautions (including: sterile gown, sterile gloves, surgical mask, hat, and large sterile drape)	c) At a minimum, if the dressing is damp, soiled, or loose change dressing aseptically and disinfect the skin around the insertion site with an appropriate antiseptic (eg, 2% chlorhexidine, 70% alcohol)
d) Disinfect skin with appropriate antiseptic (eg, 2% chlorhexidine, 70% alcohol) before catheter insertion	d) Develop and use standardized intravenous tubing setup and changes
e) Use either a sterile transparent semipermeable dressing or sterile gauze to cover the insertion site	e) Maintain aseptic technique when changing intravenous tubing and when entering the catheter including "scrub the hub"
	f) Daily review of catheter necessity with prompt removal when no longer essential

Adapted with permission from Schulman, et al.[1]
Editor's Note: Please refer to original journal article for full references.

rate ratio: 0.04, $P < .0005$) to 1 site with greatly increased risk (incidence rate ratio: 2.87, $P < .0005$).

Conclusions.—Although standardizing central-line care elements led to a significant statewide decline in NICU CLABSIs, site of care remains an independent risk factor. Using maintenance checklists reduced CLABSIs (Table 1).

▶ Overall, infection rates range from 21% to 30% of very low birth weight admissions to the neonatal intensive care unit (NICU) with more infections seen in the smallest, least-mature infants. Prolonged antibiotic exposure not only renders these infants more vulnerable to fungal infections, but also death. This report from Shulman et al on behalf of the New York State Regional Perinatal Centers is very encouraging because I am of the strong opinion that it is reproducible in other states. The bundle (Table 1) is generalizable and the concept of using checklists is gaining traction. Medicine needs to follow the example of the airline industry, with using extensive checklists to improve patient safety, and that includes preventing nosocomial infections from central lines. The investigators have documented that applying standardized evidence-based central-line care across all regional referral NICUs in New York State significantly reduced central line—acquired blood stream infection (CLABSI) rates. Additionally, site of care affects CLABSI risk. Recognition of sites with increased rates of infection will permit a structured approach to remedy the problem. Furthermore, the increased use of checklists within the network was associated with lower CLABSI rates. It is now clear that infection is not inevitable in low birth weight infants but represents instances of preventable harm. See Baley's commentary with Kaplan article.

A. A. Fanaroff, MD, FRCPE, FRCP&CH

Fluconazole Prophylaxis in Extremely Low Birth Weight Infants and Neurodevelopmental Outcomes and Quality of Life at 8 to 10 Years of Age
Kaufman DA, Cuff AL, Wamstad JB, et al (Univ of Virginia School of Medicine, Charlottesville; et al)
J Pediatr 158:759-765, 2011

Objective.—To examine the long-term effects of fluconazole prophylaxis in extremely low birth weight infants.

Study Design.—Neurodevelopmental status and quality of life of survivors from a randomized, placebo-controlled trial of fluconazole prophylaxis were evaluated at 8 to 10 years of life using the Vineland Adaptive Behavior Scales-II (VABS-II) and the Child Health Questionnaire Parent-Completed Form 28 (CHQ-PF28), respectively.

Results.—VABS-II Domain Scores for the fluconazole-treated (n = 21; 9.1 ± 0.7 years) compared with the placebo group (n = 17; 9.3 ± 0.8 years) were similar for communication [94.6 (± 14.8) versus 92.6 (± 12.6), $P = .65$], daily living skills [87.9 (± 10.6) versus 87.4 (± 9.3), $P = .89$], socialization [97.2 (± 9.2) versus 94.4 (± 7.9), $P = .31$], and motor skills [92.1 (± 17.8) versus 95.1 (± 14.6), $P = .57$]. Internalizing and externalizing behaviors and maladaptive behavior index were also similar. The CHQ-PF28 revealed no differences between the two groups regarding quality of life. Survivors were also happy or satisfied with school (90% versus 100%, $P = .49$), friendships (90%versus 88%, $P = 1.00$), and life (95%versus 100%, $P = 1.00$). Self esteem scores were 87.3 ± 15.7 versus 89.7 ± 10.4 ($P = .59$). There were also no differences between groups regarding emotional difficulties or behavior problems.

Conclusions.—Fluconazole prophylaxis for the prevention of invasive *Candida* infections is safe in extremely low birth weight infants and does not appear to be associated with any long-term adverse effects on neurodevelopment and quality of life at 8 to 10 years of life.

▶ The cohort in the above report was enrolled in a single-center, randomized clinical trial of fluconazole prophylaxis against fungal colonization and infection in preterm infants.[1] The trial demonstrated a significantly lower rate of both fungal colonization and invasive fungal infection when infants were treated with prophylactic fluconazole. In the current study, the investigators examined the outcome in childhood of enrolled infants.

It is surprising that there was no difference in reported outcomes between the 2 groups, despite a significantly higher rate of fungal infection in the placebo group. This finding may be partially explained by the limited nature of the study. Less than 50% of the surviving infants enrolled in the original study were evaluated (47% fluconazole-treated; 42% placebo), and the follow-up rate for surviving children who were reported to have a fungal infection as infants is not included. In addition, neurodevelopment and quality-of-life data relied on parent report questionnaires. In the discussion, the authors state that the study demonstrates fluconazole prophylaxis is safe and not associated with adverse outcomes. Better-quality data are needed before this conclusion can be accepted with certainty.

L. A. Papile, MD

Reference

1. Kaufman D, Boyle R, Hazen KC, Patrie JT, Robinson M, Donowitz LG. Fluconazole prophylaxis against fungal colonization and infection in preterm infants. *N Engl J Med.* 2001;345:1660-1666.

Saliva Polymerase-Chain-Reaction Assay for Cytomegalovirus Screening in Newborns
Boppana SB, for the National Institute on Deafness and Other Communication Disorders CHIMES Study (Univ of Alabama at Birmingham; et al)
N Engl J Med 364:2111-2118, 2011

Background.—Congenital cytomegalovirus (CMV) infection is an important cause of hearing loss, and most infants at risk for CMV-associated hearing loss are not identified early in life because of failure to test for the infection. The standard assay for newborn CMV screening is rapid culture performed on saliva specimens obtained at birth, but this assay cannot be automated. Two alternatives — real-time polymerase-chain-reaction (PCR)–based testing of a liquid-saliva or dried-saliva specimen obtained at birth — have been developed.

Methods.—In our prospective, multicenter screening study of newborns, we compared real-time PCR assays of liquid-saliva and dried-saliva specimens with rapid culture of saliva specimens obtained at birth.

Results.—A total of 177 of 34,989 infants (0.5%; 95% confidence interval [CI], 0.4 to 0.6) were positive for CMV, according to at least one of the three methods. Of 17,662 newborns screened with the use of the liquid-saliva PCR assay, 17,569 were negative for CMV, and the remaining 85 infants (0.5%; 95% CI, 0.4 to 0.6) had positive results on both culture and PCR assay. The sensitivity and specificity of the liquid-saliva PCR assay were 100% (95% CI, 95.8 to 100) and 99.9% (95% CI, 99.9 to 100), respectively, and the positive and negative predictive values were 91.4% (95% CI, 83.8 to 96.2) and 100% (95% CI, 99.9 to 100), respectively. Of 17,327 newborns screened by means of the dried-saliva PCR assay, 74 were positive for CMV, whereas 76 (0.4%; 95% CI, 0.3 to 0.5) were found to be CMV-positive on rapid culture. Sensitivity and specificity of the dried-saliva PCR assay were 97.4% (95% CI, 90.8 to 99.7) and 99.9% (95% CI, 99.9 to 100), respectively. The positive and negative predictive values were 90.2% (95% CI, 81.7 to 95.7) and 99.9% (95% CI, 99.9 to 100), respectively.

Conclusions.—Real-time PCR assays of both liquid- and dried-saliva specimens showed high sensitivity and specificity for detecting CMV infection and should be considered potential screening tools for CMV in newborns. (Funded by the National Institute on Deafness and Other Communication Disorders.)

▶ Similar to many metabolic diseases, congenital cytomegalovirus (CMV) infection is usually clinically silent in the immediate newborn period and frequently is not diagnosed until irreversible injury has occurred. The ability to screen newborns for congenital CMV would permit the early identification of at-risk infants and allow targeted monitoring and early intervention. Previous attempts to develop a sensitive and specific screening test using dried-blood-spot polymerase chain reaction (PCR) assay showed that the test failed to identify the majority of CMV-infected newborns.[1] In this study, the authors evaluated the usefulness of real-time PCR assay of saliva specimens for CMV screening. The rationale for using saliva samples related to the ease of sample collection and the high titers of CMV that are shed in the saliva of infected infants. Both wet and air-dried samples were evaluated, since dried specimens are easier to store and transport. The results of the PCR assay were compared with those of rapid viral culture, considered the gold standard for the diagnosis of CMV. The wet saliva sample identified all babies infected with CMV, and 97% of infected neonates were identified when a dried saliva sample was used. The excellent sensitivity (> 97%), specificity (99.9%), and false-positive rate (< 0.03%) indicate that the saliva PCR assays will identify most infants with congenital CMV infection.

It is estimated that approximately one-quarter of sensorineural hearing loss in childhood is caused by congenital CMV infection. Because the hearing loss associated with congenital CMV can develop after the neonatal period and continue to progress during early childhood, a substantial proportion will not be diagnosed by means of newborn hearing screening. The saliva PCR assay appears to be a reasonable approach to large-scale screening to identify newborns with congenital CMV infection. The cost-benefit ratio of this approach is being evaluated in a separate trial in which children identified with congenital CMV are being screened for hearing loss every 6 months until 4 years of age.

L. A. Papile, MD

Reference

1. Boppana SB, Ross SA, Novak Z, et al. Dried blood spot real-time polymerase chain reaction assays to screen newborns for congenital cytomegalovirus infection. *JAMA.* 2010;303:1375-1382.

Repeat lumbar puncture in infants with meningitis in the neonatal intensive care unit

Greenberg RG, Benjamin DK Jr, Cohen-Wolkowiez M, et al (Duke Univ, Durham, NC)
J Perinatol 31:425-429, 2011

Objective.—The purpose of this study is to examine the results of repeat lumbar puncture in infants with initial positive cerebrospinal fluid (CSF) cultures in order to determine the clinical characteristics and outcomes of infants with repeat positive cultures.

Study Design.—Cohort study of infants with an initial positive CSF culture undergoing repeat lumbar puncture between 1997 and 2004 at 150 neonatal intensive care units managed by the Pediatrix Medical group. We compared the clinical outcomes of infants with repeat positive cultures and infants with repeat negative cultures.

Result.—We identified 118 infants with repeat CSF cultures. Of these, 26 infants had repeat positive cultures. A higher proportion with repeat positive cultures died compared with those with repeat negative cultures, 6/23 (26%) vs. 6/81 (7%), respectively (P=0.02).

Conclusion.—Among infants with a positive CSF culture, a repeat positive CSF culture is common. The presence of a second positive culture is associated with increased mortality.

▶ Meningitis remains a significant cause of mortality and morbidity in the neonatal population. It is often difficult to diagnose because the signs are subtle in neonates, and up to one-third of infants have negative blood cultures. The diagnosis of meningitis must be made by cerebrospinal fluid (CSF) examination. Identification of bacteria or fungal agents causing meningitis may influence the choice of drug and length of therapy.

In this retrospective study, Greenberg et al showed that among infants with a positive CSF culture, there was a higher mortality rate in the infants with a repeat positive CSF culture. The study supports the recommendation by Polin and Harris[1] and Heath et al[2] that repeat CSF evaluation is recommended at 48 to 72 hours. This follow-up may have both therapeutic and prognostic significance. Delayed clearance of an organism is suggestive of antimicrobial resistance or the presence of an occult focus of disease such as subdural empyema, obstructive ventriculitis, or multiple small vessel thrombi. Furthermore, a repeat lumbar puncture may be useful in determining the duration of therapy, since duration is often based on the time of sterilization of CSF. The study also showed that many infants whose CSF cleared never had normalized CSF protein, glucose, and white blood cell counts. Thus, the duration of therapy cannot be based on CSF parameters.

The study suggests that a repeat lumbar puncture is indicated in the management of neonates with meningitis.[3]

F. Akita, MB, ChB

References

1. Polin RA, Harris MC. Neonatal bacterial meningitis. *Semin Neonatol.* 2001;6: 157-172.
2. Heath PT, Nik Yusoff NK, Baker CJ. Neonatal meningitis. *Arch Dis Child Fetal Neonatal Ed.* 2003;88:F173-F178.
3. Garges HP, Moody MA, Cotten CM, et al. Neonatal meningitis: what is the correlation among cerebrospinal fluid cultures, blood cultures, and cerebrospinal fluid parameters? *Pediatrics.* 2006;117:1094-1100.

10 Labor and Delivery

Antenatal corticosteroids for preterm birth: dose-dependent reduction in birthweight, length and head circumference
Norberg H, Stålnacke J, Heijtz RD, et al (Karolinska Institutet, Stockholm, Sweden; Stockholm Univ, Sweden; et al)
Acta Paediatr 100:364-369, 2011

Aim.—This study was undertaken to evaluate the effects of repeated courses of antenatal corticosteroids (ACS) on foetal growth.
Methods.—We studied 94 infants exposed to 2–9 courses of ACS. Mean gestational age (GA) at first exposure was 29 and at birth 34 weeks. Exposure data were retrieved from case record files. Information on potential confounders was collected from the Swedish Medical Birth Registry. Standard deviation scores (SDS) for birthweight (BW), birthlength (BL) and head circumference (HC) were calculated and considered as outcomes.
Results.—GA at start of ACS did not affect outcome. BW-SDS, BL-SDS and HC-SDS were −0.21, −0.19 and +0.25 in infants exposed to two courses, compared to −1.01, −1.04 and −0.23 in infants exposed to ≥4 courses of ACS (p = 0.04−0.07). In multiple regression analyses, ≥4 courses were associated with lower BW-SDS, BL-SDS and HC-SDS (p = 0.007−0.04) compared to SDS after 2−3 courses. The effects from ≥4 courses on BW and BL were comparable to reduction in birth size seen in twins and on HC to that observed after maternal smoking.
Conclusions.—Multiple courses of ACS are associated with a dose-dependent decline in foetal growth, which may affect later development and health (Fig 1).

▶ Preterm infants with a mean gestational age of 30 to 31 weeks at the time of birth who received multiple doses of antenatal glucocorticoids were evaluated for growth. Birth weight, length, and head circumferences did not differ in relation to the number of antenatal steroid courses unless the analysis also took into account gestational age at birth and sex: then all 3 were negatively associated with the number of courses and total dose of glucocorticoid. For weight, the relationship seemed to be linear (Fig 1). As stated by the authors, similar findings have been seen in other studies. Furthermore, longer-term outcomes are needed. Although only briefly mentioned in this study, antenatal glucocorticoids may affect IGF, a highly epigenetically programmed gene. Furthermore, studies in animals suggest that epigenetic regulation may occur with antenatal glucocorticoids.[1] This growth restriction was comparable to that found in twins.

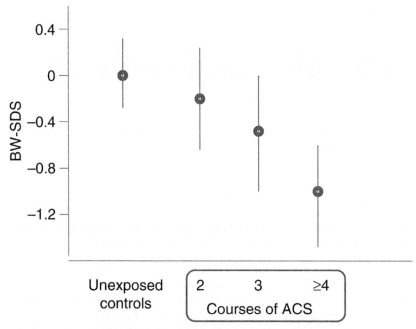

FIGURE 1.—Standard deviation scores for birthweight in unexposed controls and in relation to 2, 3 or ≥4 weekly courses of antenatal corticosteroids. Data are mean [95% confidence intervals]. (Reprinted form Norberg H, Stålnacke J, Heijtz RD, et al. Antenatal corticosteroids for preterm birth: Dose-dependent reduction in birthweight, length and head circumference. *Acta Paediatr.* 2011;100:364-369. Reprinted with permission of John Wiley & Sons, Inc.)

Head circumference growth restriction with multiple doses (greater than 4 compared with 2) was comparable to the restriction with maternal smoking. The fact that concerns about side effects, especially on growth, have been raised has resulted in less use of multiple doses. However, do we know that even when only 1 dose is given that this may not have long-lasting programming effects? Antenatal glucocorticoids have been commonly used for about 2 decades, but has a dose-effect response ever been performed? This study suggests that dose may be important for growth restriction. The same may hold true for programming effects. The very common use of this therapy strongly underlines the need for more information about the most appropriate dose (perhaps it could be much lower than commonly used) and long-term effects.

J. Neu, MD

Reference

1. Meaney MJ, Szyf M, Seckl JR. Epigenetic mechanisms of perinatal programming of hypothalamic-pituitary-adrenal function and health. *Trends Mol Med.* 2007;13: 269-277.

A Proposed Evidence-Based Neonatal Work-up to Confirm or Refute Allegations of Intrapartum Asphyxia

Muraskas JK, Morrison JC (Loyola Univ Med Ctr, Maywood, IL; Univ of Mississippi Med Ctr, Jackson)
Obstet Gynecol 116:261-268, 2010

Objective.—To propose a clinical work-up in term and near-term newborns to address the nine American College of Obstetricians and Gynecologists (the College) and American Academy of Pediatrics criteria to define an acute intrapartum event sufficient to cause cerebral palsy.

Methods.—We examined our experience as neonatal expert witnesses in 103 closed claims of alleged intrapartum asphyxia with poor newborn outcome over a 21-year period from 1987 to 2008. We estimated how often the clinical components of this proposed work-up were not obtained or recorded in the medical record.

Results.—Cord arterial blood gases and placental pathology were not obtained or sent in 38% and 32% of the 103 cases, respectively. Routine neonatal laboratory tests, including a complete blood count with differential, nucleated red blood cells, electrolytes, calcium, coagulation profile, and renal and liver function tests, were frequently absent. Cranial imaging in ultrasonograms, computed tomography, and magnetic resonance imaging were absent in more than 50% of the cases reviewed and were often not scheduled at optimal times.

Conclusion.—The medical record of newborns with poor outcomes frequently has a paucity of objective, evidence-based data. This leads to speculation and unethical expert testimony. The protocol will assist in confirming or refuting allegations of intrapartum asphyxia.

Level of Evidence.—III.

▶ This is an interesting and important article that attempts to examine the frequency of inclusion of key components of the workup of an infant suspected to have sustained intrapartum asphyxia, using the criteria suggested by American College of Obstetricians and Gynecologists/American Academy of Pediatrics. It is based on 103 cases in which the authors were personally involved as expert witnesses, so there may be a selection bias, and it is not known if this is a representative sample. Nevertheless, the authors found a large number of cases in which important objective data, such as cord arterial blood gases and placental examination, had not been obtained. They underscore the need for obtaining and documenting data necessary to confirm or refute the allegation that intrapartum asphyxia was the cause of cerebral palsy.

While we could argue about the validity of the criteria, the article clearly demonstrates the all-too-common lack of sufficient information available to expert witnesses and defense attorneys in trying to defend malpractice litigation.

It would be interesting to know if these data have changed over time. The cases spanned 22 years, and one would hope that we have learned from past experiences.

S. M. Donn, MD

A Proposed Evidence-Based Neonatal Work-up to Confirm or Refute Allegations of Intrapartum Asphyxia

Muraskas JK, Morrison JC (Loyola Univ Med Ctr, Maywood, IL; Univ of Mississippi Med Ctr, Jackson)
Obstet Gynecol 116:261-268, 2010

Objective.—To propose a clinical work-up in term and near-term newborns to address the nine American College of Obstetricians and Gynecologists (the College) and American Academy of Pediatrics criteria to define an acute intrapartum event sufficient to cause cerebral palsy.

Methods.—We examined our experience as neonatal expert witnesses in 103 closed claims of alleged intrapartum asphyxia with poor newborn outcome over a 21-year period from 1987 to 2008. We estimated how often the clinical components of this proposed work-up were not obtained or recorded in the medical record.

Results.—Cord arterial blood gases and placental pathology were not obtained or sent in 38% and 32% of the 103 cases, respectively. Routine neonatal laboratory tests, including a complete blood count with differential, nucleated red blood cells, electrolytes, calcium, coagulation profile, and renal and liver function tests, were frequently absent. Cranial imaging in ultrasonograms, computed tomography, and magnetic resonance imaging were absent in more than 50% of the cases reviewed and were often not scheduled at optimal times.

Conclusion.—The medical record of newborns with poor outcomes frequently has a paucity of objective, evidence-based data. This leads to speculation and unethical expert testimony. The protocol will assist in confirming or refuting allegations of intrapartum asphyxia.

Level of Evidence.—III (Table 2).

▶ These authors propose a standardized template for clinical evaluation of infants with acute neonatal encephalopathy potentially attributable to perinatal

TABLE 2.—Proposed Clinical Work-up of Newborns Older Than 34 Weeks of Gestation With Alleged Perinatal Asphyxia in the First Week of Life

Clinical Work-up	Days of Life			
	1	2	3	7
1. Arterial cord gas	×			
2. Apgar scores at 10 and 15 (if 5 min-score is 6 or lower)	×			
3. Physical examination: newborn weight, length, and head circumference	×			
4. Placental pathology	×			
5. Complete blood count with differential, platelets, blood cultures	×			
6. Head ultrasonography	×	×		
7. NRBC	×	×	×	
8. PT, PTT, fibrinogen, LFT, creatinine, electrolytes, glucose, calcium, ECHO	×			
9. EEG	×			
10. Head MRI				×

NRBC, nucleated red blood cell; PT, prothrombin time; PTT, partial thromboplastin time; LFT, liver function tests; ECHO, echocardiogram; EEG, electroencephalogram; MRI, magnetic resonance imaging.

asphyxia (Table 2). Although the rationale for a few of the recommended items (clotting times and echocardiography) may not be compelling, the concept of a uniform and systematic approach to evaluation of these infants is. Additional studies for inborn errors of metabolism (serum acylcarnitine levels and urine organic acids, in particular), if they are not included in routine newborn screening, should also be considered. Using a convenience sample of infants whose cases came to litigation, the authors document stunningly low rates of collection of these essential data elements. If that sample is representative, current practice is seriously deficient. If the sample is not representative because most evaluations are in fact comprehensive, these observations would suggest that inadequate diagnostic assessment may actually lead to litigation. Facile attribution of encephalopathy to intrapartum asphyxia or inability to help parents understand the cause of their infant's disability—both more likely with incomplete diagnostic investigation—certainly predispose to litigation. Either way, efforts to implement these important recommendations should be considered urgent.

W. E. Benitz, MD

Apparent Life-Threatening Events in Presumably Healthy Newborns During Early Skin-to-Skin Contact
Andres V, Garcia P, Rimet Y, et al (La Conception Univ Hosp, Marseille, France; Regional Hosp, Aix en Provence, France; et al)
Pediatrics 127:e1073-e1076, 2011

The death or near death of a presumably healthy newborn in the delivery room is uncommon. We report here 6 cases of apparent life-threatening events (ALTEs) in the delivery room during the first 2 hours of life. In each case, the incident occurred in a healthy infant who was in a prone position on his or her mother's abdomen during early skin-to-skin contact. In most cases, the mother was primiparous, and in all cases the mother and infant were not observed during the initiation of skin-to-skin contact and breastfeeding. There are many benefits of early skin-to-skin contact and breastfeeding in the delivery room. However, in view of the risk of a rare but significant ALTE, we suggest that surveillance of newborns is needed. Although many ALTEs are apparently caused by obstruction, we suggest that a standardized investigational workup be performed after an ALTE.

▶ Here, 6 healthy newborns (all having had Apgar scores of 10 and 10 at 1 and 5 minutes, respectively), all undergoing skin-to-skin (kangaroo) care shortly after birth, suffered unexpected acute life-threatening episodes (ALTEs) that resulted in varying outcomes that included no known immediate detrimental outcomes in a couple of these infants and severe neurologic damage to death in others. Of interest is that these infants also experienced these episodes in the prone position, supporting the advantage of the supine position. Although there are many benefits of skin-to-skin contact and breast-feeding in the delivery room, this report underlines that during the immediate newborn period, even if the baby has excellent Apgar scores and initially appears very healthy, close observation is still in order. This may be accomplished with new nonintrusive monitoring or simply close direct observation by trained medical personnel in these first delicate hours after birth. The ALTEs in these babies do not argue against skin-to-skin care shortly after birth, but they do beg for close observation.

J. Neu, MD

Apparent Life-Threatening Events in Presumably Healthy Newborns During Early Skin-to-Skin Contact

Andres V, Garcia P, Rimet Y, et al (La Conception Univ Hosp, Marseille, France; Regional Hosp, Aix en Provence, France; et al)
Pediatrics 127:e1073-e1076, 2011

The death or near death of a presumably healthy newborn in the delivery room is uncommon. We report here 6 cases of apparent life-threatening events (ALTEs) in the delivery room during the first 2 hours of life. In each case, the incident occurred in a healthy infant who was in a prone position on his or her mother's abdomen during early skin-to-skin contact. In most cases, the mother was primiparous, and in all cases the mother and infant were not observed during the initiation of skin-to-skin contact and breast-feeding. There are many benefits of early skin-to-skin contact and breast-feeding in the delivery room. However, in view of the risk of a rare but significant ALTE, we suggest that surveillance of newborns is needed. Although many ALTEs are apparently caused by obstruction, we suggest that a standardized investigational workup be performed after an ALTE.

▶ Skin-to-skin contact for mothers and their healthy newborns soon after birth is an increasingly popular practice. Potential benefits include improved breast-feeding outcomes and cardiorespiratory stability and reduction in infant crying. It is also presumed to promote mother-infant attachment.

In the above clinical report, the authors describe 6 cases of acute life-threatening events (ALTEs) that occurred in presumably healthy newborns within 2 hours of birth during skin-to-skin contact. After normal physical examination findings, each of the infants had been placed in direct skin-to-skin contact with their mothers while in the prone position in the delivery room, and breast-feeding was initiated. The neonates were then left unsupervised with their mothers. Four of the infants required resuscitation, of which 3 incurred hypoxic-ischemic encephalopathy and subsequently died. Evaluations for an infectious, metabolic, cardiac, or central nervous system abnormality were unremarkable in each of the infants.

The most likely cause of ALTEs in the above cases was airway obstruction, which highlights the need to medically supervise newborns during early skin-to-skin contact to ensure proper positioning of the infant.

L. A. Papile, MD

Benefits of introducing universal umbilical cord blood gas and lactate analysis into an obstetric unit

White CRH, Doherty DA, Henderson JJ, et al (The Univ of Western Australia, Crawley, Australia; et al)

Aust N Z J Obstet Gynaecol 50:318-328, 2010

Background.—Current evidence suggests that umbilical arterial pH analysis provides the most sensitive reflection of birth asphyxia. However, there's debate whether umbilical cord blood gas analysis (UC-BGA) should be conducted on some or all deliveries.

Aim.—The aim of this study was to evaluate the impact of introducing universal UC-BGA at delivery on perinatal outcome.

Methods.—An observational study of all deliveries ≥20 weeks' gestation at a tertiary obstetric unit between January 2003 and December 2006. Paired UC-BGA was performed on 97% of deliveries ($n = 19,646$). Univariate and adjusted analysis assessed inter-year UC-BGA differences and the likelihood of metabolic acidosis and nursery admission.

Results.—There was a progressive improvement in umbilical artery pH, pO_2, pCO_2, base excess and lactate values in univariate and adjusted analyses ($P < 0.001$). There was a significant reduction in the newborns with an arterial pH <7.10 (OR = 0.71; 95%CI 0.53—0.95) and lactate >6.1 mmol/L (OR = 0.37; 95%CI 0.30—0.46). Utilising population specific 5th and 95th percentiles, there was a reduction in newborns with arterial pH less than 5th percentile (pH 7.12; OR = 0.75; 95%CI 0.59—0.96) and lactate levels greater than 95th percentile (6.7 mmol/L; OR = 0.37; 95%CI 0.29—0.49). There was a reduction in term (OR = 0.65; 95%CI 0.54—0.78), and overall (OR = 0.75; 95%CI 0.64—0.87) nursery admissions. These improved perinatal outcomes were independent of intervention rates.

Conclusions.—These data suggest that introduction of universal UC-BGA may result in improved perinatal outcomes, which were observed to be independent of obstetric intervention. We suggest that these improvements might be attributed to provision of biochemical data relating to fetal acid-base status at delivery influencing intrapartum care in subsequent cases.

▶ This report describes significant improvements in immediate postnatal measures of neonatal outcomes following introduction of universal umbilical cord blood gas analyses in a regional obstetrical unit. Among infants for whom cord blood gas results were validated, rates of acidosis (pH < 7.1 or < 5th percentile) and elevated lactate levels (> 6.1 mEq/L or > 95th percentile) were reduced. These effects remained significant after correction for potential obstetrical and intrapartum confounders. The proportion of infants for whom samples were validated increased between 2003 and 2006 (odds ratio [OR], 1.17; 95% confidence interval [CI], 1.07-1.27), but this did not account for improvement in pH or lactate levels, as more infants who required instrumental deliveries or neonatal intensive care unit (NICU) admission had valid samples as the staff gained experience. Comparison of the entire birth cohorts for 2003 and 2006 reveals that there were fewer infants with Apgar scores <4 at 5 minutes (OR, 0.26; 95% CI, 0.17-0.41) and fewer admissions to the nursery (OR, 0.88; 95% CI, 0.80-0.96) or special care nursery (OR, 0.81; 95% CI, 0.73-0.90). There were no changes in use of suction, oxygen, intubation, or cardiac massage in the delivery room or in the rate of NICU admission. However, use of bag-mask ventilation in the delivery room increased (OR, 1.28; 95% CI, 1.15-1.43). The authors consider alternative explanations for these associations but make a cogent case for a causal relationship. Immediate feedback on the physiological state of newborn infants may have had subtle but important effects on care practices, perhaps including more timely, but not more frequent, obstetrical interventions. The authors intend to test this hypothesis in additional hospitals.

W. E. Benitz, MD

Comparison of 5 experts and computer analysis in rule-based fetal heart rate interpretation
Parer JT, Hamilton EF (Univ of California, San Francisco; PeriGen, Princeton, NJ)
Am J Obstet Gynecol 203:451.e1-451.e7, 2010

Objective.—The purpose of this study was to measure agreement among 5 expert clinicians and a computerized method with the use of a strict fetal heart rate classification method.

Study Design.—Five providers independently scored 769 8-minute segments from the last 3 hours of 30 tracings with the use of a 5-tier color-coded framework that contains pattern descriptions and proposals for management. Computer analysis was performed with PeriCALM Patterns (PeriGen, Princeton, NJ) to detect and classify patterns.

Results.—The clinicians agreed exactly with the majority opinion in 57% (95% confidence interval [CI], 49–64%) of the segments and were within 1 color code in 89% (95% CI, 81–96%). The average proportion of agreement was 0.83 (95% CI, 0.73–0.94). Weighted Kappa scores averaged 0.58 (range, 0.48–0.68). The computer-based results were not statistically different: 0.87 and 0.52, respectively.

Conclusion.—These 5 clinicians achieved moderate-to-substantial levels of agreement overall using a strictly defined method to classify fetal heart rate tracings. The result of the computerized method was similar to the conclusions of these clinicians.

▶ Despite its many limitations and vagaries of interpretation, electronic fetal heart rate monitoring continues to be the primary method used for fetal assessment in the United States. Standardization of nomenclature associated with this perinatal technology continues to evolve, and the current nomenclature recommended by the National Institute of Child Health and Human Development (NICHD) has been adopted by professional perinatal organizations as the agreed-upon method for professional communication and documentation.[1] In 2008, the Eunice Kennedy Shriver NICHD, the American College of Obstetricians and Gynecologists, and the Society for Maternal-Fetal Medicine sponsored a second research planning workshop to review and clarify the 1997 definitions; to propose a standard classification system for fetal heart rate (FHR) tracings; to introduce, in consensus form, key concepts of intrapartum FHR interpretation; and to make recommendations for future research.[2] The second publication endorsed the definitions and the findings of the prior workshop, without making changes in the terminology. The various FHR patterns were classified into categories: I (normal), II (indeterminate), and III (abnormal); these were approximately the same gradations that were used in the clinical statement in the 1997 document. This has been called the 3-tier system, and it was espoused on the basis of simplicity and ease of teaching. These categories have been endorsed in the American College of Obstetrics and Gynecology practice bulletin of 2009.[3] Commenting on the updated guidelines Parer et al[4] suggested:

"The middle tier, called indeterminate Category II, which contains the variant FHR patterns seen most frequently, is vast and heterogeneous. We propose that this category can be subcategorized at least tentatively, based on evidence available from previously published studies. Such subcategorization will allow the organizations proposing management recommendations to more readily set up guidelines for graded interventions and clinical responses to the spectrum of FHR patterns, with the aim of minimizing fetal acidemia without excessive obstetric intervention. Such management algorithms will need to be tested by appropriately designed clinical studies."

Indeed, because of the difficulties in interpreting the indeterminate tier, some countries have moved on to a 5-tier system.

Computerized analysis of the fetal electrocardiogram has also been developed during the past 40 years. Software compatible with the previous definitions is available and was used to compare the computer interpretation of the FHR tracings with 5 experts in the previously mentioned report. As noted, "these 5 clinicians achieved moderate-to-substantial levels of agreement overall using a strictly defined method to classify fetal heart rate tracings."[4] There was exact agreement on only 57% of the records. However, there is the perception that adding computerized evaluation of electronic fetal heart tracings adds some degree of a safety net, and in the future, perhaps computer analysis will help identify aspects that are not visually apparent using mathematical models.

A. A. Fanaroff, MD, FRCPE, FRCP&CH

References

1. Electronic fetal heart rate monitoring: research guidelines for interpretation. National Institute of Child Health and Human Development Research Planning Workshop. *Am J Obstet Gynecol.* 1997;177:1385-1390.
2. Macones GA, Hankins GDV, Spong CY, Hauth J, Moore T. The 2008 National Institute of Child Health and Human Development Workshop Report on

Electronic Fetal Monitoring: update on definitions, interpretation, and research guidelines. *Obstet Gynecol.* 2008;112:661-666.
3. American College of Obstetricians and Gynecologists. ACOG Practice Bulletin No. 106: Intrapartum fetal heart rate monitoring: nomenclature, interpretation, and general management principles. *Obstet Gynecol.* 2009;114:192-202.
4. Parer JT, Ikeda T, King TL. The 2008 National Institute of Child Health and Human Development report on fetal heart rate monitoring. *Obstet Gynecol.* 2009;114:136-138.

Cord coiling, umbilical cord insertion and placental shape in an unselected cohort delivering at term: Relationship with common obstetric outcomes

Pathak S, Hook E, Hackett G, et al (Cambridge Univ Hosps NHS Foundation Trust, UK; Cambridge Univ Hosp NHS Trust, UK; et al)
Placenta 31:963-968, 2010

Background.—The position of the placental cord insertion, its shape and cord coiling are thought to be associated with perinatal outcome. This study derives indices describing the relationship of cord insertion to the placental centre, the shape of the placenta and cord coiling in placentas from unselected term pregnancies. Further, we investigate these indices in pregnancies affected by pre-eclampsia (PET), pregnancy induced hypertension (PIH), gestational diabetes mellitus (GDM) and delivery of a small for gestational age (SGA) baby.

Design/Methodology.—Eight hundred and sixty one unselected women with singleton pregnancy delivering at 37–42 weeks were prospectively recruited to this study. Placental axes and their relationship with the cord insertion were measured using digital photography and proprietary software. From these, the cord centrality (distance of umbilical cord insertion from the centre) and placental eccentricity (deviation of the placental shape from circular) were derived. The cord coiling index (number of coils in the cord divided by the length of cord in cm) was also calculated from manual measurements.

Results.—The mean value of cord centrality index was 0.36 (SD = 0.21) and of placental eccentricity 0.49 (SD = 0.17). Left direction of umbilical cord coiling was more common than right (79% vs 16.4%). The mean cord coiling index was 0.20 (SD = 0.09) coils/cm. The indices were constant between 37 and 42 weeks and were no different in the non-affected population compared to women with pre-eclampsia ($n = 17$), PIH, ($n = 27$), GDM ($n = 38$) or delivery of an SGA baby ($n = 54$).

Conclusion.—The cord centrality index that we derive suggests that the cord insertion is most commonly 'off centre', and eccentricity index that the placental shape is elliptical. Therefore, contrary to widely held belief, the cord does not normally insert centrally nor is the placenta normally round in shape. There is a preponderance of left sided coiling. There was no difference for any of the indices between the non-affected

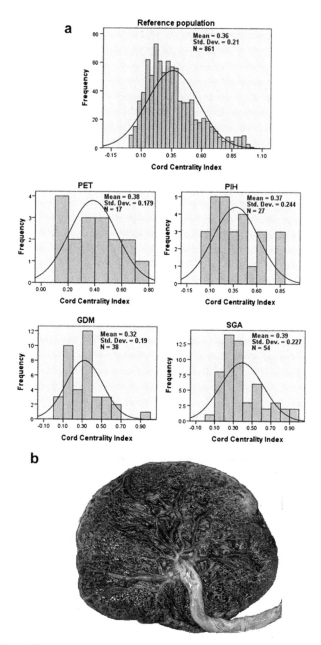

FIGURE 3.—(a) Frequency histograms of cord centrality index at 37–42 weeks; (b) explanatory photograph of a placenta showing cord centrality index of 0.36. (Reprinted from Pathak S, Hook E, Hackett G, et al. Cord coiling, umbilical cord insertion and placental shape in an unselected cohort delivering at term: relationship with common obstetric outcomes. *Placenta.* 2010;31:963-968 with permission from Elsevier.)

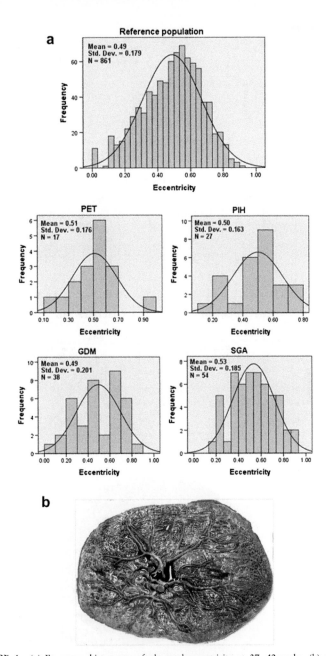

FIGURE 4.—(a) Frequency histograms of placental eccentricity at 37–42 weeks; (b) explanatory photograph of a placenta showing eccentricity of 0.49. (Reprinted from Pathak S, Hook E, Hackett G, et al. Cord coiling, umbilical cord insertion and placental shape in an unselected cohort delivering at term: relationship with common obstetric outcomes. *Placenta*. 2010;31:963-968 with permission from Elsevier.)

pregnancies and pregnancies affected by pre-eclampsia, PIH, GDM and SGA (Figs 3 and 4).

▶ This is an interesting article that focuses on the macroelements rather than the microelements of the placenta and umbilical cord. It is a companion article from the same team that published about placental weight, digitally derived placental dimensions at term, and their relationship to birth weight. They reported that there is close, although not perfect, agreement between the manual and digital placental measurements. Birth weight is strongly correlated with placental weight and circumference at term.

In the previously mentioned article,[1] mathematical modeling is used to determine the shape of the placenta, insertion of the cord, and the degree and direction of coiling of the cord (Figs 3 and 4). The authors are confident that their data

"dispel the widely held beliefs that the placenta is, in its natural and normal state, circular, and that the cord normally inserts into its center. Further, coiling index, cord centrality index and eccentricity in this study was not any different in the adverse pregnancy outcomes (pregnancy induced hypertension, preeclampsia, gestational diabetes and intra-uterine growth retardation) that we have defined compared to the data from pregnancies, which were not affected by those outcomes."

Much attention has been devoted to coiling, or lack thereof, of the umbilical cord. Both hypocoiling and excessive or hypercoiling of the cord have been associated with adverse perinatal outcome. Hypocoiling has been associated with trisomies, gestational diabetes, preterm delivery, fetal death, and increased intrapartum complications as well as interventional deliveries for fetal distress, velamentous cord insertion, single umbilical artery, and neonatal depression requiring resuscitation. Hypercoiling has mainly been associated with intra-uterine growth restriction, gestational diabetes, and fetal asphyxia. Abnormal cord coiling has also been found with thrombotic problems in the placenta and cord. The umbilical cord coiling index that we report is the equivalent of a coil every 5 cm, with a preponderance of left-sided coiling (79%), similar to the published literature. Coiling index is probably one of the most frequently reported umbilical cord—related parameters in high-risk pregnancies. Preeclampsia and gestational diabetes have been suggested as maternal risk factors for abnormal data; however, they showed no significant difference in umbilical cord coiling index with preeclampsia, PIH, GDM, or SGA compared with the reference population.

A. A. Fanaroff, MD, FRCPE, FRCP&CH

Reference

1. Pathak S, Jessop F, Hook L, Sebire NJ, Lees CC. Placental weight, digitally derived placental dimensions at term and their relationship to birth weight. *J Matern Fetal Neonatal Med.* 2010;23:1176-1182.

Cost-effectiveness of elective induction of labor at 41 weeks in nulliparous women

Kaimal AJ, Little SE, Odibo AO, et al (Harvard Med School, Boston, MA; Washington Univ in St Louis, MO; et al)
Am J Obstet Gynecol 204:137.e1-137.e9, 2011

Objective.—To investigate the cost-effectiveness of elective induction of labor at 41 weeks in nulliparous women.

Study Design.—A decision analytic model comparing induction of labor at 41 weeks vs expectant management with antenatal testing until 42 weeks in nulliparas was designed. Baseline assumptions were derived from the literature as well as from analysis of the National Birth Cohort dataset and included an intrauterine fetal demise rate of 0.12% in the 41st week and a cesarean rate of 27% in women induced at 41 weeks. One-way and multiway sensitivity analyses were conducted to examine the robustness of the findings.

Results.—Compared with expectant management, induction of labor is cost-effective with an incremental cost of $10,945 per quality-adjusted life year gained. Induction of labor at 41 weeks also resulted in a lower rate of adverse obstetric outcomes, including neonatal demise, shoulder dystocia, meconium aspiration syndrome, and severe perineal lacerations.

Conclusion.—Elective induction of labor at 41 weeks is cost-effective and improves outcomes.

▶ Increasing awareness of the adverse fetal consequences of prolonged gestation during the 1980s led to the adoption of strategies for more intensive fetal monitoring regimens or induction of labor when gestation reached 41 weeks. By the early 1990s, randomized trials had demonstrated lower rates of cesarean section and of cesarean section performed because of fetal distress in women managed by induction at 41 weeks rather than with serial antenatal monitoring.[1] However, sample sizes were not sufficient to demonstrate a reduction in perinatal mortality. With accrual of additional data in the last decade, meta-analysis demonstrated a statistically significant reduction in perinatal mortality with labor induction at or after 41 weeks' gestation (odds ratio [OR], 0.30; 95% confidence interval [CI], 0.09-0.99). This may be attributable to a reduced incidence of meconium aspiration syndrome (OR, 0.39; 95% CI, 0.21-0.75).[2] The recent American Congress of Obstetricians and Gynecologists Clinical Management Guidelines on Management of Postterm Pregnancy[3] (reaffirmed in 2009) noted that, "data suggest that routine induction at 41 weeks of gestation has fetal benefit without incurring the additional maternal risks of a higher rate of cesarean delivery. This conclusion has not been universally accepted." This decision analysis represents an attempt to promote broader acceptance of that conclusion and more general adoption of labor induction at 41 completed weeks of gestation. These authors conclude that labor induction is cost-effective, but not cost-saving, in postterm pregnancies. However, the cost analysis model predicts a 98% reduction in perinatal mortality, which is at the upper margin of the estimates of efficacy obtained from the meta-analysis.[2] This may cast some doubt on the main conclusions of this modeling, which are likely to be strongly dependent on the magnitude of this benefit. While it may be true that nothing good happens after 41 weeks, as many of us believe, there is still room for doubt that outcomes are improved by a policy of routine induction at 41 weeks. If prolonged gestation is a sign of fetal compromise rather than a risk factor, induced labor or even cesarean delivery cannot be expected to modify the underlying pathology. Until these questions can be more definitively resolved, obstetrical management of post-term pregnancies is likely to remain heterogeneous and subject to patient preferences for expectant management.

W. E. Benitz, MD

References

1. Hannah ME, Hannah WJ, Hellmann J, Hewson S, Milner R, Willan A. Induction of labor as compared with serial antenatal monitoring in post-term pregnancy. A randomized controlled trial. The Canadian Multicenter Post-term Pregnancy Trial Group. *N Engl J Med.* 1992;326:1587-1592.
2. Gülmezoglu AM, Crowther CA, Middleton P. Induction of labour for improving birth outcomes for women at or beyond term. *Cochrane Database Syst Rev.* 2006;4. CD004945.
3. ACOG Committee on Practice Bulletins-Obstetrics. ACOG Practice Bulletin. Clinical management guidelines for obstetricians-gynecologists. Number 55, September 2004. Management of Postterm Pregnancy. *Obstet Gynecol.* 2004;104:639-646.

Crying and Breathing by Extremely Preterm Infants Immediately After Birth

O'Donnell CPF, Kamlin COF, Davis PG, et al (The Royal Women's Hosp, Melbourne, Victoria, Australia)

J Pediatr 156:846-847, 2010

We reviewed videos of 61 extremely preterm infants taken immediately after birth. The majority cried (69%) and breathed (80%) without intervention. Most preterm infants are not apneic at birth.

▶ Until recently, in many centers the prevailing practice was to intubate and deliver surfactant to preterm infants less than 29 weeks' gestation. This was not the practice in Melbourne, Australia, where digital videotaping of the infants who were anticipated to need resuscitation was performed. In this way, the events and procedures could be well documented and correlated with the status of the infant. The clinical observations were hence derived from review of these tapes.

This is only a brief report; nonetheless, it is an important report since it debunks popular myths regarding the respiratory efforts of extremely immature and low birth weight infants. The video camera has become commonplace in the delivery room, and it is not only in the hands of the parents or relatives. More and more investigators are using this technique to provide feedback on the quality of resuscitation and to do research. Contrary to popular belief,

O'Donnell et al demonstrate that 80% of babies delivered at less than 28 weeks' gestation and a birth weight less than 1000 g were crying (69%) or breathing without assistance at delivery. Indeed they noted that many infants were intubated even though they were breathing and had a heart rate greater than 100 bpm on continuous positive airway pressure (CPAP). It was the heavier, more mature infants delivered vaginally that exhibited this behavior. These data should slow down those who rush to intubate, ventilate, and administer surfactant to all extremely preterm infants and provide equipoise for the ongoing studies comparing early CPAP with surfactant administration, when intubation and mechanical ventilation became necessary, to intubation and surfactant administration with the goal of rapid extubation. In the Study to Understand Prognoses and Preferences for Outcomes and Risks of Treatments (SUPPORT) trial,[1] Finer et al reported a lower mortality during hospitalization in the 24 to 25 weeks' strata for the CPAP infants (24%) versus 32% for the surfactant/intubation group, and more CPAP infants were alive and off mechanical ventilation by day 7 of life. Fewer in the CPAP group required intubation or postnatal steroids. They concluded that the study provided support for the use of CPAP in preterm infants as an alternative to intubation and surfactant.

A. A. Fanaroff, MD, FRCPE, FRCP&CH

Reference

1. SUPPORT Study Group of the Eunice Kennedy Shriver NICHD Neonatal Research Network, Finer NN, Carlo WA, Walsh MC, et al. Early CPAP versus surfactant in extremely preterm infants. *N Engl J Med.* 2010;362:1970-1979.

Delivery mode shapes the acquisition and structure of the initial microbiota across multiple body habitats in newborns
Dominguez-Bello MG, Costello EK, Contreras M, et al (Univ of Puerto Rico, San Juan; Univ of Colorado, Boulder; Venezuelan Inst for Scientific Res, Caracas, Venezuela; et al)
Proc Natl Acad Sci U S A 107:11971-11975, 2010

Upon delivery, the neonate is exposed for the first time to a wide array of microbes from a variety of sources, including maternal bacteria. Although prior studies have suggested that delivery mode shapes the microbiota's establishment and, subsequently, its role in child health, most researchers have focused on specific bacterial taxa or on a single body habitat, the gut. Thus, the initiation stage of human microbiome development remains obscure. The goal of the present study was to obtain a community-wide perspective on the influence of delivery mode and body habitat on the neonate's first microbiota. We used multiplexed 16S rRNA gene pyrosequencing to characterize bacterial communities from mothers and their newborn babies, four born vaginally and six born via Cesarean section. Mothers' skin, oral mucosa, and vagina were sampled 1 h before delivery, and neonates' skin, oral mucosa, and nasopharyngeal aspirate were sampled <5 min, and meconium 24 h, after delivery. We found that in direct contrast to the highly differentiated communities of their mothers, neonates harbored bacterial communities that were undifferentiated across multiple body habitats, regardless of delivery mode. Our results also show that vaginally delivered infants acquired bacterial communities resembling their own mother's vaginal microbiota, dominated by *Lactobacillus, Prevotella,* or *Sneathia spp.*, and C-section infants harbored bacterial communities similar to those found on the skin surface, dominated by *Staphylococcus, Corynebacterium,* and *Propionibacterium spp.* These findings establish an important baseline for studies tracking the human microbiome's successional development in different body habitats following different delivery modes, and their associated effects on infant health.

▶ In the United States, the rate of cesarean delivery has risen 48% since 1996, reaching a level of 31.8% in 2007.[1] This trend is reflected in many parts of the world, with the most populous country in the world, China, approaching 50%[2] and some private clinics in Brazil approaching 90%.[3] While many of these cesarean deliveries are indicated for medical reasons, many are clearly being done for nonmedical indications. Are there unseen consequences to all these potentially unnecessary deliveries? The article by Dominguez-Bello et al uses newly developed non—culture-based techniques to identify acquisition of microbes in newborns delivered by vaginal versus cesarean delivery. Additional evidence is accumulating that the early exposure of microbes to the newborn is highly consequential in terms of development of the immune system and subsequent illness. Is it possible that the increasing delivery rate by cesarean delivery could have long-lasting consequences? Epidemiologic data are beginning to support this concept with odds ratios of allergies, asthma, and celiac disease being significantly higher in children who were delivered by cesarean delivery.[4-6] There may be numerous confounding factors including early exposure to antibiotics in cesarean-delivered infants as well as subsequent differences in lifestyle that contribute to these increases. Nevertheless, the findings of altered microbiota in vaginal- versus cesarean-delivered infants, coupled to the epidemiologic findings, should cause alarm. If a causal link actually exists between cesarean delivery and these conditions, the subsequent morbidity incurred needs to go into the decision-making process. In addition, the high financial burden required to care for these conditions needs to be considered in subsequent cost analyses and policy decisions on reimbursement for cesarean deliveries.

J. Neu, MD

References

1. Hamilton BE, Martin JA, Ventura SJ. Births: preliminary data for 2007. *Natl Vital Stat Rep.* 2009;57:1-21.
2. Lumbiganon P, Laopaiboon M, Gülmezoglu M, et al. Method of delivery and pregnancy outcomes in Asia: the WHO global survey on maternal and perinatal health 2007-08. *Lancet.* 2010;375:490-499.

3. Rebelo da Rocha F, da Rocha CM, Cortes TR, Dutra CL, Kac G. High cesarean prevalence in a national population-based study in Brazil: the role of private practice. *Acta Obstet Gynecol Scand.* 2010;89:903-908.
4. Björkstén B. Effects of intestinal microflora and the environment on the development of asthma and allergy. *Springer Semin Immunopathol.* 2004;25:257-270.
5. Negele K, Heinrich J, Borte M, et al. Mode of delivery and development of atopic disease during the first 2 years of life. *Pediatr Allergy Immunol.* 2004;15:48-54.
6. Debley JS, Smith JM, Redding GJ, Critchlow CW. Childhood asthma hospitalization risk after cesarean delivery in former term and premature infants. *Ann Allergy Asthma Immunol.* 2005;94:228-233.

Effect of the interval between onset of sustained fetal bradycardia and cesarean delivery on long-term neonatal neurologic prognosis

Kamoshita E, Amano K, Kanai Y, et al (Kitasato Univ, Sagamihara City, Kanagawa, Japan)

Int J Gynaecol Obstet 111:23-27, 2010

Objective.—To examine the effect of the interval between onset of sustained fetal bradycardia and cesarean delivery on long-term neonatal neurologic prognosis.

Method.—A retrospective observational case-series performed with patients who had sudden-onset and sustained (<100 beats per minute) fetal bradycardia during labor. Fetal heart rate was monitored closely until cesarean delivery. The effect of the interval between the onset of bradycardia and delivery on neonatal neurologic prognosis was examined.

Results.—Among 2267 deliveries in 2002−2003 at Kitasato University Hospital, 19 pregnancies met the inclusion criteria. Episodes of fetal bradycardia were due to umbilical cord prolapse (n = 5), placental abruption (n = 4), uterine rupture (n = 3), maternal respiratory failure (n = 1), and other causes (n = 6). Mean onset of fetal bradycardia to delivery interval (BDI) was 20.5 ± 8.9 minutes. Mean decision-to-cesarean delivery interval was 11.4 ± 3.9 minutes. BDI was negatively correlated with umbilical arterial pH at delivery. There were 3 postnatal deaths. Neurologic assessment at the age of 2 years revealed that 15 of 16 children were neurologically normal. When the BDI was less than 25 minutes, all term pregnancies led to normal neonatal neurologic development.

Conclusion.—In the event of sustained intrapartum fetal bradycardia, delivery by emergency cesarean within 25 minutes improved long-term neonatal neurologic outcome.

▶ The prognostic implications of a prolonged fetal bradycardia leading to emergency delivery are of interest to treating physicians, to new parents, and too often to the medicolegal process. This article adds to the regrettably sparse literature on the matter, which essentially consists of only one prior publication.[1] Addition of the 19 infants in this report brings the total number of subjects described to 74. Although the authors of the earlier report stated that "significant neonatal morbidity occurred when ≥18 minutes elapsed between the onset of prolonged deceleration and delivery," examination of their data indicates that the probability of neurological injury or death exceeds 50% only after an interval of 21 minutes or more. Those data are largely consistent with this report, which suggests that good outcomes can be expected after intrapartum bradycardia episodes up to 25 minutes in duration. The small difference may result from use of a different criterion for defining the onset of bradycardia (fetal heart rate < 100 beat per minute in the more recent series vs < 90 in the earlier one). As previously reported, acidemia and increased base deficit were associated with increased risk of adverse outcomes, but neither pH < 6.9 nor base deficit > 20 mEq/L had a positive predictive value > 50%. More data on these relationships would be quite valuable.

W. E. Benitz, MD

Reference

1. Leung AS, Leung EK, Paul RH. Uterine rupture after previous cesarean delivery: maternal and fetal consequences. *Am J Obstet Gynecol.* 1993;169:945-950.

Effects of shoulder dystocia training on the incidence of brachial plexus injury

Inglis SR, Feier N, Chetiyaar JB, et al (Jamaica Hosp, Med Ctr, NY)
Am J Obstet Gynecol 204:322.e1-322.e6, 2011

Objective.—We sought to determine whether implementation of shoulder dystocia training reduces the incidence of obstetric brachial plexus injury (OBPI).

Study Design.—After implementing training for maternity staff, the incidence of OBPI was compared between pretraining and posttraining periods using both univariate and multivariate analyses in deliveries complicated by shoulder dystocia.

Results.—The overall incidence of OBPI in vaginal deliveries decreased from 0.40% pretraining to 0.14% posttraining $(P < .01)$. OBPI after shoulder dystocia dropped from 30% to 10.67% posttraining $(P < .01)$. Maternal body mass index $(P < .01)$ and neonatal weight $(P = .02)$ decreased and head-to-body delivery interval increased in the posttraining period $(P = .03)$. Only shoulder dystocia training remained associated with reduced OBPI $(P = .02)$ after logistic regression analysis. OBPI remained less in the posttraining period $(P = .01)$, even after excluding all neonates with birthweights >2 SD above the mean.

Conclusion.—Shoulder dystocia training was associated with a lower incidence of OBPI and the incidence of OBPI in births complicated by shoulder dystocia.

▶ Shoulder dystocia is an uncommon (1 in 1500 deliveries) but potentially catastrophic intrapartum event. Although risk factors such as maternal diabetes, obesity, and macrosomia can be identified, shoulder dystocia in most patients occurs without identifiable risk factors. It is thus crucial that the obstetric team be well trained and coordinated to take care of the emergency if and when it arises, as the consequences (injury to the brachial plexus) can be devastating and permanent.

Development of and research into simulation-based medical education have evolved and matured over the past 40 years. McGaghie et al[1] have reviewed the key elements that include (1) feedback, (2) deliberate practice, (3) curriculum integration, (4) outcome measurement, (5) simulation fidelity, (6) skill acquisition and maintenance, (7) mastery learning, (8) transfer to practice, (9) team training, (10) high-stakes testing, (11) instructor training, and (12) educational and professional context. Goffman et al[2] have demonstrated that obstetric emergency simulation training can improve physicians' communication skills, at all levels of training, and should be incorporated into labor and delivery quality improvement measures. Crofts et al[3] investigated completeness and accuracy of record keeping by comparison of documentation and actual events, recorded on video and through a force-monitoring device, during simulated shoulder dystocia. Thirty-nine physicians and 71 midwives documented their management of a shoulder dystocia simulation on paper used in their hospital (simple notepaper or preformatted form). Documentation was compared with video recording of each simulation and an electronic record of force applied during delivery. To no one's surprise, maneuvers performed were well documented. However, head-to-body delivery interval and force applied were not documented accurately in most simulated deliveries. Use of a preformatted sheet appeared to improve completeness, but not accuracy, of documentation.

Given all these theoretical and practical training sessions, it is encouraging to read that Inglis et al were able to reduce the incidence of brachial plexus injury 3-fold by incorporating simulation training. This despite delivering bigger babies from heavier mothers.

As the simulation technology advances, we must take advantage of the new models. However, ultimately it is the team-building skills and communication that will make a difference when emergencies occur.

A. A. Fanaroff, MD, FRCPE, FRCP&CH

References

1. McGaghie WC, Issenberg SB, Petrusa ER, Scalese RJ. A critical review of simulation-based medical education research: 2003-2009. *Med Educ.* 2010;44: 50-63.
2. Goffman D, Heo H, Pardanani S, Merkatz IR, Bernstein PS. Improving shoulder dystocia management among resident and attending physicians using simulations. *Am J Obstet Gynecol.* 2008;199:294.e1-294.e5.
3. Crofts JF, Bartlett C, Ellis D, Fox R, Draycott TJ. Documentation of simulated shoulder dystocia: accurate and complete? *BJOG.* 2008;115:1303-1308.

Heat Loss Prevention in Very Preterm Infants in Delivery Rooms: A Prospective, Randomized, Controlled Trial of Polyethylene Caps
Trevisanuto D, Doglioni N, Cavallin F, et al (Univ of Padua, Italy)
J Pediatr 156:914-917, 2010

Objective.—To evaluate in preterm infants whether polyethylene caps prevent heat loss after delivery better than polyethylene occlusive wrapping and conventional drying.

Study Design.—This was a prospective, randomized, controlled trial of infants <29 weeks' gestation including 3 study groups: (1) experimental group in which the heads of patients were covered with a polyethylene cap; (2) polyethylene occlusive skin wrap group; and (3) control group in which infants were dried. Axillary temperatures were compared at the time of admission to the neonatal intensive care unit (NICU) immediately after cap and wrap removal and 1 hour later.

Results.—The 96 infants randomly assigned (32 covered with caps, 32 wrapped, 32 control) completed the study. Mean axilllary temperature on NICU admission was similar in the cap group (36.1°C ± 0.8°C) and wrap group (35.8°C ± 0.9°C), and temperatures on admission to the NICU were significantly higher than in the control group (35.3°C ± 0.8°C; $P < .01$). Infants covered with polyethylene caps (43%) and placed in polyethylene bags (62%) were less likely to have a temperature <36.4°C on admission to the NICU than control infants (90%). In the cap group, temperature 1 hour after admission was significantly higher than in the control group.

Conclusions.—For very preterm infants, polyethylene caps are comparable with polyethylene occlusive skin wrapping to prevent heat loss after delivery. Both these methods are more effective than conventional treatment.

▶ Thermal regulation immediately after delivery remains a critical component of the care of preterm infants in particular. Despite the evidence and desire to keep babies warm, many still get chilled in the delivery room and are cool on admission to the neonatal intensive care unit. As previously reported, Trevisanuto et al conducted a well-designed prospective randomized trial and concluded that for very preterm infants, polyethylene caps are comparable to polyethylene occlusive skin wrapping to prevent heat loss after delivery. Both these methods are more effective than conventional treatment; however, many babies are still admitted with low temperatures. Perhaps we need to combine these 2 methods?

McCall et al[1] performed a Cochrane review to assess the efficacy and safety of interventions designed for the prevention of hypothermia in preterm or low birth weight infants applied within 10 minutes after birth in the delivery suite compared with routine thermal care.

Barriers to heat loss such as plastic wraps or bags were effective in reducing heat losses in infants less than 28 weeks' gestation but not in infants between 28 to 31 weeks' gestation. Plastic caps were effective in reducing heat losses in infants less than 29 weeks' gestation. There was insufficient evidence to suggest that either plastic wraps or plastic caps reduce the risk of death within the hospital stay. There was no evidence of significant differences in other clinical outcomes for either the plastic wrap/bag or the plastic cap comparisons. Stockinet caps were not effective in reducing heat losses.

Also, external heat sources including a transwarmer mattress and skin-to-skin care (SSC) were shown to be effective in reducing the risk of hypothermia when compared with conventional incubator care.

The authors concluded that plastic wraps or bags, plastic caps, SSC, and transwarmer mattresses all keep preterm infants warmer, leading to higher temperatures on admission to neonatal units and less hypothermia. However, the small numbers of infants and studies and the absence of long-term follow-up mean that firm recommendations for clinical practice cannot be given.

Simon et al[2] compared thermal mattresses (sodium acetate) with a plastic wrap for extremely low gestational age newborns (ELGANs) between 24 and 28 weeks' gestation with a birth weight less than 1250 g. Although the mattress was superior to the plastic wrap and both improve the thermal status of ELGANs, they concluded that all current interventions fall short of fully protecting all these vulnerable patients from thermal stress. So we are forced to conclude that keeping vulnerable preterm infants warm is problematic even when recommended routine thermal care guidelines are followed in the delivery suite. We need to try harder, and a good starting point might be to warm the delivery rooms.

A. A. Fanaroff, MD, FRCPE, FRCP&CH

References

1. McCall EM, Alderdice F, Halliday HL, Jenkins JG, Vohra S. Interventions to prevent hypothermia at birth in preterm and/or low birthweight infants. *Cochrane Database Syst Rev.* 2010;(3). CD004210.
2. Simon P, Dannaway D, Bright B, et al. Thermal defense of extremely low gestational age newborns during resuscitation: exothermic mattresses vs polyethylene wrap. *J Perinatol.* 2011;31:33-37.

Management of Intrapartum Fetal Heart Rate Tracings
American College of Obstetricians and Gynecologists
Obstet Gynecol 116:1232-1240, 2010

Intrapartum electronic fetal monitoring (EFM) is used for most women who give birth in the United States. As such, clinicians are faced daily with the management of fetal heart rate (FHR) tracings. The purpose of this document is to provide obstetric care providers with a framework for evaluation and management of intrapartum EFM patterns based on the new three-tiered categorization (Box 1).

▶ A workshop sponsored by the National Institutes of Health, American College of Obstetricians and Gynecologists (ACOG), and the Society for

---

Box 1: Three-Tiered Fetal Heart Rate Interpretation System

Category I

- Category I FHR tracings include all of the following:
- Baseline rate: 110–160 beats per minute
- Baseline FHR variability: moderate
- Late or variable decelerations: absent
- Early decelerations: present or absent
- Accelerations: present or absent

Category II

Category II FHR tracings includes all FHR tracings not categorized as Category I or Category III. Category II tracings may represent an appreciable fraction of those encountered in clinical care. Examples of Category II FHR tracings include any of the following:

Baseline rate
- Bradycardia not accompanied by absent baseline variability
- Tachycardia

Baseline FHR variability
- Minimal baseline variability
- Absent baseline variability with no recurrent decelerations
- Marked baseline variability

Accelerations
- Absence of induced accelerations after fetal stimulation

Periodic or episodic decelerations
- Recurrent variable decelerations accompanied by minimal or moderate baseline variability
- Prolonged deceleration more than 2 minutes but less than10 minutes
- Recurrent late decelerations with moderate baseline variability
- Variable decelerations with other characteristics such as slow return to baseline, overshoots, or "shoulders"

Category III

Category III FHR tracings include either
- Absent baseline FHR variability and any of the following:
  — Recurrent late decelerations
  — Recurrent variable decelerations
  — Bradycardia
- Sinusoidal pattern

Abbreviation: FHR, fetal heart rate.
Macones GA, Hankins GD, Spong CY, Hauth J, Moore T. The 2008 National Institute of Child Health and Human Development workshop report on electronic fetal monitoring: update on definitions, interpretation, and research guidelines. Obstet Gynecol 2008;112:661–6.

Maternal-Fetal Medicine in 2008 led to publication of revised recommendations for terminology describing and classifying fetal heart rate monitoring findings.[1] The revised nomenclature (Box 1) scrupulously avoids terms with potential unintended implications (eg, fetal distress, nonreassuring). This new practice guideline from ACOG provides recommendations for management of fetal heart rate tracings in each of the 3 newly defined categories of fetal heart rate findings. Category I findings are normal and require no intervention. Category II findings, including all tracings not classified as category I or III, require evaluation for underlying causes, measures to correct those as indicated, continued monitoring, and reevaluation. Category III tracings are abnormal, reflecting an increased probability of fetal acidemia, neonatal encephalopathy, and subsequent cerebral palsy (although the predictive value for neurodevelopment impairment is low). In these instances, timely initiation of intrauterine resuscitation measures should be accompanied by preparation for prompt delivery if the category III findings remain unresolved. To ensure accurate communication with our obstetrical colleagues, neonatologists must become familiar with this terminology and its implications.

W. E. Benitz, MD

Reference

1. Macones GA, Hankins GD, Spong CY, Hauth J, Moore T. The 2008 National Institute of Child Health and Human Development workshop report on electronic fetal monitoring: update on definitions, interpretation, and research guidelines. *Obstet Gynecol.* 2008;112:661-666.

Milking Compared With Delayed Cord Clamping to Increase Placental Transfusion In Preterm Neonates: A Randomized Controlled Trial
Rabe H, for the Brighton Perinatal Study Group (Brighton and Sussex Univ Hosps, UK; et al)
Obstet Gynecol 117:205-211, 2011

Objective.—To compare two strategies to enhance placento-fetal blood transfusion in preterm neonates before 33 weeks of gestation.

Methods.—We recruited women at risk for singleton preterm deliveries. All delivered before 33 completed weeks of gestation. In this single-center trial, women were randomized to either standard treatment (clamping the cord for 30 seconds after delivery) or repeated (four times) milking of the cord toward the neonate. Exclusion criteria included inadequate time to obtain consent before delivery, known congenital abnormalities of the fetus, Rhesus sensitization, or fetal hydrops.

Results.—Of 58 neonates included the trial, 31 were randomized to cord clamping and 27 were randomized to repeated milking of the cord. Mean birth weight was 1,263 ± 428 g in the clamping group and 1,235 ± 468 g in the milking group, with mean gestational age of 29.2 ± 2.3 weeks and 29.5 ± 2.7 weeks, respectively. Mean hemoglobin values for each group at 1 hour after birth were 17.3 g/L for clamping and 17.5 g/L for milking ($P = .71$). There was no significant difference in number of neonates undergoing transfusion (clamping group, 15; milking group, 17; $P = .40$) or the median number of transfusions within the first 42 days of life (median [range]: clamping group 0 [0–7]; milking group 0 [0–20]; $P = .76$).

Conclusion.—Milking the cord four times achieved a similar amount of placento-fetal blood transfusion compared with delaying clamping the cord for 30 seconds.

Clinical Trial Registration.—National Research Register UK, www.nihr.ac.uk/Pages/default.aspx, N0051177741 (Fig 3 and Box 1).

▶ The timing of umbilical cord clamping at birth is still controversial. In the modern era of medicine, the cord has been clamped early to facilitate resuscitation and stabilization of infants; recently, however, delayed cord clamping has been supported by physicians because it allows for the physiological transfer of blood from the placenta to the infant. Most deliveries take place in the

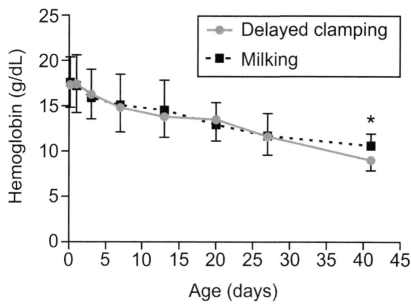

Age (days)

FIGURE 3.—Hemoglobin values during the first 6 weeks of life. Values are analyzed only until the neonate's first transfusion (if any). No significant differences were identified between the groups except for infants aged 42 days ($P=.01$), which was confirmed by repeated-measures analysis of variance. (Reprinted from Rabe H, Jewison A, Alvarez RF, et al. Milking compared with delayed cord clamping to increase placental transfusion in preterm neonates: a randomized controlled trial. *Obstet Gynecol.* 2011;117:205-211. Copyright © 2011 by the American College of Obstetricians and Gynecologists.)

Box 1: Local Unit Guidelines for Prevention of Anemia of Prematurity Including Thresholds for Donor Blood Transfusions*

General Preventive Measures to Avoid Blood Transfusions in Preterm Neonates Before 34 Weeks of Gestation

Delayed cord clamping time 30 seconds at birth (entered into labor ward protocol as first step of prevention)
Start parenteral nutrition as early as possible (12—36 hours)
Start oral iron 6 mg/kg if milk tolerated at 5 mL/kg per feed from day 7 to 10 onward
No Rh erythropoietin

Transfusion Algorithm: Hemoglobin Threshold for Transfusions (g/L)[†]

Neonates aged younger than 7 days: artificial ventilation 115; spontaneous breathing 100
Neonates aged 8 to 14 days: artificial ventilation 100; spontaneous breathing 85
Neonates aged older than 14 days: artificial ventilation 85; spontaneous breathing 80

*These guidelines were used during the study period.
[†]Data from Kirpalani H, Whyte RK, Andersen C, Asztalos EV, Heddle N, Blajchman MA, et al. The Premature Infants in Need of Transfusion (PINT) study: a randomized, controlled trial of a restrictive (low) compared with liberal (high) transfusion threshold for extremely low birth weight infants. J Pediatr 2006;149:301—7.

---

home and in rural areas where there is no rush to clamp the cord; however, in developed countries, with almost a third of deliveries being by cesarean section, the cord is clamped and cut early, mainly for convenience. Some would argue that the practice of early clamping of the cord relates to facilitating resuscitation, but in the absence of a placental separation with abruption or known blood group incompatibilities, there is no urgency to clamp the cord. Indeed delayed cord clamping has continued to show benefits and little, if any, risk in preterm infants.[1,2] The benefits of delayed cord clamping in preterm infants include increased blood volume,[1,3] improved circulatory and respiratory function, reduced need for blood transfusions, improved cerebral oxygenation, and reduced intraventricular hemorrhage and sepsis.[4] The cord blood of extremely preterm infants is a rich source of hematopoietic progenitor cells, such as hematopoietic stem cells, endothelial cell precursors, mesenchymal progenitors, and multipotent/pluripotent lineage stem cells; hence, the merit of delayed cord clamping has been magnified. Tolosa et al[5] referred to this aspect of delayed cord clamping as "realizing mankind's first stem cell transfer and propose that it should be encouraged in normal births." The extra endowment of progenitor cells resulting from delayed cord clamping has the potential to both increase red blood cell (RBC) production and boost host immune defenses through production of leukocytes. Furthermore, delayed cord clamping has a wide benefit-to-harm ratio, as no adverse effects of delayed cord clamping for preterm infants have been identified, except higher peak serum bilirubin concentration.[2] Delayed cord clamping does not affect survival of preterm infants.[1] Regrettably, there has been only one report examining the impact of delayed cord clamping on neurodevelopmental outcome.[6] The investigators found evidence of improved motor scores at 7 months corrected age in preterm infants who had received delayed cord clamping at birth.

There has been a shift in thinking to explore milking of the umbilical cord as an alternative to delayed cord clamping that may provide the same benefits without the need to delay resuscitation.[7,8] Hosono et al,[7] after a small randomized trial, reported that the milked group was less likely to have needed RBC transfusion, and those who needed transfusions had a decreased number (mean [SD]) of RBC transfusions (milked group 1.7 [3.0] vs controls 4.0 [4.2]; $P = .02$). The initial mean (SD) hemoglobin value was higher in the milked group (165 [14] g/L) than in the controls (141 [16] g/L; $P < .01$). Mean (SD) blood pressure at admission was significantly higher in the milked group (34 [9] mm Hg) than in the controls (28 [8] mm Hg; $P = .03$). There was no significant difference in mortality between the groups. The milked group had a shorter duration of ventilation or supplemental oxygen than the control group. In a subsequent report,[8] Hosono et al documented that the blood pressure was higher in the first 6 hours of life and urine output was greater in the cord-milked group. No adverse outcomes were reported.[8]

Rabe et al have expanded the experience with their single-center comparative trial documenting equivalent outcomes with milking and delayed clamping of the cord (30 seconds). Box 1, which delineates measures to reduce the need for transfusions and the criteria for blood transfusions, is a rational approach to transfusions in preterm infants. Fig 3 documents a statistically higher hemoglobin in the cord-milked group at age 42 days. The stage has now been set for the next set of randomized trials, which need to be adequately powered to answer the various questions posed. Rabe et al have leaned toward cord milking. My opinion is that whereas the results are encouraging, too few babies have been studied and I would favor comparing delayed clamping with milking in future studies, with, of course, prolonged follow-up.

A. A. Fanaroff, MD, FRCPE, FRCP&CH

References

1. Rabe H, Reynolds G, Diaz-Rossello J. A systematic review and meta-analysis of a brief delay in clamping the umbilical cord of preterm infants. *Neonatology*. 2008;93:138-144.
2. Reynolds GJ. Beyond sweetness and warmth: transition of the preterm infant. *Arch Dis Child Fetal Neonatal Ed*. 2008;93:F2-F3.
3. Strauss RG, Mock DM, Johnson KJ, et al. A randomized clinical trial comparing immediate versus delayed clamping of the umbilical cord in preterm infants: short-term clinical and laboratory endpoints. *Transfusion*. 2008;48:658-665.
4. Mercer JS, Vohr BR, McGrath MM, Padbury JF, Wallach M, Oh W. Delayed cord clamping in very preterm infants reduces the incidence of intraventricular hemorrhage and late-onset sepsis: a randomized, controlled trial. *Pediatrics*. 2006;117:1235-1242.
5. Tolosa JN, Park DH, Eve DJ, Klasko SK, Borlongan CV, Sanberg PR. Mankind's first natural stem cell transplant. *J Cell Mol Med*. 2010;14:488-495.
6. Mercer JS, Vohr BR, Erickson-Owens DA, Padbury JF, Oh W. Seven-month developmental outcomes of very low birth weight infants enrolled in a randomized controlled trial of delayed versus immediate cord clamping. *J Perinatol*. 2010;30:11-16.
7. Hosono S, Mugishima H, Fujita H, et al. Umbilical cord milking reduces the need for red cell transfusions and improves neonatal adaptation in infants born at less than 29 weeks' gestation: a randomised controlled trial. *Arch Dis Child Fetal Neonatal Ed*. 2008;93:F14-F19.
8. Hosono S, Mugishima H, Fujita H, et al. Blood pressure and urine output during the first 120 h of life in infants born at less than 29 weeks' gestation related to umbilical cord milking. *Arch Dis Child Fetal Neonatal Ed*. 2009;94:F328-F331.

Neonatal and Neurodevelopmental Outcomes of Very Low Birth Weight Infants with Histologic Chorioamnionitis

Hendson L, Russell L, Robertson CMT, et al (Univ of Alberta, Edmonton, Canada; Women and Children's Health Res Inst, Edmonton, Alberta, Canada; et al)
J Pediatr 158:397-402, 2011

Objective.—To determine survival and neurodevelopmental outcomes at 18 months corrected age among very low birth weight infants ≤32 weeks gestation with histologic chorioamnionitis.

Study Design.—Observational, regionalized, single-center cohort study with prospective follow-up.

Results.—Of the 628 infants meeting the selection criteria, 303 (48%) were born to mothers with evidence of histologic chorioamnionitis. Neonates with histologic chorioamnionitis were of lower gestational age and birth weight. On univariate analysis, they were more likely to have hypotension, bronchopulmonary dysplasia, severe intraventricular hemorrhage, severe retinopathy of prematurity, early-onset sepsis, and death. Infants with histologic chorioamnionitis were more likely to have any neurodevelopmental impairment, specifically, mental delay with a lower mental developmental index. When adjusting for perinatal variables, histologic chorioamnionitis had a protective effect on mortality rates (adjusted OR = 0.44, 95% CI: 0.24-0.8; $P = .01$; n = 619), had a nonsignificant effect on neurodevelopmental impairment (adjusted odds ratio = 1.33, 95% CI: 0.82-2.17; $P = .25$; n = 496), and was associated with a 4-point lower mental developmental index at 18-months follow-up (adjusted difference -3.93, 95% CI: -7.52 to -0.33; $P = .03$; n = 496).

Conclusions.—Although infants with histologic chorioamnionitis were at an increased risk for death and neurodevelopmental impairment, after multivariate analyses, histologic chorioamnionitis was not associated with adverse long-term outcomes. Results suggest fetal protection from treatment-responsive maternal infection and inflammation.

▶ This article was chosen for review because of the implication derived by the authors that histologic chorioamnionitis is protective against subsequent mortality and neurodevelopmental delays. This seems to be a counterintuitive outcome.

In this study, a large number of very low birth weight infants' placentas (n = 670) were analyzed to detect the presence or absence of histologic chorioamnionitis and to relate this outcome using univariate and multivariate statistical methods to subsequent death and various morbidities, including neurodevelopmental outcomes. A univariate comparison was also made between babies with chorioamnionitis alone and those with chorioamnionitis and a fetal inflammatory response (defined by polymorphonuclear leucocytes invading the umbilical cord or vasculitis of the umbilical cord or chorion). The univariate analysis showed that chorioamnionitis was associated with increased mortality and mental delays. Those babies who also had fetal inflammatory response had higher mortality and worse neurodevelopmental outcomes than those with chorioamnionitis alone. This was then analyzed in a multiple regression model adjusting for 7 confounders, such as peripartum antibiotic exposure, antenatal corticosteroids, mode of delivery, etc. When the multiple regressions were done taking the confounders into consideration, the results surprisingly showed lower mortality in those babies with chorioamnionitis. The authors state "after adjusting for 7 perinatal covariates, histologic chorioamnionitis was protective for death." This statement implies causality, and the mechanism of chorioamnionitis being by itself protective is difficult to understand. One possible explanation is that mild disease may induce a chronic stress response that stimulates protection against other factors such as respiratory distress and infection. Could the chorioamnionitis, when mild and not associated with a full-blown fetal inflammatory response, actually be protective through conditioning the infant against subsequent insults? One explanation offered by the authors is that this may occur via the adrenocortical axis by stimulating cortisol. Could an alternative explanation be via other mechanisms such as tolerization through toll-like receptor pathways? The fact that fetal inflammatory response resulted in worse outcomes than chorioamnionitis alone supports the notion that this is a spectrum, and if a little inflammation confined to the placental might be associated with protection, when this becomes amplified in a fetal inflammatory response, it appears to be detrimental.

J. Neu, MD

Neonatal medical admission in a term and late-preterm cohort exposed to magnesium sulfate
Greenberg MB, Penn AA, Thomas LJ, et al (Stanford Univ, CA; Univ of Missouri School of Medicine, St Louis; et al)
Am J Obstet Gynecol 204:515.e1-515.e7, 2011

Objective.—The purpose of this study was to estimate neonatal intensive care unit and special care unit (NICU) admission rates and care needs among term and late-preterm neonates who are exposed to antenatal magnesium sulfate.

Study Design.—We conducted a retrospective cohort study of all singleton neonates of ≥35 weeks' gestation who were exposed immediately antenatally to magnesium sulfate for maternal eclampsia prophylaxis (August 2006 through July 2008).

Results.—Fifty-one of 242 neonates (21.1%) who, at ≥35 weeks' gestation, had been exposed to antenatal magnesium sulfate were admitted to the NICU. NICU admission was associated in a dose-dependent fashion with total hours and mean dose of magnesium: >12 hours exposure, odds ratio, 2.81 (95% confidence interval, 1.31−6.03); >30 g exposure, odds ratio, 2.59 (95% confidence interval, 1.22−5.51). Infants in NICU who were diagnosed with hypermagnesemia required fluid or nutritional support more frequently (91.3% vs 39.3%; *P* < .001) than those without hypermagnesemia.

Conclusion.—Antenatal magnesium sulfate exposure is associated with NICU admission among term and late-preterm neonates in a dose-dependent fashion. Fluid and nutritional assistance commonly are needed in this cohort.

▶ I am becoming convinced that magnesium is the second most abundant element on earth after oxygen. At least it seems that way in the delivery room.

This retrospective cohort study examined the relationship of antenatal magnesium sulfate exposure in mothers with preeclampsia (with pregnancies of 35 weeks or longer) to subsequent hospitalization of their babies in the neonatal intensive care unit (NICU). Not surprisingly, more than 20% of the babies required neonatal intensive care, and there was a dose-dependent response (both total dose and exposure time > 12 hours). In addition, infants with hypermagnesemia required more frequent administration of intravenous fluids and parenteral nutrition.

Neonatal diagnoses related to magnesium exposure included respiratory distress (35%), hypotonia (12%), and hypothermia (8%). Data were analyzed to look for a relationship between the total magnesium sulfate dose received by the mother and the probability of an NICU admission of the infant.

The results of the study clearly support the notion that magnesium sulfate is a respiratory and gastrointestinal depressant and if neonatal serum levels are high enough, ventilatory support and parenteral fluids and nutrition will be necessary. Since there seems to be 1 NICU admission for every 5 to 6 neonates exposed to magnesium sulfate above the thresholds of 30 g or 12 hours, these data are very useful for decision making in the delivery room.

The number needed to harm was 5; this is concerning, not only for term and late-preterm infants but maybe even more so for the very preterm infants who are being exposed to antenatal magnesium for neuroprotection. It will be incumbent upon us to evaluate magnesium-related morbidities in this population.

S. M. Donn, MD

Neonatal morbidity after documented fetal lung maturity in late preterm and early term infants
Kamath BD, Marcotte MP, Defranco EA (Cincinnati Children's Hosp Med Ctr, OH; Univ of Cincinnati School of Medicine, OH)
Am J Obstet Gynecol 204:518.e1-518.e8, 2011

Objective.—Fetal lung maturity often is used as the sole criterion that late preterm infants are ready for postnatal life. We therefore tested the hypothesis that fetal lung maturity testing does not predict the absence of morbidity in late preterm infants.

Study Design.—We performed a retrospective cohort study to examine 152 infants who were born in the late preterm (34 0/7 to 36 6/7 weeks) and early term (37 0/7 to 38 6/7 weeks) periods after mature fetal lung indices and compared them with 262 infants who were born at ≥39 weeks' gestation and who were matched by mode of delivery.

Results.—Despite documented fetal lung maturity, infants who were born at <39 weeks had significantly higher rates of neonatal morbidities compared with infants who were born at ≥39 weeks' gestation. After adjustment for significant covariates, we found that infants who were born at <39 weeks' gestation had an increased risk of composite adverse outcome (odds ratio, 3.66; 95% confidence interval, 1.48−9.09; $P < .01$).

Conclusion.—Fetal lung maturity testing is insufficient to determine an infant's readiness for postnatal life.

▶ It has always troubled me when an obstetrical colleague proclaims that "The baby is 'mature,'" based solely on indices of fetal lung maturation. I wish I had gotten a dollar for every time in the last 30 years that I have argued the contrary.

This study confirms what every neonatologist has known: "Fetal lung maturity testing is insufficient to determine an infant's readiness for postnatal life." The authors performed a retrospective cohort study on 152 infants who were either late preterm (34-36 6/7 weeks) or term (37-38 6/7 weeks) delivered after obtaining amniotic fluid analysis predictive of lung maturity and compared them with randomly selected babies 39-40 6/7 weeks.

The rate of composite adverse neonatal outcome was statistically significantly higher in both the late preterm and term strata compared with the control group. Other neonatal complications, including hypoglycemia, need for intravenous fluids, gavage feeding, phototherapy, sepsis evaluation, neonatal intensive care unit admission, and supplemental oxygen, were also statistically higher.

Although retrospective cohort studies are often criticized for selection bias, it is still reassuring to see some scientific support for something we have all observed and known.

S. M. Donn, MD

Significant effects on neonatal morbidity and mortality after regional change in management of post-term pregnancy
Grunewald C, Håkansson S, Saltvedt S, et al (Karolinska Inst, Stockholm, Sweden; Umeå Univ Hosp, Sweden; et al)
Acta Obstet Gynecol Scand 90:26-32, 2011

Objective.—To evaluate the effects on neonatal morbidity of a regional change in induction policy for post-term pregnancy from 43^{+0} to 42^{+0} gestational weeks (GWs).

Design and Setting.—Nationwide retrospective register study between 2000 and 2007.

Population.—All singleton pregnancies with a gestational age of $>41^{+2}$ GW ($n = 119,198$).

Methods.—All Swedish counties were divided into three groups where study group allocation was designated by the proportion of pregnancies $>42^{+2}$ GW among all pregnancies of $>41^{+2}$ GW. Stockholm county formed a separate group.

Main Outcome Measures.—Perinatal morbidity.

Results.—In counties with the most active management, 19% of pregnancies $>41^{+2}$ GW were delivered at $>42^{+2}$ GW during 2000—2004 compared to 7.1% in 2005—2007. In the least active counties, corresponding figures were 21.0% compared to 19.4%. During 2005—2007, the odds ratios for meconium aspiration and 5-minute Apgar score of ≤6 in the least compared to most active counties, were 1.55 (95% CI: 1.03—2.33) and 1.26 (95% CI: 1.06—1.51). In Stockholm $>42^{+2}$ GW seen among pregnancies of $>41^{+2}$ GW decreased from 21.0% in 2000—2004 to 5.9% in 2005—2007. Reduced perinatal death risks by 48%, meconium aspiration of 51% and low Apgar scores by 31% in 2005—2007 compared with 2000—2004 were observed. Rates of operative deliveries at $>41^{+2}$ GW in Stockholm were unaltered.

Conclusion.—A significant reduction in perinatal morbidity was found, with no influence on operative delivery rates for post-term pregnancy in

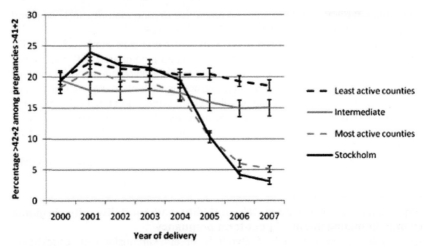

FIGURE 2.—The proportion of pregnancies >42^{+2} gestational weeks among all pregnancies >41^{+2} gestational weeks by study group and year of delivery. The vertical bars represent 95% confidence intervals. (Reprinted from Grunewald C, Håkansson S, Saltvedt S, et al. Significant effects on neonatal morbidity and mortality after regional change in management of post-term pregnancy. *Acta Obstet Gynecol Scand.* 2011;90:26-32. Reprinted by permission of the publisher [Taylor & Francis Ltd, http://www.tandf.co.uk/journals].)

Stockholm. We advocate a nationwide change toward more active management of post-term pregnancies (Fig 2).

▶ Where randomized trials, meta-analyses, and decision analyses have failed to provide definitive answers, these investigators from Sweden describe quasiexperimental results that take advantage of a well-implemented regional change in obstetrical practices within their integrated health care delivery system. In 2005, the 5 obstetrical services in Stockholm adopted a policy of offering induction of labor at 42 + 0/7 weeks rather than 43 + 0/7 weeks of gestation. In several other regions of Sweden, including Västra Götaland, the most populous county, management patterns (induction at 43 + 0/7 weeks) did not change. This afforded an opportunity to compare outcomes both between eras (before and after the practice change) and across counties (classified as most, least, and intermediately active adopters of earlier labor induction). The results are illuminating.

The proportion of women who remained pregnant at 41 + 2/7 weeks who were undelivered at 42 + 2/7 weeks declined slightly in the least active counties and modestly in the intermediate counties, but quite markedly in the counties that adopted earlier induction most aggressively (Fig 2). In Stockholm, this proportion was reduced by about 80%, so that 97% of women undelivered at 41 + 2/7 weeks were delivered within 1 week by 2007. Rates of meconium aspiration and 5-minute Apgar score less than or equal to 6 were not different in high and low adopter counties in 2000 to 2004, and did not differ between 2000 to 2004 and 2005 to 2007 in low adopter counties, but were significantly lower in high adopter counties in 2005 to 2007 (both as compared with the earlier era and to low adopter counties). In Stockholm, adoption of earlier induction was associated with lower rates of meconium aspiration (odds ratio [OR] 0.50, 95% confidence interval [CI] 0.30-0.83), 5-minute Apgar score less than or equal to 6 (OR 0.70, 95% CI 0.56-0.88), and death before 45 weeks postmenstrual age (OR 0.52, 95% CI 0.32-0.85). Similar results were obtained for the high adopter counties collectively, but were not seen in the low adopter regions. These conclusions were not altered when the data were stratified by maternal age, parity, and smoking. Notably, the Stockholm results were achieved without any increase in cesarean section or instrumental vaginal delivery rates.

The authors calculate that active management of 585 and 243 pregnancies would be needed to prevent 1 case of meconium aspiration or low Apgar score, respectively. A similar calculation might suggest a number-needed-to-treat (NNT) of approximately 800 to prevent 1 perinatal death. That estimate should be met with caution because a similar (but not statistically significant) decline in early mortality also occurred in low adopter counties. These large NNT estimates leave the question of cost-efficacy unresolved. These data also do not address the matter of induction at 41 rather than 42 weeks' gestation.[1] Nonetheless, this work constitutes a substantial step forward by providing robust evidence that intervention to induce delivery when pregnancies go past term can improve neonatal outcomes.

W. E. Benitz, MD

Reference

1. Kaimal AJ, Little SE, Odibo AO, et al. Cost-effectiveness of elective induction of labor at 41 weeks in nulliparous women. *Am J Obstet Gynecol.* 2011;204: 137.e1-137.e9.

Sudden Deaths and Severe Apparent Life-Threatening Events in Term Infants Within 24 Hours of Birth

Poets A, Steinfeldt R, Poets CF (Univ Hosp, Tuebingen, Germany)
Pediatrics 127:e869-e873, 2011

Objective and Design.—To determine the incidence of and possible risk factors for unexpected sudden infant deaths (SID) and severe apparent life-threatening events (S-ALTE) that occurred within 24 hours of birth. This was a monthly epidemiologic survey.

Patients and Methods.—Throughout 2009, every pediatric department in Germany was asked to report such cases of unexplained SID or S-ALTE in term infants after a good postnatal adaptation (10-minute Apgar score ≥8) to the Surveillance Unit for Rare Pediatric Conditions in Germany. The latter has a capture rate of > 95%. S-ALTE was defined as acute cyanosis/pallor and unconsciousness, requiring bagging, intubation and/or cardiac compressions. Hospitals that reported a case were asked to return an anonymized questionnaire and discharge letter as well as the autopsy protocol in SID cases.

Results.—Of 43 cases reported, 17 fulfilled entry criteria, yielding an incidence of 2.6 in 100 000 live births. There were 7 deaths (ie, 1.1/ 100 000); 6 of the 10 S-ALTE infants were neurologically abnormal at discharge. Twelve infants were found lying on their mother's chest or abdomen, or very close to and facing her. Nine events occurred in the first 2 hours after birth; 7, were only noticed by a health professional despite the mother being present and awake.

Conclusions.—SID or S-ALTE may occur in the first 24 hours after birth, particularly within the first 2 hours. Events seem often related to a potentially asphyxiating position. Parents may be too fatigued or otherwise not able to assess their infant's condition correctly. Closer observation during these earliest hours seems warranted.

▶ Immediate Kangaroo Mother Care (KMC), an intervention following childbirth whereby the newborn is placed skin-to-skin (STS) on the mother's chest to promote thermal regulation, breast-feeding, and maternal-newborn bonding, is being taught in very low-income countries to improve newborn health and survival. The expert group of the International Network on KMC concluded:

> "Current evidence allows the following general statements about KMC in affluent and low-income settings: KMC enhances bonding and attachment; reduces maternal postpartum depression symptoms; enhances infant physiologic stability and reduces pain, increases parental sensitivity to infant cues; contributes to the establishment and longer duration of breastfeeding and has positive effects on infant development and infant/parent interaction. Therefore, intrapartum and postnatal care in all types of settings should adhere to a paradigm of non separation of infants and their mothers/families."[1]

This is the general consensus, and KMC has become very popular. It is thus very disturbing to read that early STS contact in the prone position in primigravidas may be associated with an apparent life-threatening event (ALTE). In fact, this rather old-fashioned—looking article with detailed case descriptions gives food for thought and reminds us that we really need to be very vigilant when newly born infants are with first-time mothers so soon after birth. This is another report from France, but I am reasonably certain these happenings are occurring throughout the world. The other report from France was from Dageville et al,[2] who prospectively evaluated the incidence of neonatal ALTEs and sudden unexpected deaths during the first 2 hours after birth over a 1-year period in all the maternities of the French region of Provence, Alpes, Côte d'Azur, which included all presumably healthy full-term neonates. Among 62 968 live births, there were 2 neonatal ALTEs and no neonatal sudden unexpected death. The overall rate of neonatal ALTEs and unexpected deaths was, thus, 0.032 per 1 000 live births. Three potential risk factors were identified: STS contact, primiparous mother, and mother and baby alone in the delivery room. They concluded that rather than inhibiting early STS contact, the maternity staff must be prepared to pay particular attention to an STS infant when left alone with its primiparous mother.

We would concur with Poets et al that standardized investigations be implemented after the occurrence of ALTEs to better identify the risk factors. It is, of course, bizarre to consider that the newborn baby lying face down on the mother's chest is at risk of dying. The risk is minute, but it is greater than zero.

A. A. Fanaroff, MD, FRCPE, FRCP&CH

References

1. Nyqvist KH, Anderson GC, Bergman N, et al. Expert Group of the International Network on Kangaroo Mother Care. State of the art and recommendations. Kangaroo mother care: application in a high-tech environment. *Breastfeed Rev.* 2010;18:21-28.
2. Dageville C, Pignol J, De Smet S. Very early neonatal apparent life-threatening events and sudden unexpected deaths: incidence and risk factors. *Acta Paediatr.* 2008;97:866-869.

11 Miscellaneous

A critical review of premature infants with inguinal hernias: optimal timing of repair, incarceration risk, and postoperative apnea
Lee SL, Gleason JM, Sydorak RM (Harbor-UCLA Med Ctr, Torrance, CA; Los Angeles Med Ctr, CA)
J Pediatr Surg 46:217-220, 2011

Background/Purpose.—This study evaluated the optimal timing for repair, incarceration risk, and postoperative apnea rate in premature infants with inguinal hernias.

Methods.—This was a retrospective review of premature infants undergoing inguinal hernia repairs from 2006 to 2008.

Results.—One hundred seventy-two patients were identified. Mean gestational age was 30.7 weeks, and mean birth weight was 1428 g. At repair, mean postconceptional age was 46.6 weeks with mean weight of 3688 g. Elective repairs were performed on 127 patients. Thirty-five patients were discharged with a known hernia, and none developed incarceration. No postoperative apnea episodes occurred in any of these 127 patients. Forty-five patients had herniorrhaphy before discharge from the neonatal intensive care unit (NICU) with a median postoperative hospitalization of 8 days (2-51 days). Thirteen percent required prolonged (>48 hours) intubation after repair. Of 172 patients, 8 (4.6%) developed incarcerated hernia. Five incarcerations occurred in the NICU before discharge, and 3 patients had incarceration as their initial presentation.

Conclusions.—There is minimal risk of postoperative apnea for premature infants undergoing elective inguinal hernia repair. The risk of incarceration in premature infants discharged from the NICU with a known hernia is low. Herniorrhaphy before discharge from the NICU was associated with a prolonged hospital stay.

▶ Inguinal hernias occur in 1% to 3% of all children. They occur more often in premature infants, in boys much more frequently than girls, and more often on the right side than the left side, but they can also occur on both sides. Hernias occur more often in children with a parent or sibling who had a hernia as an infant, or in children with cystic fibrosis, developmental dysplasia of the hip, undescended testes, or urethral abnormalities. A hernia needs to be differentiated from a hydrocele, although both may occur together.

Inguinal hernia repair is one of the most common surgical procedures performed on premature infants. Improved survival rates in the neonatal intensive care unit (NICU) have led to an increase in the incidence of premature infants with inguinal hernias. My impression has been that with the new bronchopulmonary dysplasia (BPD) the giant inguinal hernias so prevalent with the old barotrauma-induced BPD have become less frequent. The report from Lee et al is indeed a critical review of their experience. Above all, the decision to perform herniorrhaphy before or after discharge from the NICU was based on the surgeon's preference. Thus, these 2 study groups potentially represented a quite dissimilar cohort of patients. Additionally, this retrospective study did not examine the rate of testicular atrophy or gonadal necrosis, usually 1% to 4% atrophy rate. Lee et al have not followed the group so they do not know recurrence rates. Another weakness was that few patients had regional anesthesia, which may have affected the apnea rate, although a recent meta-analysis showed no difference in regional versus general anesthesia in former preterm infants undergoing herniorrhaphy.[1] "Finally, reasons for the prolonged intubation in infants undergoing repair before NICU discharge were not clearly documented and we were not able to determine the true apnea rate in this subset of patients" (Lee et al).

Murphy et al[2] reported on a 5-year, retrospective chart review of all premature infants undergoing inguinal hernia repair. Because the literature suggested that postoperative apneas occurred in up to 49% of premature infants undergoing anesthesia for inguinal hernia repair, their practice is to monitor all of these babies in the intensive care unit (ICU) overnight after surgery. In addition to the considerable expense to the health care system, these cases are cancelled if no ICU bed is available. Murphy et al[2] reported that only 5 (4.7%) of 126 had apnea after the repair. (This is similar to Lee et al's experience.) All 5 had a previous history of significant apnea, and these babies were less mature with a more complicated hospital course than the other babies in the study. Murphy et al[2] concluded that selective use of postoperative ICU monitoring for high-risk patients could result in significant resource and cost savings to the health care system.

Melo-Filho et al[3] analyzed the role of BPD in the outcome of premature infants who underwent herniorrhaphy. Unfortunately, they included only 17 babies with BPD in their total series of 52 patients. They found no difference between the group with BPD and the group without BPD with regard to postoperative respiratory complications.

Overall, the encouraging finding in Lee et al's study is that the risk of incarceration in preterm babies sent home with a hernia is very low; however, it is necessary to carefully instruct the families regarding management of the hernia, teach them how to reduce it, and to come immediately for help if it cannot be reduced.

A. A. Fanaroff, MD, FRCPE, FRCP&CH

References

1. Craven PD, Badawi N, Henderson-Smart DJ, et al. Regional (spinal, epidural, caudal) versus general anesthesia in preterm infants undergoing inguinal herniorrhaphy in early infancy. *Cocharane Database Syst Rev.* 2003;(3). CD003669.
2. Murphy JJ, Swanson T, Ansemino M, Milner R. The frequency of apneas in premature infants after inguinal hernia repair: do they need overnight monitoring in the intensive care unit? *J Pediatr Surg.* 2008;43:865-868.

3. Melo-Filho AA, de Fátima Assunção Braga A, Calderoni DR, et al. Does broncho-pulmonary dysplasia change the postoperative outcome of herniorrhaphy in premature babies? *Paediatr Anaesth.* 2007;17:431-437.

A structured review of the recent literature on the economic consequences of preterm birth

Petrou S, Eddama O, Mangham L (Univ of Oxford, Headington, UK; London School of Hygiene and Tropical Medicine, UK)
Arch Dis Child Fetal Neonatal Ed 96:F225-F232, 2011

Although survival rates for preterm infants have greatly improved over the last three to four decades, these infants remain at risk of developing a broad range of short-term and long-term complications. Despite the large body of work on the clinical sequelae of preterm birth, relatively little is known about its economic consequences. This paper represents a structured review of the recent scientific literature on the economic consequences of preterm birth for the health services, for other sectors of the economy, for families and carers and, more broadly, for society. A total of 2497 studies were identified by a pretested literature search strategy, 52 of which were included in the final review. Of these 52 studies, 19 reported the costs associated with the initial period of hospitalisation, 35 reported costs incurred following the initial hospital discharge (without providing costs for the entire remaining period of childhood), four of which also reported costs associated with the initial period of hospitalisation, while two reported costs incurred throughout childhood. The paper highlights the variable methodological quality of this body of literature. The results of the studies included in the review are summarised and critically appraised. The paper also highlights gaps in our current knowledge of the topic and identifies requirements for further research in this area.

▶ The authors searched through computerized databases to identify a group of 52 studies on the economic impact of preterm birth. All studies based their estimates on preexisting accounting, clinical, or administrative data. Despite heterogeneous study samples and methodology, several trends were evident. Costs were inversely related to gestational age, rising dramatically for the smallest preterm survivors (< 26 weeks' gestation). As expected, the cost of the initial hospitalization of infants who survived was more than that of those who died; surgery also added to the expense. Postdischarge costs were related to travel, lost income, rehospitalizations, and the costs of caring for an infant with chronic disability. Some of the cost estimates had large variances associated with the influence of outliers, that is, extremely ill infants who survived with severe disabilities. Overall, despite the high individual costs for the smallest and sickest babies, the bulk of total cost through childhood resided among modestly premature infants, who are much more common. None of this is surprising to a neonatologist; instead, one wonders if these measurable dollar amounts do not pale beside the emotional and social burdens borne by the families of small preterm infants. In their summary, the authors note that "cost data alone cannot identify the most efficient allocation of finite health resources. Rather, it is information of incremental costs and incremental health gains" that should be used to maximize benefit.

D. A. Bateman, MD, MS

Closely Spaced Pregnancies Are Associated With Increased Odds of Autism in California Sibling Births
Cheslack-Postava K, Liu K, Bearman PS (Columbia Univ, NY)
Pediatrics 127:246-253, 2011

Objective.—To determine whether the interpregnancy interval (IPI) is associated with the risk of autism in subsequent births.

Methods.—Pairs of first- and second-born singleton full siblings were identified from all California births that occurred from 1992 to 2002 using birth records, and autism diagnoses were identified by using linked records of the California Department of Developmental Services. IPI was calculated as the time interval between birth dates minus the gestational age of the second sibling. In the primary analysis, logistic regression models were used to determine whether odds of autism in second-born children varied according to IPI. To address potential confounding by unmeasured family-level factors, a case-sibling control analysis determined whether affected sibling (first versus second) varied with IPI.

Results.—An inverse association between IPI and odds of autism among 662 730 second-born children was observed. In particular, IPIs of <12, 12 to 23, and 24 to 35 months were associated with odds ratios (95% confidence intervals) for autism of 3.39 (3.00–3.82), 1.86 (1.65–2.10), and 1.26 (1.10–1.45) relative to IPIs of ≥36 months. The association was not mediated by preterm birth or low birth weight and persisted across categories of sociodemographic characteristics, with some attenuation in the oldest and youngest parents. Second-born children were at increased risk of autism relative to their firstborn siblings only in pairs with short IPIs.

Conclusions.—These results suggest that children born after shorter intervals between pregnancies are at increased risk of developing autism; the highest risk was associated with pregnancies spaced <1 year apart.

▶ An apparent epidemic of autism has captured the interest of the lay public as well as pediatricians and clinical and laboratory scientists. Epidemiological studies have been fueled by the recognition that environmental factors might play a more prominent role than does genetics. In this publication, Dr Cheslack-Postava and colleagues, in analyses of California Birth Master Files of more than 600 000 children born in California between 1992 and 2002, demonstrate an increased risk of autism in the second-born of pairs of singleton children linked by short interpregnancy intervals (IPI) of fewer than 24 months, with the greatest risk for those born at IPIs of fewer than 12 months. The association persisted across sociodemographic factors and was not explained by increased rates of prematurity or low birth weight. This study adds another to the list of known risks of short IPI, including fetal growth restriction,[1] birth defects,[2] preterm delivery and low birth weight,[3] and gestational diabetes[4] in the second pregnancy.

L. J. Van Marter, MD, MPH

References

1. Salihu HM, August EM, Mbah AK, et al. The impact of birth spacing on subsequent feto-infant outcomes among community enrollees of a federal healthy start project. *J Community Health*. 2011 Jun 9 [Epub ahead of print].
2. Kwon S, Lazo-Escalante M, Villaran MV, Li CI. Relationship between interpregnancy interval and birth defects in Washington State. *J Perinatol*. 2011 May 5 [Epub ahead of print].
3. de Weger FJ, Hukkelhoven CW, Serrooyen J, Te Velde ER, Smits LJ. Advanced maternal age, short interpregnancy interval, and perinatal outcome. *Am J Obstet Gynecol*. 2011;204:421.e1-421.e9.
4. Ehrlich SF, Hedderson MM, Feng J, Davenport ER, Gunderson EP, Ferrara A. Change in body mass index between pregnancies and the risk of gestational diabetes in a second pregnancy. *Obstet Gynecol*. 2011;117:1323-1330.

Does Timing Matter? A National Perspective on the Risk of Incarceration in Premature Neonates with Inguinal Hernia
Lautz TB, Raval MV, Reynolds M (Northwestern Univ, Chicago, IL)
J Pediatr 158:573-577, 2011

Objectives.—To determine the incidence of inguinal hernia in premature neonates and identify risk factors for incarceration.

Study Design.—The 2003 and 2006 Kids' Inpatient Databases were queried for diagnoses indicative of premature birth and inguinal hernia.

Results.—Inguinal hernia was diagnosed during the birth hospitalization in 1463 ± 87 of 49 273 ± 1561 premature neonates (3%). Male sex, gestational age, birth weight, and prolonged mechanical ventilation were associated with inguinal hernia (all $P < .01$). Incarceration occurred in 176 of 1123 premature neonates (16%) who underwent hernia repair during the birth hospitalization. Delaying repair beyond 40 weeks postconceptual age doubled the risk of incarceration (21%), as compared with 36 to 39 weeks (9%) or <36 weeks (11%, $P = .002$). Sex, race, and insurance were not associated with incarceration.

Conclusion.—The risk of incarceration is doubled in premature neonates with inguinal hernia when repair is delayed beyond 40 weeks postconceptual age. This increased incarceration risk should be one of the factors considered when deciding on the optimal timing of inguinal hernia repair.

▶ Decisions about timing of inguinal hernia repair in preterm infants are often based on preferences of individual surgeons, albeit informed by experience and historical data. This review of data extracted from a national administrative data set provides additional information to guide these choices. The data reflect the well-known practice heterogeneity: of 2009 preterm infants with inguinal hernia diagnosed during their initial hospitalization, repair was performed during that hospital stay in 1123 (55.9%) and during a subsequent hospitalization in 886 (44.1%). Infants with incarceration were more likely to have undergone repair at ≥40 weeks' postmenstrual age (PMA) and after the initial hospital discharge. Because the rate of incarceration after 40 weeks' PMA (21%) was double that in infants who underwent repair earlier, there appears to be an advantage for repair before the initial hospital discharge. Repair before 40 weeks' PMA may be advisable for infants who remain hospitalized beyond their expected date of delivery. That potential benefit must be balanced against potential adverse effects of anesthesia and surgery in these infants, whose prolonged hospitalization likely reflects significant comorbidities and therefore increased risks of perioperative complications.

W. E. Benitz, MD

Early Weaning From Incubator and Early Discharge of Preterm Infants: Randomized Clinical Trial
Zecca E, Corsello M, Priolo F, et al (Catholic Univ of the Sacred Heart, Rome, Italy)
Pediatrics 126:e651-e656, 2010

Objective.—The goal was to assess the feasibility of earlier weaning from the incubator for preterm infants.

Methods.—This was a prospective, randomized study with preterm infants with birth weights of <1600 g who were admitted to a neonatal subintensive ward. Findings for 47 infants who were transferred from an incubator to an open crib at >1600 g (early transition group) were compared with those for 47 infants who were transferred from an incubator to an open crib at >1800 g (standard transition [ST] group). The primary outcome of the study was length of stay. Secondary outcomes were the number of infants returned to an incubator, the growth velocity in an open crib and during the first week at home, the proportions of breastfeeding at discharge and during the first week at home, and the hospital readmission rate.

Results.—The length of stay was significantly shorter in the early transition group than in the standard transition group (23.5 vs 33 days; *P* =.0002). No infants required transfer back to the incubator. Only 1 infant in the standard transition group was readmitted to the hospital during the first week after discharge. Growth velocities and individual amounts of breastfeeding were similar between the 2 groups.

Conclusion.—In this study, weaning of moderately preterm infants from incubators to open cribs at 1600 g was safe and resulted in earlier discharge.

▶ Even the apparently most mundane of our daily decisions in the nurseries bear examination under the microscope of a randomized controlled trial. This report documents the advantages of earlier weaning of preterm infants from incubator care. Infants were randomly assigned to weaning to an open crib when they reached a weight of either 1600 g (early transition) or 1800 g (standard transition). Discharge criteria were full feeding competency (breast or bottle sucking), normal weight gain in an open crib, axillary temperature of ≥36.5°C after 72 hours, and no apneic episodes after 72 hours without caffeine. The shorter length of stay in the early transition group resulted in discharge at a postmenstrual age of 35.6 ± 1.5 weeks versus 37.0 ± 1.1 weeks in the standard transition group (P = .0006). Both groups spent a mean of 6 days in an open crib before discharge, so those in the early group were, on the average, discharged before those in the standard group transitioned to an open crib. Because there were no differences between groups with respect to other criteria for discharge, the authors speculate that later weaning from the incubator was associated with a delay in achievement of feeding competency. This suggests that remaining in an incubator may have caused caretakers to doubt feeding readiness and that earlier weaning removed this barrier to cue-based feeding rehabilitation. Whatever the explanation, weaning infants born at 30 to 35 weeks gestation from an incubator to an open crib at weights as low as 1600 g significantly shortened hospitalization without apparent adverse effects.

W. E. Benitz, MD

Economic Outcomes in Young Adulthood for Extremely Low Birth Weight Survivors

Goddeeris JH, Saigal S, Boyle MH, et al (Michigan State Univ, East Lansing; McMaster Univ, Hamilton, Ontario, Canada)
Pediatrics 126:e1102-e1108, 2010

Objective.—The goal was to compare educational attainment and labor market outcomes in young adulthood (21—26 years of age) for a Canadian, population-based cohort of 149 extremely low birth weight (ELBW) (<1000 g) survivors and a normal birth weight (NBW) cohort of 133 young adults from the same geographic area who were matched to the ELBW cohort in childhood.

Methods.—We estimated the effects of ELBW status, according to gender, on continuous outcomes through least-squares regression and those on binary outcomes through logistic regression. We controlled for family background and considered neurosensory impairment and IQ as mediating variables.

Results.—Controlling for family background, ELBW male subjects were less likely to complete high school or to attend a university than were their NBW counterparts, and their educational attainment was reduced by >1 year. Among subjects who were working, weekly earnings were ~27% lower. ELBW female effects on education were not significant, but ELBW female subjects were less likely than NBW subjects to be employed or in school and they also seemed to experience lower earnings.

Conclusion.—Our findings suggested that ELBW survivors are somewhat less productive as adults, on average, than are subjects born NBW and that effects are not confined to subjects with severe neurosensory impairments. In accord with other studies, however, we found that productivity deficits for most ELBW subjects were not large.

▶ The study population described in the observational report is remarkable for several reasons. The extremely low birth weight (ELBW) cohort has been systematically tracked and evaluated since birth in the mid 1980s and the matched term control cohort has been followed since 8 years of age. The follow-up rate in young adulthood for these cohorts is a remarkable 90% and 92%, respectively. In addition, the ELBW cohort is population based and, as such, eschews the bias inherent in single-center or network follow-up studies.

The educational achievement and earning capacity described in the report adds credence to an emerging body of evidence garnered from national databases in Scandinavia that suggests survivors born preterm achieve lower educational attainment and poorer labor market outcomes than those born at term. Unlike previous reports, this study delineates outcomes by sex. The impact of being born ELBW affected males and females differently. For males, there was a significant difference in educational achievement with a 14% probability of not completing high school and 22% probability of not attending university. As to productivity, ELBW males had a 9% probability of either not working or attending school. For those who were working, there was a significant 27% reduction in earning power. In contrast, ELBW did not appear to have an adverse effect on educational attainment for females. The probability of not completing high school was unaffected and the probability of not attending university was only 7%. Despite attaining the same level of education as their term counterparts, females were less likely to be employed. This could not be attributed to either marriage or having children.

A perceived weakness of longitudinal studies of graduates of the neonatal intensive care unit is that the medical care rendered to the follow-up cohort differs markedly from that currently practiced; however, even with a noticeable improvement in the survival rate of ELBW subjects since the mid 1980s, the rate of neurosensory impairment in early childhood has not changed substantially.

L. A. Papile, MD

Morbidity and Discharge Timing of Late Preterm Newborns
Pulver LS, Denney JM, Silver RM, et al (Univ of Utah, Salt Lake City)
Clin Pediatr 49:1061-1067, 2010

Late preterm newborns (LPNs), those with gestational ages (GAs) between 34 weeks and 36 weeks 6 days, account for 70% of preterm births. Because they have a mature appearance and are often cared for in a well baby nursery (WBN), parents may anticipate that the nursery course will be similar to that of a term infant and that their newborn will be discharged with his/her mother. How frequently their hospitalizations are prolonged beyond that of their mothers and the morbidities associated with prolonged hospitalization (PH) have not been well described. The objectives of the study were to (1) determine the proportion of LPNs with a PH and (2) describe the most common morbidities in LPNs and identify those associated with PH. The authors conducted retrospective chart reviews of the neonatal courses of LPNs born between December 2002 and April 2007 at the University of Utah Hospital. They compared maternal and newborn discharge dates to determine the proportion of LPNs with a PH and calculated frequencies of conditions and interventions indicating morbidity and identified associations between each of the conditions/interventions and PH. Of 235 LPNs, 94 (40%) had a PH; 75% of 34-week LPNs had a PH compared with 50% of those with GAs of 35 weeks and 25% of those with GAs of 36 weeks. The most common conditions/interventions were an oxygen need, phototherapy for jaundice, and hypothermia requiring an isolette. A need for nasogastric feeding and antibiotic administration for >3 days was consistently associated with a PH. LPNs whose only intervention was phototherapy for jaundice or IV antibiotics for <3 days did not have a PH. As a group, two thirds of LPNs experienced one or more conditions/interventions indicating morbidity, and 40% had a PH. Both were much more common in LPNs with GAs of 34 weeks compared with LPNs with GAs of 36 weeks. Nursery clinicians should counsel parents of LPNs regarding the likely possibility of morbidity and PH.

▶ Late preterm (LPT) births were the first group of premature infants who neonatologists treated successfully. Over time, with the very low birth weight infants surviving and demanding many resources, the near-term infants were relatively ignored and unfortunately, by many health care providers, no longer considered to be of high risk. The resurgence of interest in this group, renaming them *late preterm* resulted from the recognition that they were indeed the largest subpopulation of preterm infants, had an increased mortality when compared with term infants, and had increased morbidity, including transient tachypnea of newborn (TTN), respiratory distress syndrome (RDS), persistent pulmonary hypertension, respiratory failure, apnea, temperature instability, jaundice, hypoglycemia, feeding difficulties, and a prolonged neonatal intensive care unit stay.[1-3] Furthermore, they have an increased prevalence of cognitive and neurodevelopmental problems and a greater rate of readmission to hospital in the first weeks after discharge than term births.

Pulver et al confirm the morbidity in LPT births but also present data by week of gestational age. The data reveal that each extra week in utero is important, and prolonged hospitalization, evident in 40% of their late preterm population, is much more common at 34 than 36 weeks. The most common morbidity was a need for supplemental oxygen, found in 35%, of whom 9% required continuous positive airway pressure and 5% required mechanical ventilation, underscoring the respiratory immaturity as a significant cause of morbidity in this population. Hibbard et al[4] noted that in a contemporary cohort, late preterm birth, compared with term delivery, was associated with increased risk of respiratory distress syndrome and other respiratory morbidity. The incidence of RDS was 10.5% for infants born at 34 weeks' gestation versus 0.3% at 38 weeks. Similarly, the incidence of TTN was 6.4% for those born at 34 weeks versus 0.4% at 38 weeks, pneumonia was 1.5% versus 0.1%, and respiratory failure was 1.6% versus 0.2%.

Other significant causes of morbidity included jaundice requiring phototherapy in 35%, hypothermia requiring care in an Isolette in 31%; and hypoglycemia requiring intravenous dextrose in 27% of this cohort of LPT births. Infants requiring nasogastric feeding were more likely to have a prolonged hospital stay. Ruled-out sepsis was not necessarily associated with prolonged hospitalization.

Radtke[5] attempted to synthesize the published research pertaining to breast-feeding establishment and outcomes among late preterm infants and to describe the state of the science on breast-feeding within this population. Among late preterm mother/infant dyads, breast-feeding initiation appears to be approximately 59% to 70% (US), whereas the odds of breast-feeding beyond 4 weeks or to the recommended 6 months (exclusive breast-feeding) appears to be significantly less than for term infants, and possibly even less for infants ≤34 to 35 weeks' gestation. Breast-feeding exclusivity is not routinely reported in articles. Rehospitalization, often related to jaundice and poor feeding, is nearly twice as common among late preterm breast-fed infants as breast-fed term or nonbreast-fed late preterm infants.

So the evidence mounts on the increased morbidity in LPT infants. Next steps must be to reduce the number of unnecessary LPT deliveries.

A. A. Fanaroff, MD, FRCPE, FRCP&CH

References

1. Raju TN, Higgins RD, Stark AR, Leveno KJ. Optimizing care and outcome for late-preterm (near-term) infants: a summary of the workshop sponsored by the National Institute of Child Health and Human Development. *Pediatrics.* 2006; 118:1207-1214.
2. Engle WA, Tomashek KM, Wallman C; Committee on Fetus and Newborn, American Academy of Pediatrics. "Late-preterm" infants: a population at risk. *Pediatrics.* 2007;120:1390.
3. Ramachandrappa A, Jain L. Health issues of the late preterm infant. *Pediatr Clin North Am.* 2009;56:565-577.
4. Consortium on Safe Labor, Hibbard JU, Wilkins I, Sun L, et al. Respiratory morbidity in late preterm births. *JAMA.* 2010;304:419-425.
5. Radtke JV. The paradox of breastfeeding-associated morbidity among late preterm infants. *J Obstet Gynecol Neonatal Nurs.* 2011;40:9-24.

Subcutaneous Fat Necrosis as a Complication of Whole-Body Cooling for Birth Asphyxia
Oza V, Treat J, Cook N, et al (Children's Hosp of Philadelphia, PA; et al)
Arch Dermatol 146:882-885, 2010

Background.—Subcutaneous fat necrosis (SCFN) of the newborn is a form of panniculitis that affects full-term neonates who often have suffered either birth asphyxia or hypothermia. The induction of hypothermia in newborns is becoming frequently used to reduce the neurologic sequelae associated with birth asphyxia. The risk of SCFN in neonates undergoing this therapy is unknown.

Observation.—We describe a neonate who developed an abscesslike presentation of SCFN and subsequent asymptomatic hypercalcemia after undergoing whole-body cooling for hypoxic-ischemic encephalopathy.

Conclusions.—Hypothermia protocols may be placing newborns at increased risk for the development of SCFN. Clinicians should recognize this association, and newborns who undergo therapeutic cooling should have frequent dermatologic assessments.

▶ This article presents a single-case report of a newborn who underwent therapeutic hypothermia after a placental abruption at term. He subsequently developed a lesion that was determined to be subcutaneous fat necrosis with suppuration. Since subcutaneous fat necrosis was well described in asphyxiated infants long before the implementation of whole-body cooling for neonatal hypoxic-ischemic encephalopathy, it is impossible to determine in this case whether the lesion arose from the underlying asphyxia, therapeutic hypothermia, or a combination of the 2. Accordingly, I was about to delete this article from my assigned list, but instead, I would like to draw your attention to the color photograph of the lesion and the accompanying photomicrographs from the biopsy specimen in the original article. Since subcutaneous fat necrosis is unusually rare, this might be a good opportunity to see such a lesion.

S. M. Donn, MD

Necrotizing Enterocolitis is Associated With *Ureaplasma* Colonization in Preterm Infants

Okogbule-Wonodi AC, Gross GW, Sun C-CJ, et al (Univ of Maryland School of Medicine, Baltimore; et al)

Pediatr Res 69:442-447, 2011

The study objective was to determine whether *Ureaplasma* respiratory tract colonization of preterm infants <33 wk gestation is associated with an increased risk for necrotizing enterocolitis (NEC). One or more tracheal or nasopharyngeal aspirates for *Ureaplasma* culture and PCR were obtained during the first week of life from 368 infants <33 wk gestation enrolled from 1999 to 2003 or from 2007 to 2009. NEC Bell stage ≥2 was confirmed by radiological criteria, and pathology, if available. Cord serum samples were analyzed for IL-6 and IL-1β concentrations, and placentas were reviewed for histological chorioamnionitis in the first cohort. NEC was confirmed in 29 of 368 (7.9%) of the combined cohorts. The incidence of NEC was 2.2-fold higher in *Ureaplasma*-positive (12.3%) than *Ureaplasma*-negative (5.5%) infants <33 wk (OR, 2.43; 95% CI, 1.13−5.2; $p = 0.023$) and 3.3-fold higher in *Ureaplasma*-positive

(14.6%) than *Ureaplasma*-negative (4.4%) infants ≤28 wk (OR, 3.67; 95% CI, 1.36—9.93; $p = 0.01$). Age of onset, hematologic parameters at onset, and NEC severity were similar between *Ureaplasma*-positive and negative infants. Cord serum IL-6 and IL-1β concentrations were significantly higher in *Ureaplasma*-positive than in *Ureaplasma*-negative NEC-affected infants. *Ureaplasma* may be a factor in NEC pathogenesis in preterm infants by contributing to intestinal mucosal injury and/or altering systemic or local immune responses.

▶ Necrotizing enterocolitis is a devastating disease in preterm newborn infants and is associated with a high mortality rate and adverse neurodevelopmental outcome among survivors.[1] Prematurity has been identified as the greatest risk factor for disease development. Although no single organism has been consistently implicated, intrauterine infection with *Ureaplasma* species is a significant risk factor for prematurity, and it is associated with neonatal morbidities such as bronchopulmonary dysplasia and periventricular leukomalacia.

This is the first study to demonstrate an association between preterm respiratory tract colonization and *Ureaplasma* and necrotizing enterocolitis. However, there are multiple limitations of this study. Use of respiratory tract colonization as a proxy for intestinal mucosal exposure likely underestimates the true incidence of gastrointestinal colonization. In addition, restriction of the surveillance period to the first week of life further underestimates the prevalence of colonization. Bacterial load and colonization/infection with other organisms were not examined in this study. Colonization patterns also differ based on the feeding substrate; however, details regarding the feeding protocol were not provided. Despite these limitations, the study's summary findings highlight the need for in vitro studies and animal models to investigate whether a causal relationship exists between *Ureaplasma* colonization and necrotizing enterocolitis in the preterm very low birth weight population. As molecular techniques continue to improve, enhanced detection of organism colonization may alter the current understanding of the neonatal intestinal microbiome and the mechanisms underlying the development of necrotizing enterocolitis.[2]

J. S. Lee, MD, MPH

References

1. Neu J, Walker WA. Necrotizing enterocolitis. *N Engl J Med.* 2011;364:255-264.
2. Viscardi RM. Ureaplasma species: role in diseases of prematurity. *Clin Perinatol.* 2010;37:393-409.

12 Pharmacology

Caffeine and Brain Development in Very Preterm Infants

Doyle LW, Cheong J, Hunt RW, et al (Univ of Melbourne, Parkville, Victoria, Australia; The Royal Children's Hosp, Melbourne, Victoria, Australia; et al)
Ann Neurol 68:734-742, 2010

Objective.—Caffeine improves neurological outcome in very preterm infants, but the mechanisms responsible for this neurological benefit are unknown. The objective of this study was to assess whether caffeine influenced brain macro- or microstructural development in preterm infants.

Methods.—Seventy preterm infants <1,251 g birthweight randomly allocated to either caffeine (n = 33) or placebo (n = 37) underwent brain magnetic resonance imaging (MRI) at term-equivalent age; white and gray matter abnormalities were qualitatively scored, global and regional brain volumes were measured, and white matter microstructure was evaluated using diffusion-weighted imaging.

Results.—There were no significant differences between the groups in the extent of white matter or gray matter abnormality, or in global or regional brain volumes. In contrast, although only available in 28 children, caffeine exposure was associated with reductions in the apparent diffusion coefficient, and radial and axial diffusivity with the greatest impact in the superior brain regions. The alterations in diffusion measures were not mediated by lowering the rate of lung injury, known as bronchopulmonary dysplasia.

Interpretation.—These diffusion changes are consistent with improved white matter microstructural development in preterm infants who received caffeine.

▶ Caffeine was cautiously introduced into the neonatal arena for the treatment of apnea and has become the dominant medication for this common, frustrating, and at times perplexing disorder. In their Cochrane review, Henderson-Smart and DePaoli concluded that "Methylxanthine is effective in reducing the number of apneic attacks and the use of mechanical ventilation in the two to seven days after starting treatment. Caffeine is also associated with better longer term outcomes. In view of its lower toxicity, caffeine would be the preferred drug for the treatment of apnea."[1] Caffeine also improves the chances of successful extubation of preterm infants within 1 week of age.[2] Additionally, important neurodevelopmental outcomes are improved by methylxanthine therapy so that caffeine is becoming a magic bullet in neonatology. Furthermore, there are potential uses of caffeine in respiratory distress syndrome because lung function improves in primate models and there was a reduction in bronchopulmonary dysplasia in the caffeine-treated group.[3] Improved later outcomes at 18 to 22 months include clinically significant decreases in cerebral palsy, cognitive impairment, and severe retinopathy of prematurity in those babies who received caffeine during the neonatal period compared with non-caffeine—treated placebo neonates.[4]

Doyle commences the discussion as follows "The major finding of this study is that caffeine treatment appeared to have a substantial effect on cerebral WM diffusion measures in very preterm infants, with no obvious effects on MR-defined cerebral injury or macrostructural cerebral development, ie, qualitative WM and GM abnormalities, or segmented, parcellated, or hippocampal volumes. The reductions in apparent diffusion coefficient (ADC) and both axial and radial diffusivity represent more mature cerebral WM organization in the caffeine-treated infants." This explanation appears to be reasonable and is based on the available evidence. It remains to be seen whether this is confirmed in other studies.

The CAP trial[3,4] continues to undergo further analysis, and Dukhovny et al[5] completed an economic evaluation of caffeine for apnea of prematurity. Their results overwhelmingly favor caffeine and I loved their statistical jargon. "The mean cost per infant was $124 466 (Canadian) in the caffeine group and $133 505 in the placebo group (difference: $9039 [−14 749 to −3375]; adjusted $P = .014$). Cost-effectiveness analysis showed caffeine to be a dominant or 'win-win' therapy: in > 99% of 1000 bootstrap replications of the analysis, caffeine-treated infants had simultaneously better outcomes and lower mean costs. These results were robust to a 1000% increase in the individual resource items, including the price of caffeine citrate." Davis et al[6] noted that the benefits of caffeine may vary in subgroups. Starting caffeine early resulted in larger reductions in days of respiratory support. Furthermore, infants receiving respiratory support who received caffeine derived more neurodevelopmental benefits.

Caffeine thus becomes an all-purpose drug that decreases apnea, promotes shorter time on ventilatory support, improves success of extubation, decreases bronchopulmonary dysplasia, and enhances neurodevelopmental outcome. There is a convincing case to use it earlier and more often in preterm infants.

A. A. Fanaroff, MD, FRCPE, FRCP&CH

References

1. Henderson-Smart DJ, De Paoli AG. Methylxanthine treatment for apnoea in preterm infants. *Cochrane Database Syst Rev.* 2010;(12). CD000140.
2. Henderson-Smart DJ, Davis PG. Prophylactic methylxanthines for endotracheal extubation in preterm infants. *Cochrane Database Syst Rev.* 2010;(12). CD000139.
3. Schmidt B, Roberts RS, Davis P, et al. Caffeine for Apnea of Prematurity Trial Group. Caffeine therapy for apnea of prematurity. *N Engl J Med.* 2006;354: 2112-2121.
4. Schmidt B, Roberts RS, Davis P, et al. Caffeine for Apnea of Prematurity Trial Group. Long-term effects of caffeine therapy for apnea of prematurity. *N Engl J Med.* 2007;357:1893-1902.
5. Dukhovny D, Lorch SA, Schmidt B, et al. Caffeine for Apnea of Prematurity Trial Group. Economic evaluation of caffeine for apnea of prematurity. *Pediatrics.* 2011;127:e146-e155.

6. Davis PG, Schmidt B, Roberts RS, et al. Caffeine for Apnea of Prematurity Trial Group. Caffeine for Apnea of Prematurity trial: benefits may vary in subgroups. *J Pediatr.* 2010;156:382-387.

Intrapulmonary drug administration in neonatal and paediatric critical care: a comprehensive review

De Luca D, Cogo P, Zecca E, et al (Polytechnical Univ of Marche, Ancona, Italy; Univ of Padova, Padua, Italy; Catholic Univ of the Sacred Heart, Rome, Italy; et al)

Eur Respir J 37:678-689, 2011

Administration of drugs directly into the respiratory tree first was proposed a long time ago. Surfactant is the paradigmatic example of such therapies. Many other drugs have been used in the same way and further compounds are under investigation for this aim. In the last two decades, despite the wide number of drugs available for direct lung administration in critical care patients, few controlled data exist regarding their use in neonates and infants.

This review will focus on drugs clinically available in a critical care setting for neonates and infants, including bronchodilators, pulmonary vasodilators, anti-inflammatory agents, mucolytics, resuscitative anti-infective agents, surfactants and other drugs.

We provide an evidence-based comprehensive review of drugs available for intratracheal administration in paediatric and neonatal critical care and we examine possible advantages and risks for each proposed indication.

▶ I found this to be an interesting and informative review of intrapulmonary drug administration in neonatal and pediatric critical care. The authors did a comprehensive analysis of pharmacologic agents given by the intratracheal route, including beta$_2$-agonists, anticholinergics, epinephrine, nitric oxide, prostacyclin and analogues, pentoxifylline, steroids, cromolyn, Clara cell secretory protein, resuscitative drugs, mucolytics, ribavirin, antibiotics, heliox, furosemide, and superoxide dismutase.

Table 2 in the original article summarizes the evidence-based clinical indications and practice points for these agents. With respect to neonatal intensive care, one can find little, if any, justification for any of these beyond inhaled nitric oxide and the selected use of steroids for the prevention of bronchopulmonary dysplasia. Some agents will result in short-term improvement, but most of the evidence is level B.

Although the potential to use the lung as a drug delivery site is attractive and shows great potential, much more needs to be learned. As the authors indicate, it is a very complex field because the drug needs to be married to the device that delivers it, and better understanding of aerosolization, distribution, pharmacokinetics, efficacy, and safety will only come from more rigorous investigation.

S. M. Donn, MD

Intrapulmonary drug administration in neonatal and paediatric critical care: a comprehensive review

De Luca D, Cogo P, Zecca E, et al (Polytechnical Univ of Marche, Ancona, Italy; Univ of Padova, Padua, Italy; Catholic Univ of the Sacred Heart, Rome, Italy; et al)
Eur Respir J 37:678-689, 2011

Administration of drugs directly into the respiratory tree first was proposed a long time ago. Surfactant is the paradigmatic example of such therapies. Many other drugs have been used in the same way and further compounds are under investigation for this aim. In the last two decades, despite the wide number of drugs available for direct lung administration in critical care patients, few controlled data exist regarding their use in neonates and infants.

This review will focus on drugs clinically available in a critical care setting for neonates and infants, including bronchodilators, pulmonary vasodilators, anti-inflammatory agents, mucolytics, resuscitative anti-infective agents, surfactants and other drugs.

We provide an evidence-based comprehensive review of drugs available for intratracheal administration in paediatric and neonatal critical care and we examine possible advantages and risks for each proposed indication (Table 2).

▶ The administration of drugs by the intravenous route is usually considered the fastest and most effective means to elicit a positive response to the drug. Often the intravenous route may not be readily accessible, especially in very small infants. Furthermore, some drugs may be best administered locally so that an unwanted systemic response is not elicited. This article reviews 8 classes of drugs, according to their mechanism of action, that have been administered by the intrapulmonary route and the levels of evidence to support or refute their use. Table 2 provides a summary of these drugs and the levels of evidence supporting or refuting their use for intrapulmonary drug delivery. Some of them are clearly intrapulmonary drugs, such as inhaled nitric oxide, heliox, and surfactant. Others such as beta-agonists, adrenalin, steroids, and furosemide and superoxide dismutase are not as obvious, and the authors attempt to provide recommendations based on the best possible evidence. The authors aptly advise that some of the delivery systems (aerosolizers, ventilators, etc) need to be optimized for the drugs to be most effective.

J. Neu, MD

TABLE 2.—Evidence-Based Clinical Indications for Intrapulmonary Drug Delivery

Drugs	Practice Points
β_2-agonists and ipratropium bromide	May transiently improve lung mechanics in neonates (B). Routine use for BPD prevention is not recommended but they may be useful in bronchial obstruction or increased work of breathing (A). In neonates, ipratropium may cause transient improvements of bronchial obstruction similarly to β_2-agonists (C). Albuterol may decrease serum potassium in pre-term infants with hyperkalaemia (B) but its use as a first-line treatment for hyperkalemia cannot be recommended (A)
Adrenaline	May improve respiratory mechanics during bronchiolitis (A) or croup (C) but its clinical effect is questionable. When given for neonatal resuscitation, adrenaline may need to be given at dose 10 times higher than the intravenous one (D)
iNO	A 30-min iNO trial at 10 ppm is advisable in congenital heart disease children at risk for pulmonary hypertension: iNO may reduce ventilation time and hypertensive events (B). There are no adequate data to recommend its use in paediatric ARDS. iNO is the first-choice therapy for PPHN in term and late pre-term babies at a standard dosage of 20 ppm, although lower doses may be effective (A). In pre-term neonates, risks and benefits should be weighted in each case (B)
Epoprostenol and iloprost	May lower pulmonary pressure in congenital heart disease children (B). Epoprostenol could be useful in severe ARDS unresponsive to conventional therapies (B). In neonates, epoprostenol or iloprost could resolve PPHN in case of iNO unavailability or failure and iloprost is probably more suitable in this setting (D)
Pentoxifylline	May reduce BPD incidence ($\sim$27%) (B)
Steroids	Might be useful to prevent BPD but there is not enough evidence to recommend them (A). Surfactant-vehicled steroids may be considered for this aim (B). Inhaled steroids may achieve a faster recovery in term neonates with meconium aspiration syndrome (B)
Cromolyn	Not useful and should not be given to neonates to prevent BPD (A)
Hypertonic saline	May allow faster clinical improvement and shorter hospitalisation in bronchiolitis (A). It may also improve lung mechanics in cystic fibrosis (A).
Dornase-α	May resolve atelectasis in long-term ventilated children (B). It also allows shorter ICU stay and ventilation time in congenital heart diseases children (B). It could be useful for refractory status asthmaticus, severe atelectasis or tube plugging in children/neonates when conventional therapies failed (D)
Acetylcysteine	Nebulised heparin/acetylcysteine is able to reduce mortality in children with burns and smoke inhalation lung injury (C). Acetylcysteine might worsen respiratory mechanics and should not be used in neonates (B)
Ribavirin	May allow shorter hospital stay and ventilation time in severe bronchiolitis (B). Ribavirin coupled with palivizumab may increase survival (C)
Heliox	No definite data are available to support or refute the use of heliox in severe obstructive diseases. It could be tried, as early as possible, in intractable cases (D). Heliox may ameliorate respiratory distress symptoms due to post-extubation stridor in children (B)
Furosemide	May cause transient lung mechanics improvement in neonates with established or pending BPD but its routine use is not recommended (A)
Superoxide dismutase	May improve long-term respiratory status in pre-term neonates (B)

Letters in parentheses represent levels of evidence and grades of recommendations modified from the Scottish Intercollegiate Guidelines Network (SIGN) guidelines [163] as follows. A: at least one high-quality meta-analysis of randomised controlled trials (RCT) or a sufficiently powered high-quality RCT. B: other meta-analysis of RCTs or a high quality systematic review of case–control studies or a low grade RCT, but with high probability that the relationship is causal. C: a well conducted case–control or cohort study with a low risk of confounding bias. D: evidence from case series, case reports or expert opinion. iNO: inhaled nitric oxide; BPD: bronchopulmonary dysplasia; ARDS: acute respiratory distress syndrome; PPHN: persistent pulmonary hypertension of the neonate; ICU: intensive care unit.

Sodium Bicarbonate Administration and Outcome in Preterm Infants

Berg CS, Barnette AR, Myers BJ, et al (Washington Univ School of Medicine, St Louis, MO)

J Pediatr 157:684-687, 2010

The short-term outcomes of sodium bicarbonate therapy in preterm infants were investigated by retrospective analysis of 165 of 984 infants who received sodium bicarbonate. The infants treated with sodium bicarbonate were more immature and had greater severity of illness and more adverse outcomes. Sodium bicarbonate therapy did not improve the blood pH.

▶ Old habits die hard. This report describes a substantial reduction between 2002 and 2006 in bicarbonate use during the first postnatal week in infants < 1500 g birth weight. In 2002, nearly 40% received intravenous bicarbonate, but that rate had fallen to 10% by 2005 to 2006 ($P < .0001$). It is not clear whether this change resulted from adoption of a new policy or from a lower severity of illness. The Clinical Risk Index for Babies (CRIB) scores decreased significantly (from 5.31 in 2002 to 3.73 in 2005 to 2006) for all infants but not for the groups that did (8.30-7.34) or did not (3.37-3.33) receive bicarbonate, indicating that a smaller proportion had high CRIB scores and suggesting that fewer infants met a stable criterion for bicarbonate therapy. Neither rates of intraventricular hemorrhage (IVH) nor mortality changed during the study interval, but bicarbonate infusions were significantly associated with an increased risk of both. It appears that bicarbonate therapy did not contribute substantially to these adverse outcomes, but that bicarbonate use, IVH, and mortality were mutually covariate with severity of illness (which was not fully accounted for by the variables included in multivariate regression analysis). On the other hand, bicarbonate infusions produced only a very small increase in serum bicarbonate levels (18.5 ± 3 mEq/L before to 20.2 ± 3.7 mEq/L after) and no improvement in serum pH (7.23 ± 0.12 to 7.24 ± 0.16). The absence of demonstrable benefit supports recommendations against use of this treatment, even if adverse effects are not unambiguously attributable to it. It would be interesting to know how the rate of bicarbonate use has changed since publication of Aschner and Poland's[1] critical review of this subject in 2008.

W. E. Benitz, MD

Reference

1. Aschner JL, Poland RL. Sodium bicarbonate: basically useless therapy. *Pediatrics.* 2008;122:831-835.

Levetiracetam for Treatment of Neonatal Seizures

Abend NS, Gutierrez-Colina AM, Monk HM, et al (The Children's Hosp of Philadelphia, PA)
J Child Neurol 26:465-470, 2011

Neonatal seizures are often refractory to treatment with initial antiseizure medications. Consequently, clinicians turn to alternatives such as levetiracetam, despite the lack of published data regarding its safety, tolerability, or efficacy in the neonatal population. We report a retrospectively identified cohort of 23 neonates with electroencephalographically confirmed seizures who received levetiracetam. Levetiracetam was considered effective if administration was associated with a greater than 50% seizure reduction within 24 hours. Levetiracetam was initiated at a mean conceptional age of 41 weeks. The mean initial dose was 16 ± 6 mg/kg and the mean maximum dose was 45 ± 19 mg/kg/day. No respiratory or cardiovascular adverse effects were reported or detected. Levetiracetam was associated with a greater than 50% seizure reduction in 35% (8 of 23), including seizure termination in 7. Further study is warranted to determine optimal levetiracetam dosing in neonates and to compare efficacy with other antiseizure medications.

▶ This report is one of several that have appeared in the medical literature over the past few years regarding the use of levetiracetam in the treatment of neonatal seizures. Each of the studies was a retrospective, single-center, open-label case report or case series. All were small and most relied on chart review to gather data. The loading dose varied from 10 to 60 mg/kg and the frequency and maintenance dosage ranged from 10 to 80 mg/kg/d. Most subjects were receiving at least one other antiepileptic drug when levetiracetam was started.

The studies have several limitations. Although no adverse events were identified, the retrospective nature of chart review limited any conclusions about safety and efficacy. Second, because dosing was not standardized and there are no pharmacokinetic data, the optimal amount and dosing schedule are unknown.

Because the treatment of neonatal seizures produces limited efficacy and may lead to adverse side effects, the off-label use of antiepileptic drugs, such as levetiracetam, is increasing. In fact, recent survey data suggest that levetiracetam is commonly recommended by pediatric neurologists managing neonatal seizures, despite a paucity of data regarding safety, tolerability, and efficacy.[1] However, before levetiracetam can be recommended for the treatment of neonatal seizures, additional studies, particularly dosing finding studies, are needed.

L. A. Papile, MD

Reference

1. Silverstein FS, Ferriero DM. Off-label use of antiepileptic drugs for the treatment of neonatal seizures. *Pediatr Neurol.* 2008;39:77-79.

Multiple Courses of Antenatal Corticosteroids for Preterm Birth Study: 2-Year Outcomes
Asztalos EV, for the Multiple Courses of Antenatal Corticosteroids for Preterm Birth Study Collaborative Group (Sunnybrook Res Inst, Toronto, Ontario, Canada; et al)
Pediatrics 126:e1045-e1055, 2010

Objective.—The aim of this study was to determine the effects of repeated courses of prenatal corticosteroid therapy versus placebo on death or neurologic impairment among the children enrolled in the Multiple Courses of Antenatal Corticosteroids for Preterm Birth Study, at 18 to 24 months of age.

Methods.—A total of 2305 infants were eligible for follow-up evaluation; 2104 infants (1069 in the prenatal corticosteroid therapy group and 1035 in the placebo group) were monitored. The primary outcome was death or neurologic impairment, defined as either cerebral palsy or cognitive delay, at 18 to 24 months of age. The secondary outcomes were measurements of growth (height, weight, and head circumference).

Results.—Children exposed to multiple courses of prenatal corticosteroid therapy had similar rates of death or neurologic impairment, compared with children exposed to placebo (148 children [13.8%] vs 142 children [13.7%]; odds ratio: 1.001[95% confidence interval: 0.75–1.30]; $P=.95$). They had a mean weight of 11.94 kg, compared with 12.14 kg in the placebo group ($P=.04$), a mean height of 85.51 cm, compared with 85.46 cm ($P=.87$), and a mean head circumference of 48.18 cm, compared with 48.25 cm ($P=.45$).

Conclusions.—Multiple courses of prenatal corticosteroid therapy, given every 14 days, did not increase or decrease the risk of death or neurologic impairment at 18 to 24 months of age, compared with a single course of prenatal corticosteroid therapy. Continued follow-up monitoring of these children is necessary to assess neurobehavioral function, school performance, and possible susceptibility to disease.

► The administration of repeated doses of antenatal steroids (ANS) has been the subject of several recent randomized clinical trials and has been found to further reduce neonatal respiratory morbidity, relative to single-course ANS. However, these studies have also raised concerns about the impact of repeated doses of ANS on fetal growth and head circumference. The study design and primary outcome, namely death or developmental impairment at 18 to 24 months corrected age, have been similar across trials, and all uniformly showed that multiple courses of ANS did not contribute to improved outcomes. However, the question regarding potential harm has yet to be answered. The brain injury noted in animal models exposed to repeated doses of ANS included a reduced number of neurons and degeneration of neurons in the hippocampus, the area of the brain involved in functions that support cognition, memory, and behavior. Developmental tests at 18 to 24 months of age are unable to sufficiently measure these outcomes. It will take continued follow-up monitoring of treated infants before the potential adverse effects of this treatment are truly known. In the interim, because long-term risk/benefit is lacking, the administration of repeated doses of ANS cannot be recommended.

L. A. Papile, MD

Antenatal Corticosteroids Promote Survival of Extremely Preterm Infants Born at 22 to 23 Weeks of Gestation
Mori R, on behalf of the Neonatal Research Network Japan (The Univ of Tokyo, Japan; et al)
J Pediatr 159:110-114, 2011

Objective.—To evaluate the effectiveness of antenatal corticosteroid (ACS) to improve neonatal outcomes for infants born at <24 weeks of gestation.

Study Design.—We performed a retrospective analysis of 11 607 infants born at 22 to 33 weeks of gestation between 2003 and 2007 from the Neonatal Research Network of Japan. We evaluated the gestational age effects of ACS administered to mothers with threatened preterm birth on several factors related to neonatal morbidity and mortality.

Results.—By logistic regression analysis, ACS exposure decreased respiratory distress syndrome and severe intraventricular hemorrhage in infants born between 24 and 29 weeks of gestation. Cox regression analysis revealed that ACS exposure was associated with a significant decrease in mortality of preterm infants born at 22 or 23 weeks of gestation (adjusted hazard ratio, 0.72; 95% CI, 0.53 to 0.97; $P = .03$). This effect was also observed at 24 to 25 and 26 to 27 weeks of gestation and in the overall study population.

Conclusions.—ACS exposure improved survival of extremely preterm infants. ACS treatment should be considered for threatened preterm birth at 22 to 23 weeks of gestation.

▶ The Japanese have long had an outstanding survival rate for infants born at the cusp of viability. This study attempted to evaluate the role of antenatal corticosteroid therapy on survival and neonatal morbidities. It was a retrospective analysis of nearly 12 000 infants born between 2003 and 2007 who were included in the Neonatal Research Network of Japan database. Infants who were born alive but died in the delivery room were included, but stillbirths were not. Furthermore, decisions to support infants at 22 to 23 weeks' gestation were individualized by clinicians based on the status of the infant.

The authors concluded that steroid exposure promotes survival at 22 to 23 weeks, but their supportive evidence is soft. There was, in fact, no statistically significant difference in neonatal mortality (defined as death within the first 28 days) between infants who were or were not exposed to antenatal corticosteroid therapy. Survival to hospital discharge reached statistical significance with a fairly wide 95% confidence interval, but later deaths were not reported.

The results of this retrospective review are difficult to interpret. First, the population is relatively homogeneous, and both population characteristics and genetics may play a significant factor. Second, the decision to administer corticosteroids is in itself a selection bias.

Although this approach may be appropriate for Japan, other countries will need to carefully consider a decision to support pregnancies of 22 and 23 weeks' gestation. A recent statement by the Working Group on Prematurity of the World Association of Perinatal Medicine on the ethical dimensions of periviability suggests that a trial of intervention is not warranted at 22 weeks and that resuscitation at 23 weeks does not show a greater balance of good than harm. "The lack of appropriate long-term follow-up care in some resource-poor areas is a factor that is optimally included in the decision about resuscitation immediately after birth in the periviable gestational age range."[1]

S. M. Donn, MD

Reference

1. Skupski DW, Chervenak FA, McCullough LB, et al. Ethical dimensions of periviability. *J Perinat Med.* 2010;38:579-583.

Correlation between Serum Caffeine Levels and Changes in Cytokine Profile in a Cohort of Preterm Infants

Valdez RC, Ahlawat R, Wills-Karp M, et al (Johns Hopkins Univ School of Medicine, Baltimore, MD; Univ of Cincinnati College of Medicine, OH; et al)
J Pediatr 158:57-64, 2011

Objective.—To determine changes in cytokine levels associated with caffeine treatment in a cohort of preterm infants.

Study Design.—For this observational prospective study, we collected clinical data from 26 preterm infants ($\leq$30 weeks gestational age). In addition to caffeine levels, cytokine profiles in peripheral blood (PB) and tracheal aspirates (TA) were determined with enzyme-linked immunosorbent assay at birth, before and after (at 24 hours and 1 week) initiation of caffeine. Non-parametric statistics were applied.

Results.—Included infants were 26.9 ± 1.7 weeks gestational age and weighed 985 ± 202 g. At birth, all cytokine concentrations were significantly greater in TA than PB. Serum caffeine levels were 11.1 μg/mL (interquartile range, 1.85) at approximately 24 hours post-load and 16.4 (8.7) μg/mL at 1 week on treatment. At approximately 24 hours post-load, interleukin (IL)-10 levels decreased by 47.5% ($P = .01$) in PB and 38.5% ($P = .03$) in TA, whereas other cytokine levels remained unchanged. At 1 week, caffeine levels were correlated (U-shaped) with changes in proinflammatory tumor necrosis factor-α ($R^2 = 0.65$; $P = .0008$), interleukin (IL)-1β ($R^2 = 0.73$; $P = .0007$), and IL-6 ($R^2 = 0.59$; $P = .003$), whereas inversely correlated (linear) with the anti-inflammatory IL-10 ($R^2 = 0.64$;

$P = .0008$). Altogether, caffeine, at serum levels ≥ 20 μg/mL, was associated with a proinflammatory profile after 1 week of treatment.

Conclusions.—Caffeine treatment for apnea of prematurity correlates with changes in cytokine profile. Caffeine levels ≥ 20 μg/mL are associated with a proinflammatory profile in our cohort of preterm infants.

▶ Caffeine treatment of very preterm infants is associated with improved pulmonary[1] and neurodevelopmental[2] outcomes and might lower health care costs among survivors.[3] One of the proposed mechanisms of this association is caffeine-induced abrogation of the inflammatory response. In this article, Dr. Raul Chavez Valdez and colleagues report their analyses of the effects of caffeine administration on tracheal and peripheral blood cytokine levels. Evaluating levels after the loading dose, they found that only interleukin (IL)-10, an anti-inflammatory protein, was affected, falling in tracheal secretions and peripheral blood 1 day after the caffeine load. At a week of caffeine therapy, there was an inverse linear correlation between IL-10 and caffeine, but a U-shaped response was detected for proinflammatory proteins, IL-1-beta, 1L-6, and tumor necrosis factor-alpha, with the highest levels of these associated with the lowest and highest caffeine levels. Caffeine levels greater than 20 after a week of treatment were associated with a proinflammatory profile. It is unclear whether these analyses controlled for all potential confounding factors, including infection. Caffeine exerts an antagonistic effect on adenosine, a factor associated with tissue hypoxia and inflammation. In their review article published in *Pediatric Research*, Rivkees and Wendler describe the effects of adenosine on the embryo and newborn and the potential role of caffeine in modulating both adenosine's protective and adverse effects.[4] As is the case with many physiological processes, the intersection of physiology and pharmacology of caffeine, inflammation, and disorders of prematurity appears to be more complex than was initially appreciated.

L. J. Van Marter, MD, MPH

References

1. Schmidt B, Roberts RS, Davis P, et al. Caffeine for Apnea of Prematurity Trial Group. Caffeine therapy for apnea of prematurity. *N Engl J Med.* 2006;354: 2112-2121.
2. Schmidt B, Roberts RS, Davis P, et al. Caffeine for Apnea of Prematurity Trial Group. Long-term effects of caffeine therapy for apnea of prematurity. *N Engl J Med.* 2007;357:1893-1902.
3. Dukhovny D, Lorch SA, Schmidt B, et al. Caffeine for Apnea of Prematurity Trial Group. Economic evaluation of caffeine for apnea of prematurity. *Pediatrics.* 2011;127:e146-e155.
4. Rivkees SA, Wendler CC. Adverse and protective influences of adenosine on the newborn and embryo: implications for preterm white matter injury and embryo protection. *Pediatr Res.* 2011;69:271-278.

Economic Evaluation of Caffeine for Apnea of Prematurity

Dukhovny D, Lorch SA, Schmidt B, et al (Harvard Med School, Boston, MA; Univ of Pennsylvania School of Medicine, Philadelphia; et al)
Pediatrics 127:e146-e155, 2011

Objective.—To determine the cost-effectiveness of treatment with caffeine compared with placebo for apnea of prematurity in infants with birth weights less than 1250 g, from birth through 18 to 21 months' corrected age.

Methods.—We undertook a retrospective economic evaluation of the cost per survivor without neurodevelopmental impairment by using individual-patient data from the Caffeine for Apnea of Prematurity clinical trial (N = 1869). We included direct medical costs either to the insurance payer or the hospital but excluded costs to parents and society, such as lost productivity. We used a price of $0.21/mg of generic caffeine citrate for our base-case analysis. All costs were expressed in 2008 Canadian dollars and discounted at 3%. The time horizon for this analysis extended through 18 to 21 months' corrected age to match the clinical trial.

Results.—The mean cost per infant was $124 466 in the caffeine group and $133 505 in the placebo group (difference: $9039 [−14 749 to −3375]; adjusted $P = .014$). Cost-effectiveness analysis showed caffeine to be a dominant or "win-win" therapy: in >99% of 1000 bootstrap replications of the analysis, caffeine-treated infants had simultaneously better outcomes and lower mean costs. These results were robust to a 1000% increase in the individual resource items, including the price of caffeine citrate.

Conclusions.—In comparison with placebo, caffeine therapy for apnea of prematurity in infants weighing less than 1250 g is economically appealing for infants up to 18 to 21 months' corrected age.

▶ It was refreshing to see a cost-benefit analysis on an expensive but frequently used pharmacotherapy. All too often, drugs and devices are infused into clinical practice without consideration of cost. Methylxanthines in general, and caffeine specifically, have been used in neonatal practice for decades without much concern for safety, efficacy, or cost until the Caffeine for Apnea of Prematurity (CAP) trial. This large and robust clinical trial has generated enough data to now address all 3 issues. Caffeine (for apnea of prematurity) is a safe drug; it reduces the incidence of apnea, and treated infants are less expensive to care for through 18 to 21 months. The only downside to this trial has been the wider use of caffeine, especially to prevent chronic lung disease. Whether the results of the CAP trial can be extrapolated to these other indications remains to be seen.

Nevertheless, Dukhovny et al are to be congratulated for this undertaking, and this analysis should serve as a model for other widely used treatments in the neonatal intensive care unit.

S. M. Donn, MD

Understanding Variation in Vitamin A Supplementation Among NICUs
Kaplan HC, Tabangin ME, McClendon D, et al (Cincinnati Children's Hosp Med Ctr, OH)
Pediatrics 126:e367-e373, 2010

Objective.—We examined and characterized variation among NICUs in the use of vitamin A supplementation for the prevention of bronchopulmonary dysplasia in extremely low birth weight infants.

Methods.—An historical cohort study of extremely low birth weight infants admitted within 7 days after birth to NICUs participating in the Pediatric Health Information System database, between January 1, 2005, and March 31, 2008, was performed. NICU medical directors were surveyed to determine attitudes and decision-making regarding adoption of vitamin A supplementation. The proportion of infants receiving vitamin A at each center was measured over time. Patient and hospital characteristics associated with vitamin A use were examined.

Results.—Among 4184 eligible infants cared for in 30 NICUs, 1005 infants (24%) received vitamin A. Eighteen centers (60%) used vitamin A for some patients. Infants discharged in 2007 (odds ratio: 2.7 [95% confidence interval: 1.4−5.3]) and 2008 (odds ratio: 2.8 [95% confidence interval: 1.4−5.8]), compared with 2005, were more likely to receive vitamin A. NICU medical directors from centers using vitamin A, compared with centers that did not adopt vitamin A supplementation, reported stronger beliefs in the efficacy of vitamin A to reduce the incidence of bronchopulmonary dysplasia (83% vs 33%; $P = .03$) and in the ease with which vitamin A could be implemented (75% vs 22%; $P = .02$).

Conclusions.—Although the use of vitamin A is increasing, marked variation across NICUs remains. Provider attitudes and system characteristics seem to influence vitamin A adoption.

▶ Despite the limitations of survey-based research, I found this study interesting and timely. In this age of evidence-based clinical practice, vitamin A, one of only very few drugs with an evidence base demonstrating a statistically significant reduction in bronchopulmonary dysplasia (BPD), has still not found its way into mainstream practice. Kaplan and coinvestigators found that only a quarter of eligible babies were treated, even though 60% of surveyed neonatal intensive care unit medical directors reported that vitamin A was used in their units. There was an upward trend in utilization of vitamin A from 2005 to 2008, but variation in practice patterns persists.

The investigators tried to establish reasons for this. Centers using vitamin A had a stronger acceptance of evidence compared with those who did not use it, and difficulty in implementation of vitamin A treatment was frequently cited as a reason in units not using it.

We neonatologists are an interesting lot. We frequently use steroids, diuretics, and bronchodilators to prevent or treat BPD despite no evidence and a narrow therapeutic index, but we do not use a drug that has not only evidence for efficacy but a wide therapeutic margin as well. What are we missing?

S. M. Donn, MD

13 Postnatal Growth and Development/ Follow-up

Adult Outcome of Extremely Preterm Infants
Doyle LW, Anderson PJ (Univ of Melbourne, Victoria, Australia)
Pediatrics 126:342-351, 2010

Survival rates for extremely preterm (<28 weeks' gestational age) infants have increased and are approaching 3 in 4 with the advent of modern perinatal and neonatal intensive care. In contrast with some children with chronic diseases such as cystic fibrosis, most survivors of extreme prematurity have no ongoing health issues. However, as a group, they do have higher rates of adverse health outcomes, and more of them will present to pediatricians over time and, ultimately, to adult physicians as they grow older. Pediatricians can aid the transition to adult health care by being aware of the nutritional, cardiovascular, respiratory, motor, cognitive, psychiatric, and functional outcomes into adulthood of survivors of extreme prematurity.

▶ This review summarizes available data related to outcomes of extremely low (< 28 weeks)-gestational-age (ELGA) infants in early adulthood. Although the data are limited and reflect the results of care provided more than 2 decades ago, the authors correctly assert that they "provide the best estimates of what to expect for today's survivors, until superseded by more contemporary data." It is reassuring that most such infants have no significant health problems as young adults. There is cause for concern that they may be more likely to have reduced adult stature, lower bone density, impaired glucose tolerance, hypertension, and obstructive airways disease. Survivors of extreme prematurity have greatly increased rates of cerebral palsy, blindness, and deafness and are more likely to have intellectual impairment, but these deficits are found in a minority (11%-27%) of these subjects. ELGA infants are more likely to repeat grades and less likely to complete high school. They perform less well on cognitive testing and are at greater risk for hyperactivity and inattention. Not surprisingly, boys are at greater risk for those cognitive and behavioral impairments. Despite these limitations, preterm infants may do better in some functional areas, such as work performance. However, they are less likely to leave the parental home, experience sexual intercourse, or reproduce and are more likely to receive financial assistance because of disabilities. Importantly, self-reported quality-of-life scores are comparable with those for adults born at term. Although this review is directed to physicians who will care for survivors of extreme prematurity in adolescence or early adulthood, it provides information that will be very useful in counseling parents of the ELGA neonates about their long-term prospects.

W. E. Benitz, MD

Development of Preschool and Academic Skills in Children Born Very Preterm

Aarnoudse-Moens CSH, Oosterlaan J, Duivenvoorden HJ, et al (Sophia Children's Hosp, Rotterdam, The Netherlands; VU Univ Amsterdam, The Netherlands; Erasmus Univ Med Centre, Rotterdam, The Netherlands)
J Pediatr 158:15-20, 2011

Objective.—To examine performance in preschool and academic skills in very preterm (gestational age ≤30 weeks) and term-born comparison children aged 4 to 12 years.

Study Design.—Very preterm children (n = 200; mean age, 8.2 ± 2.5 years) born between 1996 and 2004 were compared with 230 term-born children (mean age, 8.3 ± 2.3). The Dutch National Pupil Monitoring System was used to measure preschool numerical reasoning and early linguistics, and primary school simple and complex word reading, reading comprehension, spelling, and mathematics/arithmetic. With univariate analyses of variance, we assessed the effects of preterm birth on performance across grades and on grade retention.

Results.—In preschool, very preterm children performed comparably with term-born children in early linguistics, but perform more poorly (0.7 standard deviation [SD]) in numerical reasoning skills. In primary school, very preterm children scored 0.3 SD lower in complex word reading and 0.6 SD lower in mathematics/arithmetic, but performed comparably with peers in reading comprehension and spelling. They had a higher grade repeat rate (25.5%), although grade repeat did not improve their academic skills.

Conclusions.—Very preterm children do well in early linguistics, reading comprehension, and spelling, but have clinically significant deficits in numerical reasoning skills and mathematics/arithmetic, which persist with time.

▶ The major clinical outcomes that are important to preterm infants and their families are not only survival but survival accompanied by normal long-term neurodevelopment. These goals are not easily attainable; however, the landscape has improved over the past 2 decades and there are now more intact survivors who attend mainstream schools and ultimately live independently. How to preserve brain function and permit normal brain development ex utero remains an enormous challenge. The period between 20 and 32 weeks after conception is one of rapid brain growth and development. During this time, illness, hemorrhage, ischemia, metabolic disturbances such as hypoglycemia, hyperbilirubinemia, and undernutrition, and infection may compromise neurodevelopment. Indeed, events leading to premature birth, such as chorioamnionitis, may have excited cytokines, which in turn injure the developing brain. Scores of publications continue to demonstrate inferior intellect and function in the most immature babies when compared with their term peers.

Aanoudse-Moens et al[1] completed a meta-analysis of neurobehavioral outcomes and reported that the combined effect sizes show that very preterm or very low birth weight (VLBW) children score 0.60 standard deviation (SD) lower on mathematics tests, 0.48 SD on reading tests, and 0.76 SD on spelling tests than term-born peers. Their summary statement was:

"Very preterm and/or VLBW children have moderate-to-severe deficits in academic achievement, attention problems, and internalizing behavioral problems and poor EF [executive function], which are adverse outcomes that were strongly correlated to their immaturity at birth. During transition to young adulthood these children continue to lag behind term-born peers."

Aanoudse-Moens et al report on their own cohort of 200 preterm infants that they have followed with a matched control group of term infants for 4 to 12 years. Their findings conform to the pattern of other publications. Very preterm children perform comparably with the comparison group in early linguistics, spelling, and reading comprehension; however, they have significant deficits in numerical reasoning skills and in mathematics/arithmetic. In primary school, they show catch-up with peers in reading of simple words, although they continue to lag behind peers in reading of complex words and mathematics/arithmetic. Boys appear to be even more disadvantaged in this area. It is disappointing to note that although 25% of the low birth weight babies repeat a grade, this does not seem to improve their academic skills.

Taylor et al[2] from our institution reviewed the topic of mathematic deficiencies in very low birth weight or very preterm birth. They noted that children with birth weights less than 1500 g and those with a gestational age less than 32 weeks have more mathematics disabilities or deficiencies (MD) and higher rates of mathematics learning disabilities than normal birth weight term-born children. They commented:

"MD are found even in children without global disorders in cognition or neurosensory status and when IQ is controlled, and they are associated with other learning problems and weaknesses in perceptual motor abilities and executive function. Factors related to poorer mathematics outcomes include lower birth weight and [gestational age] GA, neonatal complications, and possible abnormalities in brain structure."

Little is known about MD.

Thus, although the outcomes have improved overall, there is no room for complacency. Understanding the mechanisms of injury may help to provide the solutions since we are cognizant that neuroplasticity permits the neonatal brain to move a given function to a different location as a consequence of normal experience or brain damage.

A. A. Fanaroff, MD, FRCPE, FRCP&CH

References

1. Aarnoudse-Moens CS, Weisglas-Kuperus N, van Goudoever JB, Oosterlaan J. Meta-analysis of neurobehavioral outcomes in very preterm and/or very low birth weight children. *Pediatrics.* 2009;124:717-728.
2. Taylor HG, Espy KA, Anderson PJ. Mathematics deficiencies in children with very low birth weight or very preterm birth. *Dev Disabil Res Rev.* 2009;15:52-59.

Early Intervention Improves Cognitive Outcomes for Preterm Infants: Randomized Controlled Trial

Nordhov SM, Rønning JA, Dahl LB, et al (Univ Hosp of North Norway Trust, Tromsø, Norway; et al)
Pediatrics 126:e1088-e1094, 2010

Objective.—The goal was to examine the effectiveness of an early intervention on cognitive and motor outcomes at corrected ages of 3 and 5 years for children with birth weights (BWs) of <2000 g.

Methods.—A randomized controlled trial of a modified version of the Mother-Infant Transaction Program was performed. Outcomes were assessed with the Bayley Scales of Infant Development II and the Wechsler Preschool and Primary Scale of Intelligence-Revised at 3 and 5 years, respectively. McCarthy Scales of Children's Abilities and the grooved pegboard test were used to test motor outcomes at 5 years.

Results.—A total of 146 infants were assigned randomly (intervention group: 72 infants; control group: 74 infants). The mean BWs were 1396 ± 429 g for the intervention group and 1381 ± 436 g for the control group. After adjustment for maternal education, a nonsignificant difference in Mental Developmental Index scores at 3 years of 4.5 points (95% confidence interval: −0.3 to 9.3 points) in favor of the intervention group was found, whereas the intervention effect on full-scale IQ scores at 5 years was 6.4 points (95% confidence interval: 0.6−12.2 points). Significantly more children in the intervention group had IQ scores of ≥85 at 3 and 5 years. There were no differences between the groups with respect to motor outcomes.

Conclusion.—This modified version of the Mother-Infant Transaction Program improved cognitive outcomes at corrected age of 5 years for children with BWs of <2000 g.

▶ The Mother-Infant Transaction Program (MITP), an intervention program that uses a transactional model to facilitate maternal adjustment to the care of a low birth weight infant and indirectly enhance the child's development, was first described in 1986. Sequential neurodevelopmental assessments of the original cohort of very low birth weight infants enrolled in the pilot study suggested that the intervention was associated with a sustained positive effect on intelligence after 3 years of age.[1]

The MITP consists of 11 sessions, beginning during the final week of hospitalization and extending into the home over a 3-month period. In this randomized trial, the investigators modified the MITP to include an initial debriefing session in which parents could talk about their experiences of the hospital stay and express feelings such as grief, disappointment, or anger, and to encourage both parents to participate in the intervention. After the initial session, the intervention consisted of 1-hour daily sessions with both parents and their infant on 7 consecutive days, starting the week before planned discharge. Each session addressed aspects such as the infant's reflexes, self-regulation and interactions, signs of distress and predominant states, and how parents could bring the infants into a quiet alert state for mutual interaction. The last 2 in-hospital sessions were devoted to parents achieving sensitivity and responsiveness toward their infant through daily routines. The daily in-hospital sessions were followed by 4 home visits by the same intervention nurse at 3, 14, 30, and 90 days after discharge. The home visits addressed adjustment to the home environment, interaction between parents and the infant, how to guide and stimulate the infant, and discussion and evaluation of the intervention program. Infants were randomized to receive the intervention or usual postdischarge care.

Participants in the intervention group did not have access to the intervention nurses outside the scheduled intervention dates.

The modified MITP intervention program demonstrated increased effects over time on cognitive outcomes, culminating in significant group differences at 5 years of age. A similar pattern was noted in the original pilot study. The authors postulate that the transactional model inherent in the modified MITP creates a positive feedback loop through enhanced interaction between less stressed and more confident parents and their responsive infants. A logical next step would be to replicate the intervention program on a different sample of infants considered to be at biological risk.

L. A. Papile, MD

Reference

1. Achenbach TM, Howell CT, Aoki MF, Rauh VA. Nine-year outcome of the Vermont intervention program for low birth weight infants. *Pediatrics.* 1993;91:45-55.

Early-Childhood Neurodevelopmental Outcomes Are Not Improving for Infants Born at <25 Weeks' Gestational Age
Hintz SR, for the NICHD Neonatal Research Network (Stanford Univ School of Medicine, Palo Alto, CA; et al)
Pediatrics 127:62-70, 2011

Objective.—We compared neurodevelopmental outcomes at 18 to 22 months' corrected age of infants born with extremely low birth weight at an estimated gestational age of <25 weeks during 2 periods: 1999—2001 (epoch 1) and 2002—2004 (epoch 2).

Patients and Methods.—We conducted a multicenter, retrospective analysis of the Eunice Kennedy Shriver National Institute of Child Health and Human Development Neonatal Research Network. Perinatal and neonatal variables and outcomes were compared between epochs. Neurodevelopmental outcomes at 18 to 22 months' corrected age were evaluated with neurologic exams and Bayley Scales of Infant Development II. Logistic regression analyses determined the independent risk of epoch for adverse outcomes.

Results.—Infant survival was similar between epochs (epoch 1, 35.4%, vs epoch 2, 32.3%; $P=.09$). A total of 411 of 452 surviving infants in epoch 1 and 405 of 438 surviving infants in epoch 2 were evaluated at 18 to 22 months' corrected age. Cesarean delivery $(P=.03)$, surgery for patent ductus arteriosus $(P=.004)$, and late sepsis $(P=.01)$ were more common in epoch 2, but postnatal steroid use was dramatically reduced (63.5% vs 32.8%; $P<.0001$). Adverse outcomes at 18 to 22 months' corrected age were common in both epochs. Moderate-to-severe cerebral palsy was diagnosed in 11.1% of surviving infants in epoch 1 and 14.9% in epoch 2 (adjusted odds ratio [OR]: 1.52 [95% confidence interval (CI): 0.86−2.71]; $P=.15$), the Mental Developmental Index was <70 in 44.9% in epoch 1 and 51% in epoch 2 (OR: 1.30 [95% CI: 0.91−1.87]; $P=.15$), and neurodevelopmental impairment was diagnosed in 50.1% of surviving infants in epoch 1 and 58.7% in epoch 2 (OR: 1.4 [95% CI: 0.98−2.04]; $P=.07$).

Conclusions.—Early-childhood outcomes for infants born at <25 weeks' estimated gestational age were unchanged between the 2 periods.

▶ It is important to keep in mind that the neurodevelopmental outcomes reported in the Hintz study cannot be generalized. The cohorts consisted of surviving infants who were cared for in newborn centers that participated in the National Institute of Child Health and Human Development Neonatal Research Network (NRN), all of which are university based and, as such, serve a population of extremely low gestational age infants who are the sickest and most socially disadvantaged, factors that have been shown to have a detrimental effect on later neurodevelopment. Medicaid was the source of payment for approximately 70% in both epochs, and the rates of surgery and late-onset sepsis remained high at approximately 50% in both cohorts.

Regional cohort studies may give a more realistic approximation of neurosensory outcomes for these extremely preterm infants, because they are not confounded by referral bias. The Victoria Infant Collaborative Study Group, a regional consortium that is dedicated to the systematic follow-up of infants who are born in Victoria, Australia, and are less than 28 weeks of gestational age, recently reported a moderate/severe impairment rate of 20% at 2 years of age for the cohort born in 2005.[1] The outcome for the subset of infants less than 25 weeks of gestational age was not delineated. In a previous report from the Collaborative, the rate of moderate/severe impairment at 2 years corrected age was 39% for infants born at less than 25 weeks of gestational age in 1997, a rate that is far lower than the 50% to 59% reported in this study.[2] Both the NRN and the Collaborative studies report similar survival rates; however, neither group includes infants who were born alive, but not admitted to a neonatal intensive care unit.

L. A. Papile, MD

References

1. Doyle LW, Roberts G, Anderson PJ; Victorian Infant Collaborative Study group. Outcomes at age 2 years of infants <28 weeks' gestational age born in Victoria in 2005. *J Pediatr.* 2010;156:49-53.
2. Doyle LW; Victorian Infant Collaborative Study Group. Neonatal intensive care at borderline viability—is it worth it? *Early Hum Dev.* 2004;80:103-113.

Executive and Memory Function in Adolescents Born Very Preterm
Luu TM, Ment L, Allan W, et al (Sainte-Justine Univ Health Ctr, Montreal, Quebec, Canada; Yale Univ School of Medicine, New Haven, CT; Maine Med Ctr, Portland; et al)
Pediatrics 127:e639-e646, 2011

Background.—Many preterm children display school difficulties, which may be mediated by impairment in executive function and memory.

Objective.—To evaluate executive and memory function among adolescents born preterm compared with term controls at 16 years.

Methods.—A total of 337 of 437 (77%) adolescents born in 1989 to 1992 with a birth weight < 1250 g and 102 term controls were assessed with a battery of executive function and memory tasks. Multiple regression analyses were used to compare groups and to identify associations between selected factors and outcomes among preterm subjects.

Results.—Adolescents born preterm, compared with term controls, showed deficits in executive function in the order of 0.4 to 0.6 SD on tasks of verbal fluency, inhibition, cognitive flexibility, planning/organization, and working memory as well as verbal and visuospatial memory. After exclusion of adolescents with neurosensory disabilities and full-scale IQ < 70, significant group differences persisted on most tests. Preterm subjects, compared with term controls, were at increased risk of exhibiting problems related to executive dysfunction, as measured with the Behavior Rating Inventory of Executive Function, on the Metacognition Index (odds ratio [OR]: 2.5 [95% confidence interval (CI): 1.2—5.1]) and the Global Executive Composite (OR: 4.2 [95% CI: 1.6—10.9]), but not on the Behavioral Regulation index (OR: 1.5 [95% CI: 0.7—3.5]). Among adolescents born preterm, severe brain injury on neonatal ultrasound and lower maternal education were the most consistent factors associated with poor outcomes.

Conclusions.—Even after exclusion of preterm subjects with significant disabilities, adolescents born preterm in the early 1990s were at increased risk of deficits in executive function and memory.

▶ Follow-up of graduates from the intensive care unit has shed the orphan role it held for so long and is now a genuine and legitimate component of neonatology. Indeed, neurodevelopmental follow-up has become an integral part of the primary outcome in most prospective randomized interventional trials on both term and preterm infants. Absence of harm and normal long-term neurodevelopment are the desired outcome. This report from Luu et al is part of an emerging body of literature showing that very preterm birth is associated with executive function (EF) impairments. Their adolescent cohort of extremely immature infants demonstrates multiple deficits of EF. Of note, infants with the greatest degree of brain injury on ultrasound and those with mothers who had the least education were the most vulnerable to EF deficits. This implies that providing a more stimulating and enriched home environment may be of some benefit in averting the EF deficits.

Johnson et al[1] from Leicester in the United Kingdom similarly reported that children born extremely preterm had significantly poorer academic attainment and a higher prevalence of learning difficulties than their term peers. General cognitive ability and specific deficits in visuospatial skills or phoneme deletion (the smallest segmental unit of sound used to form meaningful contrasts between utterances) at 6 years of age were predictive of mathematics and reading attainment at 11 years in both extremely preterm and term children. Phonemic fluency skills are increasingly delayed, but phonological processing, attention, and EFs at 6 years of age were associated with academic attainment in children born extremely preterm.

Woodward et al[2] correlated neonatal MRI with executive functioning abilities at 4 years of age. Very preterm children performed less well than full-term children on measures of planning ability, cognitive flexibility, selective attention, and inhibitory control. Executive impairments at 4 years of age were confined to preterm children with mild or moderate to severe white matter abnormalities on MRI. These findings support the importance of cerebral white matter integrity for later EF.

To determine whether the EF deficits related only to abnormal neurodevelopment, Ni et al[3] from Taiwan studied 6-year-old very low birth weight children with normal early development. They were still at risk of EF deficits, including planning, cognitive flexibility, and nonverbal working memory. Both gestation age and birth weight were important covariant factors.

Mulder et al[4] were of the opinion (not necessarily shared by other investigators) that processing speed and working memory are important factors underlying academic attainment in very preterm children. Specific tests of processing speed and working memory, which together take approximately only 10 minutes to administer, could potentially be used as efficient screening instruments to assess which children are at risk of educational problems and should be referred for a full neuropsychological assessment. Time alone will determine whether they are correct, but it is vital that these EF deficits be identified as soon as possible and appropriate interventions implemented.

A. A. Fanaroff, MD, FRCPE, FRCP&CH

References

1. Johnson S, Wolke D, Hennessy E, Marlow N. Educational outcomes in extremely preterm children: neuropsychological correlates and predictors of attainment. *Dev Neuropsychol.* 2011;36:74-95.

2. Woodward LJ, Clark CA, Pritchard VE, Anderson PJ, Inder TE. Neonatal white matter abnormalities predict global executive function impairment in children born very preterm. *Dev Neuropsychol.* 2011;36:22-41.
3. Ni TL, Huang CC, Guo NW. Executive function deficit in preschool children born very low birth weight with normal early development. *Early Hum Dev.* 2011;87: 137-141.
4. Mulder H, Pitchford NJ, Marlow N. Processing speed and working memory underlie academic attainment in very preterm children. *Arch Dis Child Fetal Neonatal Ed.* 2010;95:F267-F272.

Neurodevelopment of Extremely Preterm Infants who had Necrotizing Enterocolitis with or without Late Bacteremia

Martin CR, Dammann O, Allred EN, et al (Beth Israel Deaconess Med Ctr, Boston, MA; Tufts Univ, Medford, MA; et al)

J Pediatr 157:751-756, 2010

Objective.—To evaluate neurodevelopment after necrotizing enterocolitis (NEC) and late bacteremia, alone and together.

Study Design.—Sample included 1155 infants born at 23 to 27 weeks' gestation. NEC was classified by the modified Bell's staging criteria and grouped as medical NEC or surgical NEC. Late bacteremia was defined as a positive blood culture result after the first postnatal week. Neurodevelopment was assessed at 24 months corrected age. Multivariable models estimated the risk of developmental dysfunction and microcephaly associated with medical or surgical NEC with and without late bacteremia.

Results.—Children who had surgical NEC unaccompanied by late bacteremia were at increased risk of psychomotor developmental indexes <70 (OR = 2.7 [1.2, 6.4]), and children who had both surgical NEC and late bacteremia were at increased risk of diparetic cerebral palsy (OR = 8.4 [1.9, 39]) and microcephaly (OR = 9.3 [2.2, 40]). In contrast, children who had medical NEC with or without late bacteremia were not at increased risk of any developmental dysfunction.

Conclusion.—The risk of neurodevelopmental dysfunction and microcephaly is increased in children who had surgical NEC, especially if they also had late bacteremia. These observations support the hypothesis that bowel injury might initiate systemic inflammation potentially affecting the developing brain (Fig).

▶ Neonatologists are highly aware of the challenges associated with preventing, diagnosing, and treating babies with necrotizing enterocolitis (NEC), which is one of the leading causes of mortality and morbidity in extremely low birth weight infants.[1] They are also aware of the intestinal consequences of NEC such as strictures and short gut syndrome. Over the past few years, studies such as the one by Martin et al are beginning to emphasize that infants with NEC have a high likelihood of major neurodevelopmental outcome, partially based on severity of the disease. Of interest is that babies who have higher inflammatory cytokine plasma concentrations have poorer neurodevelopmental

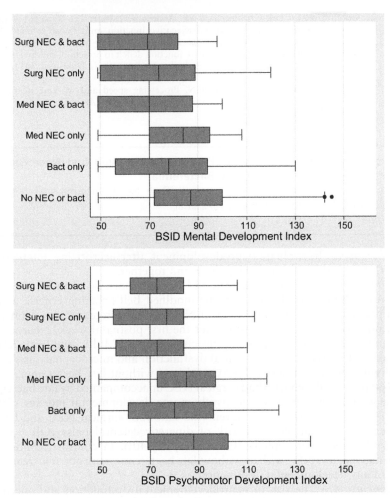

FIGURE.—In these box and whisker displays of the distribution of MDI and PDI, the median is indicated by the *vertical line* close to the middle of each box and the 25th and 75th centiles by the sides of each box. The dispersion of the MDI and PDI scores is indicated by the length of the *horizontal lines* that emanate from the *box*, as well as by the *large dots*, which identify outliers. There is a *box* for each combination of NEC and late bacteremia. (Reprinted from Journal of Pediatrics, Martin CR, Dammann O, Allred EN, et al. Neurodevelopment of extremely preterm infants who had necrotizing enterocolitis with or without late bacteremia. *J Pediatr*. 2010;157:751-756. Copyright 2010 with permission from Elsevier.)

outcomes.[2] The hypothesis that the gut is the origin of systemic inflammation in many of these situations[3] is certainly supported by these studies. In this study, the odds ratio of diparetic cerebral palsy is 8.4 for babies with surgical NEC and late bacteremia, a very worrisome outcome. There are also signals that medical NEC with bacteremia may also have neurodevelopmental consequences (Fig). One of the most important aspects of this study as so nicely pointed out in the discussion section is that these neurodevelopmental consequences of NEC are likely to be multifactorial, but the argument for gut origin inflammation that affects other organs provides a target for disease prevention that encompasses not only NEC but also distal organs that can be affected by the inflammatory state initiated in the intestine.

J. Neu, MD

References

1. Neu J, Walker WA. Necrotizing enterocolitis. *N Engl J Med.* 2011;364:255-264.
2. Lodha A, Asztalos E, Moore AM. Cytokine levels in neonatal necrotizing enterocolitis and long-term growth and neurodevelopment. *Acta Paediatr.* 2010;99: 338-343.
3. Caicedo RA, Schanler RJ, Li N, Neu J. The developing intestinal ecosystem: implications for the neonate. *Pediatr Res.* 2005;58:625-628.

Neurodevelopmental Outcomes of Triplets or Higher-Order Extremely Low Birth Weight Infants
Wadhawan R, for the Eunice Kennedy Shriver National Institute of Child Health & Human Development Neonatal Research Network (All Children's Hosp, St Petersburg, FL; et al)
Pediatrics 127:e654-e660, 2011

Background.—Extremely low birth weight twins have a higher rate of death or neurodevelopmental impairment than singletons. Higher-order extremely low birth weight multiple births may have an even higher rate of death or neurodevelopmental impairment.

Methods.—Extremely low birth weight (birth weight 401−1000 g) multiple births born in participating centers of the Neonatal Research Network between 1996 and 2005 were assessed for death or neurodevelopmental impairment at 18 to 22 months' corrected age. Neurodevelopmental impairment was defined by the presence of 1 or more of the following: moderate to severe cerebral palsy; mental developmental index score or psychomotor developmental index score less than 70; severe bilateral deafness; or blindness. Infants who died within 12 hours of birth were excluded. Maternal and infant demographic and clinical variables were compared among singleton, twin, and triplet or higher-order infants. Logistic regression analysis was performed to establish the association between singletons, twins, and triplet or higher-order multiples and death or neurodevelopmental impairment, controlling for confounding variables that may affect death or neurodevelopmental impairment.

Results.—Our cohort consisted of 8296 singleton, 2164 twin, and 521 triplet or higher-order infants. The risk of death or neurodevelopmental impairment was increased in triplets or higher-order multiples when compared with singletons (adjusted odds ratio: 1.7 [95% confidence interval: 1.29−2.24]), and there was a trend toward an increased risk when compared with twins (adjusted odds ratio: 1.27 [95% confidence: 0.95−1.71]).

TABLE 3.—Short-Term and 18- to 22-Months Outcomes by Univariate Analysis

Outcome	Singletons, n = 8296	Twins, n = 2164	Triplets or Higher-Order Births, n = 521	P, Twins vs Singletons	P, Triplets or Higher-Order Births vs Singletons	P, Triplets or Higher-Order Births vs Twins
Severe intraventricular hemorrhage, n (%)	1361 (17.0)	415 (20.4)	79 (16.0)	.0016	.61	.048
Bronchopulmonary dysplasia, n (%)[a]	3002 (47.9)	756 (50.9)	165 (44.0)	.05	.21	.038
Late-onset sepsis, n (%)	3042 (38.8)	782 (40.2)	183 (39.5)	.27	.77	.80
Necrotizing enterocolitis, n (%)	933 (11.3)	252 (11.7)	35 (6.7)	.61	.0002	.0003
Death before discharge, n (%)	2080 (25.1)	694 (32.1)	137 (26.3)	<.0001	.64	.043
Death or NDI, n (%)	4418 (53.3)	1324 (61.2)	289 (55.5)	<.0001	.44	.064
NDI, n (%)[b]	2190 (36.1)	585 (41.1)	149 (39.1)	.0018	.3341	.57

[a]Defined as supplementary oxygen at 36 weeks (yes or no) for survivors to 36 weeks.
[b]Denominator: surviving infants with complete follow-up data (singletons, n = 6068; twins, n = 1425; triplets or higher order, n = 381).

Conclusions.—Triplet or higher-order births are associated with an increased risk of death or neurodevelopmental impairment at 18 to 22 months' corrected age when compared with extremely low birth weight singleton infants, and there was a trend toward an increased risk when compared with twins (Table 3).

▶ This report from the National Institute of Child Health and Human Development (NICHD) Neonatal Research Network builds on a large body of literature on the outcomes of extremely low birth weight (ELBW) triplets that is confusing and often apparently inconsistent. This work both exemplifies and helps us understand that inconsistency. Paradoxically, the raw data from this large multicenter cohort (Table 3) indicate that ELBW twins, but not triplets, have higher rates of severe intraventricular hemorrhage, bronchopulmonary dysplasia, death, neurodevelopmental impairment (NDI), or the combined outcome of death or NDI. Triplets had less necrotizing enterocolitis than either singletons or twins. Multiple logistic regression revealed that the unexpectedly better outcomes in triplets were mediated by factors other than multiplicity of gestation, however. Mothers of triplets were more likely to be white, married, better educated, to have nongovernmental insurance, and to have received prenatal care and prenatal steroids; they were less likely to have had preeclampsia or hypertension. After adjustment for several of these variables, triplet gestation was associated with a significantly greater risk of death or NDI (odds ratio 1.7 for triplets vs singletons), confirming the suspicion that it is better not to have to share the womb with multiple roommates.

What are the practical implications of these results? First, the fact that unadjusted outcomes of triplets are comparable with those of singletons is not an argument against fetal reduction in triplet pregnancies. Lower-order gestations have the advantage of reducing the risk of having ELBW neonates, so these data are simply not cogent to those difficult and sensitive conversations. Second, these data confound use of outcomes statistics in discussing prognosis with parents of ELBW triplets. These results imply that outcomes for triplets will be better than those predicted by the NICHD Neonatal Network Outcomes Calculator,[1] for example, as the covariates that shift the data for triplets in a favorable direction (race, education, and so forth) are not accounted for in that model, but those characteristics are not shared by all triplets. Regrettably, the specifics of the regression model are not provided in this report. Until use of more sophisticated mathematical models at the bedside becomes more routine, the best that we can do is to remember to consider triplet gestation as only one among many variables relevant to prognosis for ELBW infants.

W. E. Benitz, MD

Reference

1. Tyson JE, Parikh NA, Langer J, Green C, Higgins RD. Intensive care for extreme prematurity—moving beyond gestational age. *N Engl J Med.* 2008;358:1672-1681.

Long-Term Cognitive Outcomes After Pediatric Stroke

Kolk A, Ennok M, Laugesaar R, et al (Univ of Tartu, Estonia; Tartu Univ Hosp, Estonia)
Pediatr Neurol 44:101-109, 2011

This study assessed neurocognitive and neurologic outcomes of children with neonatal and childhood strokes. Twenty-one children with neonatal (mean age, 6.86 years) and 10 children with childhood (mean age, 8.21 years) strokes, identified via the Estonian Pediatric Stroke Database (1995-2006), participated. A developmental neuropsychologic assessment was used for neurocognitive outcomes, and the Paediatric Stroke Outcome Measure for neurologic outcomes. Neuromotor impairment was evident in 62% of children with neonatal strokes, and in 70% of children with childhood strokes. Compared with control subjects, children with strokes exhibited worse attention, language, memory, and sensorimotor functions. The sensorimotor domain comprised the most impaired neurocognitive area, whereas executive functions remained intact in both stroke groups. A well-preserved executive function may account for the normal range of intelligence in children with strokes. More severe impairment in neurocognitive skills was evident after neonatal strokes, and the visuospatial domain was more impaired than in children from the childhood group. Prognoses were worse after left hemisphere strokes associated with epilepsy. Our results on emerging neurocognitive deficits in several areas underline the importance of neuropsychologic testing and the follow-up of children with pediatric strokes.

▶ Early outcome studies indicate that neonatal stroke adversely affects motor function, but usually spares general cognitive function; however, a recent longitudinal study found a statistically significant decline in overall intellectual ability between early childhood and school age with subtle deficits in higher-level cognitive skills noted.[1]

In this observational study, the authors evaluated neurocognitive functions of 21 children with neonatal stroke at a mean age of 8.21 years and compared their outcome to that of an age- and sex-matched cohort of healthy children. The stroke cohort had an IQ greater than 80 and the school-aged children attended a normal school and class appropriate for their age. Nine of the children with stroke had epilepsy and received antiepileptic medication. A comprehensive neuropsychological battery (NEPSY) that measures attention and executive functions, language, sensorimotor functions, visuospatial functions, and memory and learning was used. The stroke group performed at the same level as the control group in executive function, but there was a significant difference in attention between groups, with the greatest difference occurring in visual attention. Although the stroke group performed less well in the other 3 domains, the differences were not significant. Lesion side exerted a detectable effect on cognitive performance in the stroke group. Generally, children with a right hemisphere lesion performed better than those with a left hemisphere stroke, with significant differences noted in several visuospatial and sensorimotor functions. Children with epilepsy performed less well than children without epilepsy.

The dichotomous findings of good performance in executive functions and diffuse impairments of other functions are most likely explained by the fact that neonatal strokes do not involve the prefrontal regions of the brain. This may also be the reason children with neonatal stroke perform well on IQ tests. However, as the results of the study highlight, children with neonatal stroke need to be followed longitudinally to identify specific neuropsychological impairments early and intervene as needed.

L. A. Papile, MD

Reference

1. Westmacott R, MacGregor D, Askalan R, deVeber G. Late emergence of cognitive deficits after unilateral neonatal stroke. *Stroke.* 2009;40:2012-2019.

Long-term outcome of children with congenital toxoplasmosis
Berrébi A, Assouline C, Bessières M-H, et al (Hôpital Paule de Viguier, Toulouse, France; Hôpital des Enfants, Toulouse, France; Hôpital Rangueil, Toulouse, France)
Am J Obstet Gynecol 203:552.e1-552.e6, 2010

Objective.—Maternal toxoplasmosis infection acquired during pregnancy carries significant risk of fetal damage. We aimed to assess the long-term outcome of children and young adults with congenital toxoplasmosis diagnosed and treated in utero.

Study Design.—This was a 20 year prospective study (1985-2005). All mothers received spiramycin, alone or associated with pyrimethamine-sulfadoxine, and underwent amniocentesis and monthly ultrasound screening. Infected children were followed every 3-6 months.

Results.—Of 666 liveborn children (676 mothers), 112 (17%) had congenital toxoplasmosis. Among these, 107 were followed up for 12-250 months: 79 were asymptomatic (74%) and 28 had chorioretinitis (26%). Only 1 child had a serious neurological involvement.

Conclusion.—The percentage of chorioretinitis in treated children depends on length of follow-up, but this complication occurs mainly before the age of 5 years and almost always before the age of 10 years. Visual impairment was infrequently severe, and outcome appears consistently good. Long-term follow-up is recommended to monitor ocular and neurological prognosis, whatever the practical difficulties.

► In France, all pregnant women who are seronegative for toxoplasmosis at the beginning of pregnancy have monthly serological screenings for toxoplasmosis throughout their pregnancy. As soon as seroconversion occurs, they are treated with daily spiramycin and undergo an amniocentesis and monthly ultrasound scans.

This study included 676 women infected with toxoplasmosis who were followed at a regional center. At birth, infants underwent cranial ultrasonography, ocular examination, and serological and parasitological studies. Infants with a positive fetal diagnosis were treated with pyrimethamine and sulfadoxine until 2 years of age. Any infant whose amniotic fluid polymerase chain reaction was negative for toxoplasmosis was considered to have a fetal infection if antibodies were still present at 18 months of age. The rate of congenital toxoplasmosis was 17% (112/666).

Ultrasound screening in late pregnancy showed minor abnormalities in 6 fetuses (5%), including moderate ventricular dilatation in 4 infants and moderate intrauterine growth restriction (< 10th percentile) in 2 infants. On long-term follow-up, 4 of the 6 had normal development, 1 had language delay, and 1 developed epilepsy. The remaining 101 children had age-appropriate neurological and intellectual development and all were in age-appropriate grades in school. Chorioretinitis was noted in 28 children, with peripheral unilateral lesions found in 70%. Only 39% of infants with chorioretinitis had lesions detected in the newborn period.

Although these results are encouraging, they most likely do not represent the true spectrum of disease. Most women had relatively late seroconversion (mean gestational age was 23 ± 6 weeks) because women who had early seroconversion, the type that leads to the most serious fetal abnormalities, were not referred for treatment.

L. A. Papile, MD

Prevention and Schizophrenia—The Role of Dietary Factors
McGrath J, Brown A, St Clair D (The Park Centre for Mental Health, Wacol, Australia; College of Physicians and Surgeons of Columbia Univ, NY; Univ of Aberdeen, Foresterhill, UK)
Schizophr Bull 37:272-283, 2011

Adequate prenatal nutrition is essential for optimal brain development. There is a growing body of evidence from epidemiology linking exposure to nutritional deprivation and increased risk of schizophrenia. Based on studies from the Netherlands and China, those exposed to macronutrient deficiencies during famine have an increased risk of schizophrenia. With respect to micronutrients, we focus on 3 candidates where there is biological plausibility for a role in this disorder and at least 1 study of an association with schizophrenia. These nutrients include vitamin D, folic acid, and iron. While the current evidence is incomplete, we discuss the potential implications of these findings for the prevention of schizophrenia. We argue that schizophrenia can draw inspiration from public health interventions related to prenatal nutrition and other outcomes and speculate on relevant factors that bear on the nature, risks, impact, and logistics of various nutritional strategies that may be employed to prevent this disorder.

▶ The likely relationship of specific psychiatric disorders in offspring to dietary factors during pregnancy is raised in this article. They begin by citing data from survivors of the Dutch Famine in the Netherlands during World War II and Mao Zedong's Great Leap Forward between 1959 and 1961 who had a 2-fold risk in the development of schizophrenia. They then discuss 3 micronutrients for which there are epidemiology data for increased risk of schizophrenia and data from animals that demonstrate brain anatomical and biochemical abnormalities that may relate to deficiency of vitamin D, folate, and iron. The authors try to make it clear that the data on a causal relationship between these deficiencies remain sparse, but they present a strong case both from an epidemiologic standpoint and from a hypothetical mechanistic perspective that likelihood exists for such a relationship. Although it may seem like a simple solution to just make sure these nutrients are added to the diets of pregnant women as supplements, it is likely to be more complicated and some caution will be needed. The authors caution that some of the data on vitamin D supplementation are bimodal, showing that small supplements may decrease the risk, but higher supplements may actually increase the risk. They express concern about the epigenetic effects of folate, along with its capability to methylate important genes, such as IGF. The long-term effects of such perturbations are not yet fully known. Nevertheless, the potential for relatively low cost preventative strategies that may prevent this devastating condition using nutritional strategies beg additional attention to this area of research.

J. Neu, MD

Parent-Completed Developmental Screening in Premature Children: A Valid Tool for Follow-Up Programs

Flamant C, Branger B, Tich SNT, et al (Univ Hosp, Nantes, France; "Loire Infant Follow-up Team" (LIFT) Network, Pays de Loire, France; et al)

PLoS One 6:e20004, 2011

Our goals were to (1) validate the parental Ages and Stages Questionnaires (ASQ) as a screening tool for psychomotor development among a cohort of ex-premature infants reaching 2 years, and (2) analyse the influence of parental socio-economic status and maternal education on the efficacy of the questionnaire. A regional population of 703 very preterm infants (<35 weeks gestational age) born between 2003 and 2006 were evaluated at 2 years by their parents who completed the ASQ, by a pediatric clinical examination, and by the revised Brunet Lezine psychometric test with establishment of a DQ score. Detailed information regarding parental socio-economic status was available for 419 infants. At 2 years corrected age, 630 infants (89.6%) had an optimal neuromotor examination. Overall ASQ scores for predicting a DQ score ≤85 produced an area under the receiver operator curve value of 0.85 (95% Confidence Interval:0.82−0.87). An ASQ cut-off score of ≤220 had optimal discriminatory power for identifying a DQ score ≤85 with a sensitivity of 0.85 (95%CI:0.75−0.91), a specificity of 0.72 (95%CI:0.69−0.75), a positive likelihood ratio of 3, and a negative likelihood ratio of 0.21. The median value for ASQ was not significantly associated with socio-economic level or maternal education. ASQ is an easy and reliable tool regardless of the socio-economic status of the family to predict normal neurologic outcome in expremature infants at 2 years of age. ASQ may be beneficial with a low-cost impact to some follow-up programs, and helps to establish a genuine sense of parental involvement.

▶ Data regarding the neurodevelopmental outcome of infants who survive modern-day neonatal intensive care are essential to understanding the risk-benefit ratio of therapies and practices. However, the paradigm of formal neuro-developmental assessment at 18 to 22 months' corrected age used as the gold standard in many clinical trials is difficult to sustain for infants not enrolled in studies, because it is costly, time-consuming, and poorly compensated, at least in the United States.

In the above observational study, the authors compared the results of a formal French psychometric test (Brunet-Lezine) at 24 months' corrected age with those obtained on the Ages and Stages Questionnaire (ASQ), a parent-administered evaluation of infant development. The ASQ standard for a failed screen is failure in 1 of the 5 domains measured. Using this criterion, the sensitivity and specificity of the ASQ compared with the formal assessment were 0.88 and 0.57, respectively, for detecting a formal assessment score of ≤85 (1 SD below the mean). However, when the investigators constructed a receiver operating curve using the ASQ as a continuous variable, they noted an area under the curve of 0.85 with a cut-off score of 220 having optimal discriminatory power for identifying a formal assessment score of ≤85. The sensitivity and specificity for a score ≤220 (0.85 and 0.72, respectively) fulfill the criteria for a valid screening tool (xx sensitivity and xx specificity). An additional advantage of the ASQ was that the level of maternal education or socioeconomic status did not influence the validity of the test. These data suggest that the ASQ is an attractive, low-cost alternative to formal neurodevelopmental assessment of all high-risk infants and allows programs to conserve resources by focusing on the subset of infants who are most likely to have poor outcome.

L. A. Papile, MD

Aerobic Fitness and Physical Activity Levels of Children Born Prematurely following Randomization to Postnatal Dexamethasone

Nixon PA, Washburn LK, Mudd LM, et al (Wake Forest Univ, Winston-Salem, NC; Wake Forest Univ School of Medicine, Winston-Salem, NC; Appalachian State Univ, Boone, NC)
J Pediatr 158:113-118, 2011

Objective.—To investigate the effects of postnatal dexamethasone treatment on aerobic fitness and physical activity levels in school-aged children born with very low birth weight (VLBW).

Study Design.—This was a follow-up study of 65 VLBW infants who participated in a randomized controlled trial of dexamethasone (DEX) to reduce ventilator dependency. Aerobic fitness was determined from peak oxygen uptake (VO_{2peak}) with a cycle ergometer. Habitual physical activity was assessed by questionnaire.

Results.—A trend for a treatment with an interaction between treatment and of diagnosis of chronic lung disease (CLD) was found, with the children in the placebo group with CLD having the lowest VO_{2peak} ($P = .09$). Reduced fitness was seen in 53% of the group treated with DEX and 48% of the group given placebo. No between-group differences in physical activity were seen. Parental reports suggested that nearly two-thirds of the children participated in <1 hour per week of vigorous physical activity, which was explained in part by decreased large airway function ($r = 0.30$; $P = .03$).

Conclusions.—We found no adverse effect of postnatal DEX on aerobic fitness or habitual physical activity at school age. However, the reduced fitness and physical activity levels emphasize the need for closer follow-up and early interventions promoting physical activity to reduce the risk of chronic disease in this at-risk population.

▶ This study addresses an interesting question in a cohort of children who were born prematurely and involved in a study of dexamethasone (DEX) given for 42 days versus placebo in a randomized fashion: do the children who were treated with DEX have poorer lung function and/or decreased physical activity when compared with controls? One point of interest in the patient entry diagram is that 16 of the original 61 babies in the placebo group died, while only 7 of the original 57 babies in the DEX group died. In the DEX group, 6 children could not be enrolled because 3 had cerebral palsy, cognitive impairments, or inability to reach the pedals, whereas only 1 child was not able to enroll in the placebo group because of cognitive limitations. Nevertheless, the point of this study was to determine aerobic fitness and physical activity levels in these children. The peak oxygen uptake in preterm babies who received DEX versus placebo was not different. However, if chronic lung disease (CLD) was taken into consideration, children in the placebo group with CLD showed a slight trend toward decrease in peak oxygen uptake, whereas those who received DEX as babies did not suggest any differences. What appeared to be the most important outcome of this study was the fact that these babies as a whole (there were no differences between placebo or DEX groups) engaged in strikingly low levels of physical activity with only approximately 0.5 to 0.8 hours of vigorous activity per week. This is supported by previous studies by others that show low activity levels in young adults who were born prematurely.[1] Another study has demonstrated poor neuromuscular performance in babies born prematurely.[2] The etiology of the poor fitness levels in these children (< 80% of predicted) is unclear, and the authors suggest several hypotheses, but the sum of the studies strongly supports this finding. One possible reason that could potentially be remedied fairly simply is a perception by the parents that these children are more vulnerable and do not encourage participation in physical activities. The authors make a very important point in stating that the higher risk that these individuals have for cardiometabolic disease should provide a stimulus for parents to encourage rather than discourage physical activity in these children. Consideration should be given by neonatologists and pediatricians to discuss this with parents and encourage physical activity in these children.

J. Neu, MD

References

1. Vrijlandt EJ, Gerritsen J, Boezen HM, Grevink RG, Duiverman EJ. Lung function and exercise capacity in young adults born prematurely. *Am J Respir Crit Care Med.* 2006;173:890-896.
2. Falk B, Eliakim A, Dotan R, Liebermann DG, Regev R, Bar-Or O. Birth weight and physical ability in 5- to 8-yr-old healthy children born prematurely. *Med Sci Sports Exerc.* 1997;29:1124-1130.

14 Renal, Metabolism, and Endocrine Disorders

Acute Kidney Injury Reduces Survival in Very Low Birth Weight Infants
Koralkar R, Ambalavanan N, Levitan EB, et al (Univ of Alabama at Birmingham, AL; et al)
Pediatr Res 69:354-358, 2011

Acute kidney injury (AKI) independently predicts mortality in children and adults. Our understanding of the epidemiology of AKI in very LBW (VLBW) infants is limited to retrospective studies. After adjustment for demographics, comorbidities, and interventions, infants with AKI have decreased survival compared with those without AKI. The study was conducted in regional quaternary care NICU of the University of Alabama at Birmingham. VLBW infants were followed prospectively and were classified into a serum creatinine (SCr)-based classification for AKI. Forty-one of 229 (18%) VLBW infants developed AKI. Those with AKI were more likely to have umbilical artery catheters, assisted ventilation, blood pressure medications, and lower 1- and 5-min Apgar scores. Of the infants with AKI, 17 of 41 (42%) died compared with 9 of 188 (5%) of those without AKI ($p < 0.001$). AKI was associated with mortality with a crude hazard ratio (HR) of 9.3 (95% CI, 4.1−21.0). After adjusting for potential confounders, those with AKI had higher chance of death as the adjusted HR was 2.4 (95% CI 0.95−6.04). AKI is associated with mortality in VLBW infants. Efforts to prevent and ameliorate the impact of AKI may improve the outcomes in this vulnerable population (Tables 1, 3, and 4).

▶ Acute kidney injury (AKI) is a common clinical problem in neonatal intensive care units (NICUs) and is usually associated with a contributing condition, such as hypovolemia, hypotension, hypoxia often caused by sepsis, asphyxia, and heart failure. AKI can be anticipated in 56% of infants with perinatal asphyxia. Unfortunately, a lack of consensus definition of AKI makes the diagnosis difficult. It is important to differentiate between prerenal failure and intrinsic renal failure; the fractional sodium excretion is a valuable index in this regard. A fluid challenge with or without furosemide may help distinguish

265

TABLE 1.—Categorical Definition of Neonatal AKI

Stage	Serum Creatinine
AKI 1	↑ SCr ≥0.3 mg/dL (26.5 μmol/L) from previous value within 48 h ↑ SCr ≥150−200% from previous value
AKI 2	↑ SCr ≥200−300% from previous value
AKI 3	↑ SCr ≥300% from previous value or SCr ≥2.5 mg/dL (221.0 μmol/L) or need for dialysis

TABLE 3.—Incidence of AKI and Mortality by Birth Weight Category

Birth Weight	≤750 g (*n* = 64)	750−1000 g (*n* = 62)	1000−1250 g (*n* = 51)	1250−1500 g (*n* = 52)	*p*
No AKI	35 (18.6%)	54 (28.7%)	48 (25.5%)	51 (27.1%)	<0.001
AKI 1	6 (60%)	2 (20%)	2 (20%)	0	
AKI 2	8 (80%)	2 (20%)	0	0	
AKI 3	15 (71.4%)	4 (19%)	1 (4.8%)	1 (4.8%)	
Mortality	21 (80%)	3 (12%)	1 (4%)	1 (4%)	<0.001

TABLE 4.—Incidence of AKI and Mortality by GA Category

GA	≤26 wk (*n* = 69)	26−28 wk (*n* = 43)	28−30 wk (*n* = 63)	>30 wk (*n* = 54)	*p*
No AKI	39 (20.7%)	38 (20.2%)	59 (31.4%)	52 (27.7%)	<0.001
AKI 1	7 (70%)	1 (10%)	1 (10%)	1 (10%)	
AKI 2	9 (90%)	1 (10%)	0	0	
AKI 3	14 (56.7%)	3 (14.3%)	3 (14.3%)	1 (4.8%)	
Mortality	22 (84%)	1 (4%)	3 (12%)	0	<0.001

prerenal from intrinsic renal failure. Attention is now focused on biomarkers for AKI that might enable early recognition and prompt interventions to limit renal injury. Neutrophil gelatinase-associated lipocalin (NGAL) and specifically urinary NGAL (UNGAL) predict renal failure sooner than serum creatinine and the immunoassay can be done as quickly as creatinine.[1] There are, however, few data available in neonates.

Mortazavi et al[2] reported that the causes of AKF in neonates in Iran were intrinsic kidney failure in 52%, prerenal in 42%, and postrenal in 5%. Oliguria was observed in 72% of the patients. Perinatal asphyxia was present in 30% of the neonates, sepsis in 29%, respiratory distress syndrome in 25%, dehydration in 24%, and heart failure in 21%. Most patients (85%) had more than 1 associated contributing condition. The mortality rate was 20.5%. Most patients (76%) were discharged with normal kidney function and 3% with diminished kidney function. Initial admission to the NICU, female sex, septicemia, and the need for mechanical ventilation were associated with a higher mortality rate.

Askenazi et al[3] noted, "observational studies suggest high rates of AKI and poor outcomes in critically ill neonates. Neonates with AKI are at risk of developing chronic kidney disease and hypertension. Large prospective studies are needed to test definitions and to better understand risk factors, incidence, independent outcomes, and mechanisms that lead to poor short- and long-term outcomes. Early biomarkers of AKI need to be explored in critically ill neonates." Koralkar et al followed these recommendations with a prospective study (abstracted here) of very low birth weight (VLBW) infants (birth weight < 1500 g) to answer some of these questions. They document that 41 (18%) of 229 of these infants have AKI using a creatinine-based definition (Table 1); however, because they did not measure serum creatinine on every baby every day, this number may be an underestimate. Furthermore, they demonstrate that AKI is a serious condition and there is an independent association between AKI and mortality when looked at both by gestational age and birth weight (Tables 3 and 4). The investigators are to be congratulated on what they claim is the first prospective epidemiologic study on AKI in VLBW infants that attempts to control for potential confounders. Most infants who developed AKI were extremely premature and developed AKI within the first week of life. Sicker babies depressed at birth, requiring mechanical ventilation and blood pressure support in addition to umbilical artery catheterization, were most likely to manifest AKI. The next steps are to identify early and reliable markers of AKI, intervene appropriately, and improve outcomes. These infants all need long-term follow-up to monitor their renal function and watch for the onset of hypertension.

A. A. Fanaroff, MD, FRCPE, FRCP&CH

References

1. Mussap M, Degrandi R, Fravega M, Fanos V. Acute kidney injury in critically ill infants: the role of urine Neutrophil Gelatinase-Associated Lipocalin (NGAL). *J Matern Fetal Neonatal Med.* 2010;23:70-72.
2. Mortazavi F, Sakha SH, Nejati N. Acute kidney failure in neonatal period. *Iran J Kidney Dis.* 2009;3:136-140.
3. Askenazi DJ, Ambalavanan N, Goldstein SL. Acute kidney injury in critically ill newborns: what do we know? What do we need to learn? *Pediatr Nephrol.* 2009;24:265-274.

Increasing Supplemental Thyroid Hormone Use among Premature Infants Born at 23 to 32 weeks' Gestation
Linn M, Yoder BA, Clark RH (Univ of Utah, Salt Lake City; Pediatrix Med Group, Ft. Lauderdale, FL)
Am J Perinatol 27:731-736, 2010

We assessed the pattern of levo-thyroxine (l-thyroxine) therapy in very premature newborns over a 10-year period. We analyzed the electronic database of a large private neonatal practice group (Pediatrix, Ft. Lauderdale, FL) for 23- to 32-week gestation neonates ($n = 96,813$) managed during 1997 to 2006. L-thyroxine use was analyzed by birth year and by gestational age (GA). L-thyroxine use increased with decreasing GA (nadir 0.3% at 32 weeks, peak 8.4% at 24 weeks). L-thyroxine supplementation increased 2.6-fold over time among infants $\leq$26 weeks' GA (3.4% in 1997 to 1999 to 8.7% in 2004 to 2006), but did not change among infants born at $\geq$29 weeks' GA. The highest rate of l-thyroxine supplementation (12.8%) occurred among 24-week GA infants in 2006. Median age at start of l-thyroxine was 23 days (25 to 75%, 15 to 38 days). Only 2% of treated infants were started on day of life 1. Despite no clear evidence from randomized trials supporting thyroid supplementation, l-thyroxine treatment of very preterm infants has significantly increased over the past decade. As l-thyroxine treatment was not consistent with protocols from published randomized trials, new focused randomized controlled trials are needed.

▶ Another unproven therapy creeps into our practices. The syndrome of transient hypothyroidism of prematurity is real, distressingly common among extremely low birth weight (ELBW) infants, and associated with compromised neurodevelopmental outcomes. However, several randomized controlled trials of thyroxine (T4) replacement have failed to demonstrate any improvement in outcome. A post hoc subgroup analysis of long-term outcomes from 1 trial[1] is often cited as showing improved educational and motor outcomes in T4-supplemented infants < 28-weeks' gestation but worse outcomes in those born at 29-weeks' gestation, but those differences were not statistically significant. The ontogeny of fetal thyroid function and thyroid hormone action is complex and incompletely understood. Most maternal T4 crossing the placenta is deiodinated to inactive reverse triiodothyronine (rT3), yet a substantial proportion of the T4 in the fetal circulation is of maternal origin. Circulating fetal levels of triiodothyronine (T3) (the active form of thyroid hormone) are low throughout gestation but may be locally higher because of conversion of T4 in the developing brain. Fetal metabolism of T4 appears to shift from deiodination to rT3 (inactive) to T3 (active) during the second and early third trimester. It is difficult to predict what T4 levels might be optimal in the fetus or how the requirements for normal brain development might be altered by extreme prematurity. A deeper understanding of this physiology is needed to guide management of ELBW infants with low free-T4 levels. Until the results of the planned controlled trials are available, empirical treatment of these infants with thyroxine should be undertaken with great caution, if at all.

W. E. Benitz, MD

Reference

1. van Wassenaer AG, Westera J, Houtzager BA, Kok JH. Ten-year follow-up of children born at <30 weeks' gestational age supplemented with thyroxine in the neonatal period in a randomized, controlled trial. *Pediatrics.* 2005;116:e613-e618.

Neonatal blood glucose concentrations in caesarean and vaginally delivered term infants

Marom R, Dollberg S, Mimouni FB, et al (Lis Maternity Hosp, Tel Aviv, Israel; Tel Aviv Univ, Israel)
Acta Paediatr 99:1474-1477, 2010

Background.—Little is known about the glucose concentrations at and after birth of infants delivered by caesarean section (CS), when compared with infants born vaginally (VD).

Aim.—To compare venous cord blood glucose concentrations of term infants born after elective CS to infants born by VD. We studied the null hypothesis that mode of delivery does not affect neonatal blood glucose values.

Methods.—We compared cord blood glucose concentrations in healthy term infants born after VD (n = 16) or by elective CS (n = 21). Glucose concentrations were obtained immediately at birth from the umbilical cord. Kruskal–Wallis was used to compare glucose concentrations and demographic variables between the groups.

Results.—Gestational age was 39.6 ± 0.8 weeks in VD group vs. 38.7 ± 0.9 weeks in CS group, and birthweight was 3359 ± 494 vs. 3500 ± 528 g. Cord blood glucose concentration was higher in VD (81.3 ± 16.9 mg/dL) than CS infants (70.3 ± 9.7 mg/dL, p = 0.039). The change in blood glucose concentration over the first 2-h of life differed significantly between the two groups, being an increase in CS versus a decrease in VD infants (−3.5 ± 15.2 vs. −15.4 ± 24.6 mg/dL, p = 0.013).

Conclusions.—Glucose concentrations in VD infants are higher than in infants born by elective CS without labour.

▶ There remains a paucity of well-conducted studies on blood sugar values in babies soon after delivery, thus limiting the data available to determine the normal distribution and precluding the precise definition of hypoglycemia. This pilot study yields some provocative and in some respects contradictory data on blood sugars according to the type of delivery but does not assist in defining abnormal blood glucose. It is rather strange but true that the blood glucose at birth is higher in babies delivered vaginally, yet at 2 hours of age, the values are higher in the infants delivered operatively. We recognize that the sample size is small and that the study was terminated because of a change in policy at the institution that limited the ability of the investigators to collect blood samples at 2 hours. Furthermore, the absence of blood glucose measurements in the mother at the time of delivery hampers the interpretation of the data. Perhaps the higher glucose at birth in the vaginally delivered babies can be explained by the response to stress hormones with vaginal birth and the 6-hour lack of food intake in the mothers undergoing cesarean section. Interpreting the higher glucose on the C-section babies at 2 hours is more difficult. Normal-term infants have sufficient alternate energy stores and capacity for glucose production from glycogenolysis and gluconeogenesis to ensure normal glucose metabolism during the transition to extrauterine life and early neonatal period. The authors suggest that the stress of vaginal birth may have depleted some of these stores. This remains purely speculative. The main lesson from this well-intentioned but limited trial is that more prospective well-planned studies are required.

A. A. Fanaroff, MD, FRCPE, FRCP&CH

15 Respiratory Disorders

Airway obstruction and gas leak during mask ventilation of preterm infants in the delivery room
Schmölzer GM, Dawson JA, Kamlin COF, et al (The Royal Women's Hosp, Melbourne, Australia; et al)
Arch Dis Child Fetal Neonatal Ed 96:F254-F257, 2011

Introduction.—Preterm infants with inadequate breathing receive positive pressure ventilation (PPV) by mask with variable success. The authors examined recordings of PPV given to preterm infants in the delivery room for prevalence of mask leak and airway obstruction.

Methods and Patients.—The authors reviewed recordings of infants at <32 weeks' gestation born between February 2006 and March 2009. PPV was delivered with a T-piece or self-inflating bag and a round silicone face mask. Airway pressures and gas flow were recorded with a respiratory function monitor (RFM). Videos recorded from a web camera were used to review the resuscitation. The first 2 min of PPV were analysed for each infant. Obstruction was arbitrarily defined as a 75% reduction in delivered expired tidal volume (V_{Te}) and significant face-mask leak as >75%.

Results.—The authors analysed recordings of 56 preterm infants. Obstruction occurred in 14 (26%) recordings and leaks in 27 (51%). Both obstruction and mask leaks were seen in eight (14%) recordings, and neither was seen in 15 (27%). Obstruction occurred at a median (IQR) of 48 (24−60) s after the start of PPV. A median (range) of 22 (3−83) consecutive obstructed inflations were delivered. Face-mask leaks occurred from the first inflation in 19/27 (70%) and in the remaining eight at a median (IQR) of 30 (24−46) s after the start of PPV. A median (range) of 10 (3−117) consecutive inflations with a leak >75% were delivered.

Conclusion.—Airway obstruction and face-mask leak are common during the first 2 min of PPV. An RFM enables detection of important airway obstruction and mask leak.

▶ The recognition that the stage for bronchopulmonary dysplasia and other problems of prematurity is often set in the delivery room through errors in neonatal resuscitation, including, but not limited to, barotrauma and oxygen toxicity, has spawned important studies of delivery room management. Such work has led to improvements in technology and practice, including greater use of continuous positive airway pressure (CPAP) at birth, resuscitation with room air or blended oxygen, end-tidal carbon dioxide monitors to assess intubation success, and the use of T-piece resuscitators. In this highly informative study, Georg Schmölzer and colleagues, in work with Colin Morley and Peter Davis of Melbourne, Australia, document what many neonatologists have recognized in anecdotal experience: effective bag-mask ventilation of very preterm infants isn't so easy. Using a respiratory function monitor and video capture of the first 2 minutes of resuscitation of 106 infants born before 30 weeks of gestation, among the 56 receiving positive-pressure bag-mask ventilation, the investigators showed that airway obstruction (25%), mask leak (48%), or both (14%) were very common. In fact, only 27% of resuscitations were uncomplicated by mask leak or airway obstruction. Although recognition of face-mask leak generally was quicker, neither face-mask leak nor airway obstruction was uniformly promptly recognized; the median and ranges of leaked and obstructed breaths were 10 (3-117) and 22 (3-83), respectively. Lest the reader think these phenomena are limited to neonatal intensive care units "downunder," I recommend thinking again. These problems are likely to have predominant origins in the anatomy of the extremely preterm airway and are less likely to be associated with local practice or equipment. The so-called million dollar question is how best to address what is likely to be a widespread problem. Options include development or identification of technologies (eg, better-fitting masks) or techniques for more effectively ventilating very preterm infants, routinely using a respiratory function monitor in the delivery room to quickly identify bag-mask ventilation problems, relying on quicker use of CPAP, or more promptly intubating very preterm infants. My hope is that the solutions will be found in the first 3 options and neonatologists will continue to work toward providing more effective noninvasive support and reserving intubation and mechanical ventilation for the small group of infants in whom the need for such support is indisputable.

L. J. Van Marter, MD, MPH

Early CPAP versus Surfactant in Extremely Preterm Infants
SUPPORT Study Group of the Eunice Kennedy Shriver NICHD Neonatal Research Network (Univ of California at San Diego, CA; Univ of Alabama at Birmingham; Case Western Reserve Univ, Cleveland, OH; et al)
N Engl J Med 362:1970-1979, 2010

Background.—There are limited data to inform the choice between early treatment with continuous positive airway pressure (CPAP) and early surfactant treatment as the initial support for extremely-low-birth-weight infants.

Methods.—We performed a randomized, multicenter trial, with a 2-by-2 factorial design, involving infants who were born between 24 weeks 0 days and 27 weeks 6 days of gestation. Infants were randomly assigned to intubation and surfactant treatment (within 1 hour after birth) or to CPAP treatment initiated in the delivery room, with subsequent use of a protocol-driven limited ventilation strategy. Infants were also randomly assigned to one of two target ranges of oxygen saturation. The primary outcome was death or bronchopulmonary dysplasia as defined by the requirement for supplemental oxygen at 36 weeks (with an attempt at withdrawal of supplemental oxygen in neonates who were receiving less than 30% oxygen).

Results.—A total of 1316 infants were enrolled in the study. The rates of the primary outcome did not differ significantly between the CPAP group and the surfactant group (47.8% and 51.0%, respectively; relative risk with CPAP, 0.95; 95% confidence interval [CI], 0.85 to 1.05) after adjustment for gestational age, center, and familial clustering. The results were similar when bronchopulmonary dysplasia was defined according to the need for any supplemental oxygen at 36 weeks (rates of primary outcome, 48.7% and 54.1%, respectively; relative risk with CPAP, 0.91; 95% CI, 0.83 to 1.01). Infants who received CPAP treatment, as compared with infants who received surfactant treatment, less frequently required intubation or postnatal corticosteroids for bronchopulmonary dysplasia (P<0.001), required fewer days of mechanical ventilation (P=0.03), and were more likely to be alive and free from the need for mechanical ventilation by day 7 (P=0.01). The rates of other adverse neonatal outcomes did not differ significantly between the two groups.

Conclusions.—The results of this study support consideration of CPAP as an alternative to intubation and surfactant in preterm infants. (Clinical-Trials.gov number, NCT00233324.)

▶ The Surfactant Positive Airway Pressure and Pulse Oximetry Randomized Trial (SUPPORT) is a tour de force for which the National Institute of Child Health and Human Development (NICHD) Neonatal Research Network deserves great credit. In this randomized, multicenter trial, a strategy of treatment with continuous positive airway pressure (CPAP) and protocol-driven limited ventilation that is started in the delivery room and continued in the neonatal intensive care unit (NICU) was compared with a strategy of early intratracheal administration of surfactant (within 1 hour after birth) followed by a conventional ventilation strategy. In a 2-by-2 factorial design, infants were also randomly assigned to 1 of 2 target ranges of oxygen saturation (85% to 89% or 91% to 95%) until the infant was 36 weeks of age or no longer received ventilatory support or supplemental oxygen (this component will be discussed elsewhere). Enrollment had to take place prior to delivery and, as noted by Rich et al,[1] those mothers receiving antenatal consultation were more likely to give permission for the study and were also more likely to receive antenatal corticosteroids. Not all mothers who gave consent were eligible for the study, as they may have delivered beyond the gestational age window (24-27 [6/7] weeks). Rich et al concluded that in a trial that involved preterm infants and required prenatal consent, more than 5 women were identified as being likely to deliver in the SUPPORT gestational age window for each 1 who delivered an enrolled infant. Hats off to the coordinators who ensured the success of this complex trial. The main results are thought-provoking and may change behavior in many units where the standard practice is to administer surfactant as soon as possible to babies with a gestational age of fewer than 29 weeks. Finer[2] found no significant difference in the primary outcome of death or bronchopulmonary dysplasia between infants randomly assigned to

TABLE 3.—Selected Prespecified Outcomes*

Outcome	CPAP (N = 663)	Surfactant (N = 653)	Relative Risk with CPAP (95% CI)	Difference in Means (95% CI)	Adjusted P Value
BPD or death by 36 wk of postmenstrual age — no. (%)					
Physiological definition of BPD†	317 (47.8)	333 (51.0)	0.95 (0.85 to 1.05)		0.30
BPD defined by need for supplemental oxygen	323 (48.7)	353 (54.1)	0.91 (0.83 to 1.01)		0.07
BPD by 36 wk of postmenstrual age — no./total no. (%)					
Physiological definition of BPD†	223/569 (39.2)	219/539 (40.6)	0.99 (0.87 to 1.14)		0.92
BPD defined by need for supplemental oxygen	229/569 (40.2)	239/539 (44.3)	0.94 (0.82 to 1.06)		0.32
Death by 36 wk of postmenstrual age — no. (%)	94 (14.2)	114 (17.5)	0.81 (0.63 to 1.03)		0.09
Need for supplemental oxygen — no. of days ‡§					
Adjusted mean	62.2±1.6	65.3±1.6		−3.1 (−7.1 to 0.8)	0.12
Unadjusted median	52	56			
Interquartile range	20 to 86	27 to 91			
Need for mechanical ventilation — no. of days ‡§					
Adjusted mean	24.8±1.0	27.7±1.1		−3.0 (−5.6 to −0.3)	0.03
Unadjusted median	10	13			
Interquartile range	2 to 32	2 to 36			
Survival without need for high-frequency or conventional ventilation at 7 days — no./total no. (%)	362/655 (55.3)	318/652 (48.8)	1.14 (1.03 to 1.25)		0.01
Any air leak in first 14 days — no. (%)	45 (6.8)	48 (7.4)	0.89 (0.6 to 1.32)		0.56
Necrotizing enterocolitis requiring medical or surgical treatment — no./total no. (%)	83/654 (12.7)	63/636 (9.9)	1.25 (0.92 to 1.71)		0.15
Intraventricular hemorrhage grade 3 or 4 — no./total no. (%) ¶	92/642 (14.3)	72/628 (11.5)	1.26 (0.94 to 1.68)		0.12
Postnatal corticosteroid therapy for BPD — no./total no. (%)	47/649 (7.2)	83/631 (13.2)	0.57 (0.41 to 0.78)		<0.001
Severe retinopathy of prematurity among survivors — no./total no. (%)	67/511 (13.1)	65/473 (13.7)	0.94 (0.69 to 1.28)		0.71

Editor's Note: Please refer to original journal article for full references.

*Plus–minus values are means ±SD. BPD denotes bronchopulmonary dysplasia, CI confidence interval, and CPAP continuous positive airway pressure.

†The physiological definition of BPD includes, as a criterion, the receipt of more than 30% supplemental oxygen at 36 weeks, the need for positive-pressure support, or in the case of infants requiring less than 30% oxygen, the need for any supplemental oxygen at 36 weeks after an attempt at withdrawal of supplemental oxygen. [16,17]

‡Data are for 1098 infants who survived to discharge, transfer, or 120 days; the maximum follow-up was 120 days.

§This variable includes high-frequency ventilation and conventional ventilation.

¶There are four grades of intraventricular hemorrhage; higher grades indicate more severe bleeding.

early CPAP and those assigned to early surfactant treatment. In secondary analyses, the CPAP strategy, as compared with early surfactant treatment, resulted in a lower rate of intubation (both in the delivery room and in the NICU), a reduced rate of postnatal corticosteroid use, and a shorter duration of ventilation without an increased risk of any adverse neonatal outcome (Table 3). These data support consideration of CPAP as an alternative to routine intubation and surfactant administration in preterm infants. In secondary analyses stratified according to gestational age at birth, there was a significant reduction in the risk of death in the CPAP group, as compared with the early-intubation group, among infants born between 24 weeks 0 days and 25 weeks 6 days of gestation, but not among infants who were born at a later gestational age. The authors noted "Given the fact that there was no significant interaction between the intervention and gestational age, the post hoc nature of these analyses, and the number of secondary analyses performed, this observation must be interpreted with caution, and further testing should be performed in this immature population." My impression has been that there has been a subtle swing to a gentler approach to extremely preterm infants starting in the delivery room, and CPAP is attempted first, rather than immediate intubation and early surfactant administration. Time alone will inform us whether this approach reduces mortality and significant morbidity.

A. A. Fanaroff, MD, FRCPE, FRCP&CH

References

1. Rich WD, Auten KJ, Gantz MG, et al; National Institute of Child Health and Human Development Neonatal Research Network. Antenatal consent in the SUPPORT trial: challenges, costs, and representative enrollment. *Pediatrics.* 2010;126:e215-e221.
2. Finer NN. Nasal continuous positive airway pressure does not reduce rate of death or bronchopulmonary dysplasia in preterm infants. *J Pediatr.* 2008;153:145.

Expression of water and ion transporters in tracheal aspirates from neonates with respiratory distress

Li Y, Marcoux M-O, Gineste M, et al (Karolinska Institutet, Stockholm, Sweden; Children's Hosp, Toulouse, France)

Acta Paediatr 98:1729-1737, 2009

Aim.—The aim of the study was to determine whether neonatal respiratory distress is related to changes in water and ion transporter expression in lung epithelium.

Methods.—The study included 32 neonates on mechanical ventilation: 6 patients with normal lung X-rays (control group), eight with respiratory distress syndrome (RDS), eight with transient tachypnea of the newborn (TTN), 10 with abnormal lung X-rays (mixed group). The protein abundance of water channel AQP5, epithelial sodium channel (ENaC; α-, β- and γ-ENaC) and Na^+, K^+-ATPase $\alpha1$ were examined in tracheal aspirates using semiquantitative immunoblotting.

Results.—β-ENaC level was significantly lower in RDS group compared with infants with TTN and infants in the control group. AQP5 expression was significantly higher in TTN compared with the infants with RDS and all other infants with abnormal lung X-rays.

Conclusion.—Neonatal respiratory distress is associated with changes in β-ENaC and AQP5 expression. The lower β-ENaC expression may be one of the factors that predispose to the development of RDS. The higher AQP5 expression may provide the possibility for reabsorption of postnatal lung liquid, which contributes to quick recovery of infants with TTN.

▶ Li et al have accumulated some interesting data on the common respiratory disorders. They demonstrate that neonatal respiratory distress is associated with changes in β-epithelial sodium channel (β-ENaC) and aquaporin (AQP5) expression. The various roles of ENaC and aquaporin in respiratory distress and transient tachypnea of the newborn (TTN) serve as a reminder that it is not only surfactant, oxygen, and continuous positive airway pressure or mechanical ventilation that must be considered in the delivery room but also the shift in the function of the lung from secretion to absorption of fluid. It is fascinating to learn that AQP5 expression enhances reabsorption of postnatal lung liquid and aids in the rapid recovery of infants with TTN.

Transition for the fetus from a liquid environment with gas exchange through the placenta to air breathing must occur efficiently and effectively. Given all the physical and biochemical switching, it is a miracle that most babies accomplish this seemingly effortlessly. A key element in this transition is the clearance of lung fluid. This is accomplished by a combination of decreased secretion, increased absorption, and to a lesser extent excretion accompanying the big squeeze of the thorax during the birth process. The bulk of this fluid clearance is mediated by transepithelial sodium reabsorption through amiloride-sensitive sodium channels in the alveolar epithelial cells with only a limited contribution from mechanical factors and Starling forces. Disruption of this process can lead to retention of fluid in air spaces, setting the stage for alveolar hypoventilation. When infants are delivered near term, especially by cesarean section (repeat or primary) before the onset of spontaneous labor, the fetus is often deprived of these hormonal changes, making the neonatal transition more difficult.

At birth, the distal lung epithelium rapidly switches from secretion to absorption to adapt to air breathing. Understanding the dynamics and determinants of fluid secretion and absorption in the lung is crucial to understanding the pathophysiology of abnormal adaptation and instituting the appropriate therapy for neonates with respiratory distress. We must be aware of the various drivers of this change, such as aquaporins, the EnaC, antenatal corticosteroids, gestational age, labor including a vaginal birth, thyroid hormone, vasopressin, and stress hormones, to mention some of the key elements. Aquaporins are proteins embedded in the cell membrane that regulate the flow of water. They are the plumbing system for cells. The apical membrane of many tight epithelia contains ENaCs that are primarily characterized by their high affinity to the diuretic blocker amiloride.

Barker[1] noted that the mechanisms for lung liquid clearance during the neonatal period develop gradually during the latter part of the third trimester of pregnancy, but the phenotypic switch of the lung epithelium from net secretion to net absorption, triggered by events at birth, is sudden. Although lung liquid absorption at birth is a performance without rehearsal, the lung may be called on for an encore in later life when these same mechanisms are activated to clear accumulated edema liquid.

O'Brodovich[2] showed tremendous foresight and perception when he summarized his concepts of pulmonary fluid dynamics as follows some 16 years ago. He noted that "At birth, the mature lung switches from active Cl- (fluid) secretion to active Na+ (fluid) absorption in response to circulating catecholamines. Changes in oxygen tension augment the Na(+)-transporting capacity of the epithelium and increase gene expression for the epithelial Na+ channel (ENaC). The inability of the immature fetal lung to switch from fluid secretion to fluid absorption results, at least in large part, from an immaturity in the expression of ENaC, which can be upregulated by glucocorticosteroids. Both pharmacological blockade of the lung's epithelial Na+ channel and genetic knockout experiments using mice deficient in the ENaC pore-forming subunit have demonstrated the critical physiological importance of lung Na+ transport at birth. When Na+ transport is ineffective, newborn animals develop respiratory distress and hypoxemia, retain their fetal lung liquid and, in the case of the ENaC knockout mice, die. Bioelectrical studies of human infants' nasal epithelia demonstrate that both transient tachypnea of the newborn and respiratory distress syndrome have defective amiloride-sensitive Na+ transport. Neonatal respiratory distress syndrome has, in addition to a relative deficiency in surfactant, defective Na+ transport, which plays a mechanistic role in the development of the disease." Helve et al,[3,4] which includes O'Brodovich, confirmed that all 3 subunits of the human ENaC are low in preterm relative to full-term infants. Alpha-hENaC mRNA in respiratory epithelium is increased by therapeutic doses of glucocorticosteroid. They suggested that "Low expression of alpha-hENaC in human respiratory epithelium may play a role in the pathogenesis of respiratory distress in preterm infants." Bonanno and Wapner[5] postulated that in addition to increased surfactant production and secretion, corticosteroids facilitate clearance of fetal lung fluid. Thus, antenatal corticosteroids may prove valuable in the late preterm period and before elective cesarean delivery at term.

A. A. Fanaroff, MD, FRCPE, FRCP&CH

References

1. Barker PM, Olver R. Lung edema clearance: 20 years of progress invited review: clearance of lung liquid during the perinatal period. *J Appl Physiol*. 2002;93: 1542-1548.
2. O'Brodovich HM. Immature epithelial Na+ channel expression is one of the pathogenetic mechanisms leading to human neonatal respiratory distress syndrome. *Proc Assoc Am Physicians*. 1996;108:345-355.
3. Helve O, Pitkänen OM, Andersson S, O'Brodovich H, Kirjavainen T, Otulakowski G. Low expression of human epithelial sodium channel in airway epithelium of preterm infants with respiratory distress. *Pediatrics*. 2004;113:1267-1272.

4. Helve O, Pitkänen O, Janér C, Andersson S. Pulmonary fluid balance in the human newborn infant. *Neonatology.* 2009;95:347-352.
5. Bonanno C, Wapner RJ. Antenatal corticosteroid treatment: what's happened since Drs Liggins and Howie? *Am J Obstet Gynecol.* 2009;200:448-457.

Involvement of type II pneumocytes in the pathogenesis of chronic obstructive pulmonary disease

Zhao C-Z, Fang X-C, Wang D, et al (Zhejiang Univ, China)
Respir Med 104:1391-1395, 2010

Chronic obstructive pulmonary disease (COPD) is a leading cause of morbidity and mortality, but the cellular and molecular mechanisms are still not fully understood. Type II pneumocytes are identified as the synthesizing cells of the alveolar surfactant, which has important properties in maintaining alveolar and airway stability. Lung surfactant can reduce the surface tension and prevent alveolar collapse and the airway walls collapse. Pulmonary surfactant components play important roles in normal lung function and inflammation in the lung. Surfactant has furthermore been shown to modulate the process of innate host defense, including suppression of cytokine secretion and transcription factor activation, in the inflammatory network of COPD. Abnormalities of lung surfactant might be one of the mechanisms leading to increased airway resistance in COPD. The increased expression of Granzyme A and B was found in lung tissues of patients with COPD and type II pneumocytes was proposed to be involved in the pathogenesis of COPD. These novel findings provide new sights into the role of the type II pneumocytes in the pathogenesis of COPD.

▶ Chronic obstructive pulmonary disease (COPD) is one of the world's most urgent health care problems. COPD is currently the fourth leading cause of death in the Unites States and is the only one of the top 10 causes of death with increasing incidence and mortality.[1] Smoking and air pollution are key epidemiologic factors in the development of COPD. Histologically, COPD is characterized by mucous metaplasia, inflammation, and obstruction of the airways and emphysema.

Until recently, type II alveolar pneumocytes have been notable primarily for their role in respiratory distress syndrome, as they are the producers of pulmonary surfactant. However, the review article by Zhao et al highlights the type II alveolar epithelial cell as a potential target for intervention in COPD. The role of type II alveolar epithelial cells in the pathogenesis of COPD arises from their synthesis of surfactant, surfactant proteins, and other products, in particular the serine proteases granzyme A (GrA) and B (GrB).

First, biochemical and biophysical dysfunction of pulmonary surfactant has been reported in COPD, including decreased concentrations of total phospholipids and surface activity.[2] Surfactant is required not only to prevent alveolar collapse but also to maintain flow in narrow conducting airways.[3] Surfactant dysfunction could also increase the pressure gradient across the alveolar wall, resulting in rupture.

Second, smokers demonstrate significantly lower levels of 2 surfactant proteins, SP-A and SP-D.[4] These proteins form part of the innate immune system, and deficiencies increase the susceptibility to oxidative stress and infection.[5]

Finally, increased GrA expression has been found in the type II pneumocytes of patients with COPD compared with control subjects.[6] Numerous studies have shown these 2 enzymes, along with perforin, to be major effector molecules of CD8-positive T cells, which infiltrate the airways and lung parenchyma of patients with COPD.[7] GrA and GrB exert their proteolytic actions on extracellular matrix, thereby promoting tissue destruction and emphysema.

Aside from the production of surfactant, the potential role of the type II alveolar epithelial cell in the development of bronchopulmonary dysplasia has not been studied. Based on the recent COPD literature, further attention on this cell as a potential contributor to chronic lung disease pathogenesis in infants may be warranted.

M. B. Hershenson, MD

References

1. Jemal A, Ward E, Hao Y, Thun M. Trends in the leading causes of death in the United States, 1970-2002. *JAMA*. 2005;294:1255-1259.
2. Lusuardi M, Capelli A, Carli S, Tacconi MT, Salmona M, Donner CF. Role of surfactant in chronic obstructive pulmonary disease: therapeutic implications. *Respiration*. 1992;1:28-32.
3. Yager D, Butler JP, Bastacky J, Israel E, Smith G, Drazen JM. Amplification of airway constriction due to liquid filling of airway interstices. *J Appl Physiol*. 1989;66:2873-2884.
4. Honda Y, Takahashi H, Kuroki Y, Akino T, Abe S. Decreased contents of surfactant proteins A and D in BAL fluids of healthy smokers. *Chest*. 1996;109:1006-1009.
5. McCormack FX, Whitsett JA. The pulmonary collectins, SP-A and SP-D, orchestrate innate immunity in the lung. *J Clin Invest*. 2002;109:707-712.
6. Vernooy JH, Möller GM, van Suylen RJ, et al. Increased granzyme A expression in type II pneumocytes of patients with severe chronic obstructive pulmonary disease. *Am J Respir Crit Care Med*. 2007;175:464-472.
7. Freeman CM, Han MK, Martinez FJ, et al. Cytotoxic potential of lung CD8(+) T cells increases with chronic obstructive pulmonary disease severity and with in vitro stimulation by IL-18 or IL-15. *J Immunol*. 2010;184:6504-6513.

Minidex: very low dose dexamethasone (0.05 mg/kg/day) in chronic lung disease

Yates HL, Newell SJ (Leeds Teaching Hosps Trust, UK; St James' Univ Hosp, Leeds, UK)
Arch Dis Child Fetal Neonatal Ed 96:F190-F194, 2011

Objective.—Postnatal dexamethasone therapy is controversial. This study aimed to determine the short-term effects of Minidex (low-dose dexamethasone 0.05 mg/kg/day) on ventilator-dependent preterm babies.

Methods.—Very preterm babies (less than 30 weeks of gestation or under 1500 g) who were ventilator dependent at over 2 weeks of life and received Minidex therapy (low-dose dexamethasone 0.05 mg/kg/day for 10 days followed by alternate-day doses for 6 days) were compared retrospectively to a matched comparison group who received neither Minidex nor standard-dose dexamethasone.

Results.—50 babies who received Minidex were compared to a comparison group of 26 babies. Babies treated with Minidex extubated significantly faster than controls, Cox regression hazard ratio 6.24 (95% CI 2.34 to 16.63). By day 4, 34% of babies treated with Minidex had extubated but no controls had. Babies who received Minidex showed significant improvements in both ventilatory index and oxygen requirements, had no increased rate of clinical hypertension (OR 1.16 (95% CI 0.42 to 3.21)) or hyperglycaemia (OR 1.55 (95% CI 0.44 to 5.45)) and had a similar rate of chronic lung disease at 36 weeks' corrected age (OR 1.61 (95% CI 0.62 to 4.22)). No baby developed gastrointestinal perforation or haemorrhage.

Conclusion.—Minidex therapy facilitates extubation and is not associated with clinically significant short-term side effects. A randomised controlled trial is required to further assess efficacy and long-term outcomes.

▶ Although antenatal corticosteroids were introduced slowly into the neonatal-perinatal arena despite overwhelming evidence that they reduced mortality, respiratory distress, and intracranial hemorrhage, postnatal corticosteroids rapidly became the standard of care despite scanty data as to their benefits and no data concerning harm. Indeed, 2 major trials evaluating postnatal corticosteroids were stopped prematurely because of evidence of harm in the steroid arm of the trial.[1,2] In the National Institute of Child Health and Human Development Neonatal Research Network study,[1] the dexamethasone was administered within 24 hours after birth at a dosage of 0.15 mg/kg of body weight per day for 3 days, followed by a tapering of the dosage over a period of 7 days. The primary outcome was death or chronic lung disease at 36 weeks' postmenstrual age. The infants in the dexamethasone group were less likely than those in the placebo group to receive oxygen supplementation 28 days after birth ($P = .004$) or open-label dexamethasone, but they were more likely to have hypertension and to receive insulin treatment for hyperglycemia. During the first 14 days, spontaneous gastrointestinal perforation occurred in a larger proportion of infants in the dexamethasone group (13% vs 4% in the placebo group). Additionally, the dexamethasone-treated infants had a lower weight and a smaller head circumference at 36 weeks' postmenstrual age. They concluded: "in preterm infants, early administration of dexamethasone at a moderate dose has no effect on death or chronic lung disease and is associated with gastrointestinal perforation and decreased growth." In the Watterberg trial, mechanically ventilated infants with birth weights of 500 to 999 g were enrolled into this multicenter, randomized, masked trial between 12 and 48 hours of life. Patients received placebo or hydrocortisone: 1.0 mg/kg/d for 12 days, then 0.5 mg/kg/d for 3 days. Patient enrollment was stopped at 360 patients because of an increase in spontaneous gastrointestinal perforation in the hydrocortisone-treated group. Survival without bronchopulmonary dysplasia (BPD) was similar, as were mortality, head circumference, and weight at 36 weeks. However, for patients exposed to histological chorioamnionitis (n = 149), hydrocortisone treatment significantly decreased mortality and increased survival without BPD. These 2 trials were followed by a flurry of discussions and statements, but the overall response in the community was to decrease the utilization of postnatal corticosteroids.

In a revised policy statement from the Committee on Fetus and Newborn with Watterberg as the lead author, the group noted:

"The purpose of this revised statement is to review current information on the use of postnatal glucocorticoids to prevent or treat broncho-pulmonary dysplasia in the preterm infant and to make updated recommendations regarding their use. High-dose dexamethasone (0.5 mg/kg per day) does not seem to confer additional therapeutic benefit over lower doses and is not recommended. Evidence is insufficient to make a recommendation regarding other glucocorticoid doses and preparations. The clinician must use clinical judgment when attempting to balance the potential adverse effects of glucocorticoid treatment with those of broncho-pulmonary dysplasia."[3]

Fast-forward to the Minidex publication abstract from this article. Recognizing that standard-dosage dexamethasone, which is 0.5 mg/kg/d, facilitates extubation in ventilator-dependent preterm infants but has been associated with significant harmful short-term side effects, including hypertension, hyperglycemia, gastrointestinal hemorrhage/perforation, cardiomyopathy, poor growth, and increased risk of sepsis, in addition to neurodevelopmental problems, the authors completed what amounts to a pilot study, using one-tenth of the standard dexamethasone dosage for 10 days, followed by alternate-day therapy for 6 days in 50 patients. They found that pulmonary function improved and they did not have any undesirable side effects. Of course, they have no long-term follow-up data as of yet.

The stage is now set for the next set of randomized trials using this protocol. It is desirable that dexamethasone be compared with hydrocortisone and that long-term neurodevelopmental outcome be an important outcome variable. The problem is that huge numbers will need to be enrolled and followed long-term so the study will take a long time; however, it is the only manner in which closure can be accomplished on this complex and highly emotionally charged issue. Not only will the dose and nature of the steroid selected be important but also the timing of initiation of therapy. In their review, Doyle et al[4] commented: "The benefits of late dexamethasone may not outweigh actual or potential adverse effects. Given the evidence of both benefits and harms of treatment, and the limitations of the evidence at present, it appears prudent to reserve the use of late dexamethasone to infants who cannot be weaned from mechanical ventilation, and to minimize the dose and duration of any course of treatment." They were very negative about hydrocortisone,[5] noting: "Postnatal hydrocortisone in the doses and regimens used in the reported trials has few beneficial or harmful effects and cannot be recommended for prevention of

BPD. There are no randomized trials to substantiate the use of hydrocortisone in chronically ventilator-dependent infants with established or evolving BPD."[5]

From the available data, it would appear prudent to intervene somewhere between 7 and 14 days. I leave resolution of these issues to the various groups designing these studies.

A. A. Fanaroff, MD, FRCPE, FRCP&CH

References

1. Stark AR, Carlo WA, Tyson JE, et al; National Institute of Child Health and Human Development Neonatal Research Network. Adverse effects of early dexamethasone in extremely-low-birth-weight infants. National Institute of Child Health and Human Development Neonatal Research Network. *N Engl J Med.* 2001;344:95-101.
2. Watterberg KL, Gerdes JS, Cole C, et al. Prophylaxis of early adrenal insufficiency to prevent bronchopulmonary dysplasia: a multicenter trial. *Pediatrics.* 2004;114:1649-1657.
3. Watterberg KL, American Academy of Pediatrics. Committee on Fetus and Newborn. Policy statement—postnatal corticosteroids to prevent or treat bronchopulmonary dysplasia. *Pediatrics.* 2010;126:800-808.
4. Doyle LW, Ehrenkranz RA, Halliday HL. Dexamethasone treatment after the first week of life for bronchopulmonary dysplasia in preterm infants: a systematic review. *Neonatology.* 2010;98:289-296.
5. Doyle LW, Ehrenkranz RA, Halliday HL. Postnatal hydrocortisone for preventing or treating bronchopulmonary dysplasia in preterm infants: a systematic review. *Neonatology.* 2010;98:111-117.

Multicenter Crossover Study of Automated Control of Inspired Oxygen in Ventilated Preterm Infants

Claure N, Bancalari E, D'Ugard C, et al (Univ of Miami, FL; et al)
Pediatrics 127:e76-e83, 2011

Objective.—To determine the efficacy and safety of automated adjustment of the fraction of inspired oxygen (FIO_2) adjustment in maintaining arterial oxygen saturation (SpO_2) within an intended range for mechanically ventilated preterm infants with frequent episodes of decreased SpO_2.

Methods.—Thirty-two infants (gestational age [median and interquartile range]: 25 weeks [24–27 weeks]; age: 27 days [17–36 days]) were studied during 2 consecutive 24-hour periods, one with FIO_2 adjusted by clinical staff members (manual) and the other by an automated system (automated), in random sequence.

Results.—Time with SpO_2 within the intended range (87%–93%) increased significantly during the automated period, compared with the manual period (40% ± 14% vs 32% ± 13% [mean ± SD]). Times with SpO_2 of >93% or >98% were significantly reduced during the automated period (21% ± 20% vs 37% ± 12% and 0.7% vs 5.6% [interquartile ranges: 0.1%–7.2% and 2.7%–11.2%], respectively). Time with SpO_2 of <87% increased significantly during the automated period (32% ± 12% vs 23% ± 9%), with more-frequent episodes with SpO_2 between 80% and

86%, whereas times with SpO_2 of <80% or <75% did not differ between periods. Hourly median FIO_2 values throughout the automated period were lower and there were substantially fewer manual FIO_2 changes (10 ± 9 vs 112 ± 59 changes per 24 hours; $P < .001$), compared with the manual period.

Conclusions.—In infants with fluctuations in SpO_2, automated FIO_2 adjustment improved maintenance of the intended SpO_2 range led to reduced time with high SpO_2 and more-frequent episodes with SpO_2 between 80% and 86%.

▶ Despite many decades of oxygen supplementation for preterm infants, some very basic issues remain unresolved. A fundamental unresolved question relates to the optimal level of oxygenation at which preterm infants receiving supplemental oxygen or assisted ventilation should be maintained. This is of particular relevance for the pathogenesis of retinopathy of prematurity, which is attributed to both initial hyperoxia and subsequent episodic hypoxia.[1]

Excessive fluctuation in oxygenation is one of the most vexing problems in neonatal care. The group at the University of Miami has made considerable strides in addressing this challenge. In a small, multicenter, collaborative trial, they have documented the ability of automated control of inspired oxygen to more frequently maintain ventilated preterm infants in a tight 87% to 93% oxygen saturation range when compared with routine manual adjustment of inspired oxygen. Of interest, hyperoxic, but not hypoxic, periods were significantly reduced in the automated group.

In addition to our current uncertainty about whether episodic desaturation and the oxidant stress associated with reoxygenation are causes of significant pathophysiology, the optimal level of baseline oxygen saturation for preterm infants is unclear. The 2 phenomena are linked because we have recently shown that intermittent hypoxic episodes are significantly increased at lower (85%-89%) versus higher (90%-95%) baseline oxygen targets.[2] Two large, recently completed, multicenter trials present the neonatologist with a considerable dilemma. Preterm infants exposed to the lower of the 2 targets exhibited less retinopathy of prematurity but higher mortality.[3,4] Therefore, much work still needs to be done in both the clinical arena and in using in vivo and in vitro biologic models to unravel this issue.

Meanwhile, it is very reassuring that concurrent research initiatives are focused on optimizing delivery systems for supplemental oxygen in preterm infants. As with any new promising technology, both efficacy and safety are key, as these investigators are well aware. It is my belief that the elimination of large fluctuations in oxygenation is likely to be beneficial for this high-risk population. At a time when we are focused on avoiding excessive intubation of preterm infants, it remains to be seen whether this automated approach for supplemental oxygen administration may be adapted for CPAP or cannula-based ventilatory strategies. Potential conflict: please note that I served on the Data and Safety Monitoring Board of this trial.

R. J. Martin, MD

References

1. Chen ML, Guo L, Smith LE, Dammann CE, Dammann O. High or low oxygen saturation and severe retinopathy of prematurity: a meta-analysis. *Pediatrics.* 2010;125:e1483-e1492.
2. Di Fiore JM, Walsh M, Finer N, Carlo W, Martin RJ; SUPPORT Study Group of the NICHD Neonatal Network. Low oxygen saturation target range is associated with increased incidence of intermittent hypoxemia [abstract]. E-PAS 2011;3305.7.
3. Stenson B, Brocklehurst P, Tarnow-Mordi W. Increased 36-week survival with high oxygen saturation target in extremely preterm infants. *N Engl J Med.* 2011;364: 1680-1682.
4. SUPPORT Study Group of the Eunice Kennedy Shriver NICHD Neonatal Research Network, Carlo WA, Finer NN, Walsh MC, et al. Target ranges of oxygen saturation in extremely preterm infants. *N Engl J Med.* 2010;362:1959-1969.

Multicenter Crossover Study of Automated Control of Inspired Oxygen in Ventilated Preterm Infants

Claure N, Bancalari E, D'Ugard C, et al (Univ of Miami, FL; et al)
Pediatrics 127:e76-e83, 2011

Objective.—To determine the efficacy and safety of automated adjustment of the fraction of inspired oxygen (FIO_2) adjustment in maintaining arterial oxygen saturation (SpO_2) within an intended range for mechanically ventilated preterm infants with frequent episodes of decreased SpO_2.

Methods.—Thirty-two infants (gestational age [median and interquartile range]: 25 weeks [24—27 weeks]; age: 27 days [17—36 days]) were studied during 2 consecutive 24-hour periods, one with FIO_2 adjusted by clinical staff members (manual) and the other by an automated system (automated), in random sequence.

Results.—Time with SpO_2 within the intended range (87%—93%) increased significantly during the automated period, compared with the manual period (40% ± 14% vs 32% ± 13% [mean ± SD]). Times with SpO_2 of >93% or >98% were significantly reduced during the automated period (21% ± 20% vs 37% ± 12% and 0.7% vs 5.6% [interquartile ranges: 0.1%—7.2% and 2.7%—11.2%], respectively). Time with SpO_2 of <87% increased significantly during the automated period (32% ± 12% vs 23% ± 9%), with more-frequent episodes with SpO_2 between 80% and 86%, whereas times with SpO_2 of <80% or <75% did not differ between periods. Hourly median FIO_2 values throughout the automated period were lower and there were substantially fewer manual FIO_2 changes (10 ± 9 vs 112 ± 59 changes per 24 hours; $P < .001$), compared with the manual period.

Conclusions.—In infants with fluctuations in SpO_2, automated FIO_2 adjustment improved maintenance of the intended SpO_2 range led to reduced time with high SpO_2 and more-frequent episodes with SpO_2 between 80% and 86%.

▶ Automated systems for aircraft control, including processes as complex and sensitive as landing the aircraft, have been in use for decades. These systems reduce process variability and enhance operational safety. This report provides proof of concept for bringing similar strategies into the neonatal intensive care unit. It should not be surprising that an automatic, constantly vigilant, rule-driven system with the capacity to respond rapidly and frequently to fluctuations in pulse oximetry measurements would outperform human controllers, who cannot share those characteristics. Demonstration of a system that fulfills this expectation is nonetheless an important accomplishment. In this pilot study, a group of preterm infants were selected because of instability in pulse oximetry measurements, as reflected in having at least 4 episodes of Spo_2 < 80% in an 8-hour period during the 24 hours prior to study enrollment, while receiving positive pressure ventilation. Using a randomized crossover design, the automated system was found to be associated with more time with oxygen saturations in the target range (87%-93%) and less time below 75% or above 93%. The proportion of time with pulse oximetry above 98% while receiving supplemental oxygen was reduced from a median of 5.6% to 0.7%. Although the proportion of time at Spo_2 between 80% and 86% increased from a median of 15% to 20%, these data are consistent with substantially more stable oxygen saturations during automated management. Remarkably, auto-mated control also resulted in less oxygen exposure (median Fio_2 0.32 vs 0.37 in the manual control group). A weakness of the study is that it does not indicate whether, how, or to what extent the management protocol (auto-mated vs manual) was masked to the bedside providers, leaving open the possibility that these results simply reflect the faith of the providers in the automated system and the advantages of the consequent reluctance to intervene quickly. The authors also caution that these results should not be extrapolated to other populations, such as more stable very low birth weight infants, preterm infants, or those who do not require positive pressure ventilation. Whether greater stability of Spo_2 with reduced exposure to high Fio_2 through automated Fio_2 adjustment will result in better respiratory, ophthalmic, or neurologic outcomes remains to be demonstrated. This report does demonstrate that the time has come for systematic evaluation of such technologies in our units.

W. E. Benitz, MD

Neurodevelopmental outcome of infants with congenital diaphragmatic hernia prospectively enrolled in an interdisciplinary follow-up program
Danzer E, Gerdes M, Bernbaum J, et al (The Children's Hosp of Philadelphia, PA; The Univ of Pennsylvania School of Medicine, Philadelphia)
J Pediatr Surg 45:1759-1766, 2010

Purpose.—The purpose of the study was to evaluate the neurodevelopmental outcome in infants with congenital diaphragmatic hernia (CDH).
Methods.—Between June 2004 and September 2007, 41 CDH survivors were prospectively enrolled in an interdisciplinary follow-up program. Neurodevelopmental status was evaluated using the Bayley Scales of Infant Development II (prior 2006, n = 9), the Bayley Scales of Infant Development III (after 2006, n = 27), or the Wechsler Preschool and

Primary Scale of Intelligence III (children older than 4 years, n = 5). Scores were grouped as average, mildly delayed, and severely delayed by standard deviation intervals (115-85, 71-84, <70), and mixed if average and mildly delayed in either cognitive or language.

Results.—Median age at last assessment was 24 months (range, 6-62). Average, mixed, mildly delayed, and severely delayed scores for neurocognitive and language skills were found in 49%, 19%, 17%, and 15%, respectively. Psychomotor scores were normal, mildly delayed, and severely delayed in 46%, 23%, and 31%, respectively. Autism was present in 7%. Abnormal muscle tonicity was found in 51% (49% hypotonic, 2% hypertonic). Multivariate risk factors for borderline or delayed neurodevelopmental, neurocognitive, and/or psychomotor outcome were intrathoracic liver position ($P = .02$), presence of a right-sided CDH ($P = .02$), extracorporeal membrane oxygenation need ($P < .001$), Gore-Tex patch repair ($P = .02$), O_2 requirement at 30 days of life ($P < .01$), and hypotonicity ($P < .01$).

Conclusions.—The prospective evaluation in an interdisciplinary follow-up program uncovered striking morbidities in neurodevelopmental status in approximately half of the CDH infants. The most common neurologic sequelae are neuromuscular hypotonicity and psychomotor dysfunction. Patient-specific factors are important determinants of adverse neurologic outcome.

▶ Successful long-term management of congenital diaphragmatic hernia (CDH) has remained frustratingly elusive despite advances in prenatal diagnosis and intervention, and postnatal strategies, including delayed surgical repair, high-frequency ventilation, and extracorporeal membrane oxygenation (ECMO).

This article reports on a small series of 41 infants with CDH who survived the neonatal period and were seen at follow-up, which ranged from 6 to 62 months. Approximately half of the cohort demonstrated "striking morbidities in neurodevelopmental status," characterized primarily by disturbances in tone and psychomotor function.

Although the sample size was small, the investigators performed a multivariate logistic regression analysis and found that intrathoracic liver position, right-sided CDH, need for ECMO, Gore-Tex patch repair, need for supplemental oxygen, and hypotonicity were predictors of poor outcome.

After caring for CDH patients for more than 30 years, the results of this observation do not surprise me. However, I applaud the efforts of this group of investigators in publishing their findings. They have been at the forefront of CDH management and remind us that long-term outcomes are ultimately more important than status at discharge from the neonatal intensive care unit (NICU).

This article provides important information for counseling of parents, both prenatally and in the NICU. Unfortunately, the authors did not provide mortality rates for CDH during the period of study, so prognosis can only be stated in terms of survival. Still, less than half of surviving infants are normal at 2-year follow-up. I think we are now obligated to inform parents of such before offering invasive therapies.

The frustration continues.

S. M. Donn, MD

Oxygenation with T-Piece versus Self-Inflating Bag for Ventilation of Extremely Preterm Infants at Birth: A Randomized Controlled Trial
Dawson JA, Schmölzer GM, Kamlin COF, et al (The Royal Women's Hosp, Melbourne, Australia; et al)
J Pediatr 158:912-918, 2011

Objective.—To investigate whether infants <29 weeks gestation who receive positive pressure ventilation (PPV) immediately after birth with a T-piece have higher oxygen saturation (SpO_2) measurements at 5 minutes than infants ventilated with a self inflating bag (SIB).

Study Design.—Randomized, controlled trial of T-piece or SIB ventilation in which SpO_2 was recorded immediately after birth from the right hand/wrist with a Masimo Radical pulse oximeter, set at 2-second averaging and maximum sensitivity. All resuscitations started with air.

Results.—Forty-one infants received PPV with a T-piece and 39 infants received PPV with a SIB. At 5 minutes after birth, there was no significant difference between the median (interquartile range) SpO_2 in the T-piece and SIB groups (61% [13% to 72%] versus 55% [42% to 67%]; $P = .27$). More infants in the T-piece group received oxygen during delivery room resuscitation (41 [100%] versus 35 [90%], $P = .04$). There was no difference in the groups in the use of continuous positive airway pressure, endotracheal intubation, or administration of surfactant in the delivery room.

Conclusion.—There was no significant difference in SpO_2 at 5 minutes after birth in infants <29 weeks gestation given PPV with a T-piece or a SIB as used in this study.

▶ The recruitment of alveoli and improved functional residual capacity (FRC) by means of applied positive pressure ventilation (PPV) in the delivery room is a cautionary tale. In 1997, Björklund et al[1] observed that injury to the lung can occur following a brief period of hyperventilation in the first few minutes of life. The introduction of the T-piece resuscitator in the delivery room has removed some of the subjective feel of the infants' lungs when providing PPV with the self-inflating bag but has the advantage of delivering preset peak inflating pressure (PIP) and positive end-expiratory pressure levels. This study focused on the first 5 minutes of life and the achievement of oxygen saturation with both devices using air resuscitation unless indicated by failure to improve. While there was no statistical difference in oxygenation at 5 minutes or outcome at 28 weeks' gestation between the groups, there were differences in how the apparatus was applied, with more frequent breaths and more variable PIP in the self-inflating bag group. As the authors note, it is possible that the infants in the study might have been able to generate FRC through their own respiratory efforts and therefore improved their oxygenation regardless of the type of resuscitation device. Larger studies comparing resuscitation devices are needed.

H. M. Towers, MBBCh, FRCPI

Reference

1. Björklund LJ, Ingimarsson J, Curstedt T, et al. Manual ventilation with a few large breaths at birth compromises the therapeutic effect of subsequent surfactant replacement in immature lambs. *Pediatr Res.* 1997;42:348-355.

Perinatal management of congenital diaphragmatic hernia: when and how should babies be delivered? Results from the Canadian Pediatric Surgery Network

Safavi A, Canadian Pediatric Surgery Network (Univ of British Columbia, Vancouver, Canada)
J Pediatr Surg 45:2334-2339, 2010

Purpose.—A prenatal diagnosis of congenital diaphragmatic hernia (CDH) enables therapeutic decision making during the intrapartum period. This study seeks to identify the gestational age and delivery mode associated with optimal outcomes.

Patients and Methods.—A national data set was used to study CDH babies born between 2005 and 2009. The primary outcome was survival to discharge. Primary and secondary outcomes were analyzed by categorical gestational age (preterm, <37 weeks; early term, 37-38 weeks; late term, >39 weeks) by intended and actual route of delivery and by birth plan conformity, regardless of route.

Results.—Of 214 live born babies (gestational age, 37.6 ± 4.0 weeks; birth weight, 3064 ± 696 g), 143 (66.8%) had a prenatal diagnosis and 174 (81.3%) survived to discharge. Among 143 prenatally diagnosed pregnancies, 122 (85.3%) underwent abdominal delivery (AD) and 21 (14.6%) underwent cesarean delivery (CS). Conformity between intended and actual delivery occurred in 119 (83.2%). Neither categorical gestational age nor delivery route influenced outcome. Although babies delivered by planned CS had a lower mortality than those delivered by planned AD (2/21 and 36/122, respectively; $P = .04$), this difference was not significant by multivariate analysis. Conformity to any birth plan was associated with a trend toward improved survival.

Conclusion.—Our data do not support advocacy of any specific delivery plan or route nor optimal gestational age for prenatally diagnosed CDH.

▶ Over the recent decade, much attention has been paid to the postnatal management of infants born with congenital diaphragmatic hernia (CDH), with the identification of postnatal strategies, such as gentle ventilation, delayed repair, and the utilization of multidisciplinary treatment protocols that have been associated with improved survival rates. The scant literature surrounding intrapartum management of pregnancies with a fetus prenatally diagnosed with CDH has been conflicting in terms of the role of gestational age and route of delivery.

This study examines a recent population-based national cohort of infants with CDH born over a 4.5-year period. Not only was this study able to examine route of delivery and gestational age among both the prenatally and postnatally diagnosed infants but also it was able to examine outcomes by delivery plan and conformance to this plan for the prenatally diagnosed infants.

It is important to note that survival of the overall cohort was high (81.3%), such that even with a relatively large cohort, it is not surprising that differences in mortality did not approach statistical significance. The trend toward lower mortality in infants born by elective cesarean delivery did not reach statistical significance, but is congruent with a similar finding by the CDH study group, and may become an important factor in populations or institutions with lower overall survival.

With regard to gestational age, there was a trend toward improved survival in the early term group compared with the preterm and late term cohorts, particularly among those whose route of delivery conformed with the birth plan (87.1% in the early terms vs 66% in the preterms and 72% in the late terms, $P = .12$). Prior studies have come to conflicting conclusions, such that the role of timing of delivery among infants with CDH at term gestation remains unclear.

R. L. Chapman, MD

Pulmonary Hypertension and the Asphyxiated Newborn

Lapointe A, Barrington KJ (Université de Montréal, Québec, Canada)
J Pediatr 158:e19-e24, 2011

Persistent pulmonary hypertension of the newborn may occur with perinatal asphyxia, either because of direct effects of hypoxia/ischemia on pulmonary arterial function or indirectly because both are associated with meconium aspiration syndrome or perinatal sepsis/pneumonia. Therapies for persistent pulmonary hypertension of the newborn have the potential to affect cerebral function and cerebral perfusion in infants with hypoxic ischemic encephalopathy. Our literature review concludes that hyperventilation should be avoided, bicarbonate therapy is unproven, and hypoxia and hyperoxia should both be avoided. Nitric oxide improves pulmonary artery pressure and systemic perfusion. The effects of inotropic agents on cerebral perfusion or outcomes are uncertain.

▶ The history of the management of persistent pulmonary hypertension of the newborn (PPHN) represents an odyssey in neonatal intensive care. The late 1970s and early 1980s were characterized by the use of extreme hyperventilation and alkalosis and subsequently followed by the diametrically opposed approach of hypoventilation and hypercapnia, which polarized the neonatal community. Yet no randomized controlled trials were performed to resolve this issue, and management in the new millennium is best described as regression to the mean.

In this article, Lapointe and Barrington carefully weigh the evidence in their review of treatment for PPHN complicating asphyxia neonatorum. They present a thoughtful analysis of mechanical ventilation, alkali therapy, oxygen, and a host of vasoactive drugs, including systemic vasoconstrictors and pulmonary vasodilators.

The real importance of this review, however, is to remind us of how little we know about cerebral circulation and oxygen delivery and of the potential adverse effects of common therapies on neurodevelopmental outcomes. Primum non nocere.

S. M. Donn, MD

Randomized Controlled Trial of Lung Lavage with Dilute Surfactant for Meconium Aspiration Syndrome

Dargaville PA, on behalf of the lessMAS Trial Study Group (Royal Hobart Hosp and Univ of Tasmania, Australia; et al)
J Pediatr 158:383-389, 2011

Objective.—To evaluate whether lung lavage with surfactant changes the duration of mechanical respiratory support or other outcomes in meconium aspiration syndrome (MAS).

Study Design.—We conducted a randomized controlled trial that enrolled ventilated infants with MAS. Infants randomized to lavage received two 15-mL/kg aliquots of dilute bovine surfactant instilled into, and recovered from, the lung. Control subjects received standard care, which in both groups included high frequency ventilation, nitric oxide, and, where available, extracorporeal membrane oxygenation (ECMO).

Results.—Sixty-six infants were randomized, with one ineligible infant excluded from analysis. Median duration of respiratory support was similar in infants who underwent lavage and control subjects (5.5 versus 6.0 days, $P = .77$). Requirement for high frequency ventilation and nitric oxide did not differ between the groups. Fewer infants who underwent lavage died or required ECMO: 10% (3/30) compared with 31% (11/35) in the control group (odds ratio, 0.24; 95% confidence interval, 0.060-0.97). Lavage transiently reduced oxygen saturation without substantial heart rate or blood pressure alterations. Mean airway pressure was more rapidly weaned in the lavage group after randomization.

Conclusion.—Lung lavage with dilute surfactant does not alter duration of respiratory support, but may reduce mortality, especially in units not offering ECMO.

▶ Meconium, the fecal material that accumulates in the fetal colon throughout gestation, is a term derived from the Greek *mekoni*, meaning poppy juice or opium. Commencing with Aristotle's observation of the association between meconium staining of the amniotic fluid and a sleepy state or neonatal depression, obstetricians have been concerned about fetal well-being in the presence of meconium-stained amniotic fluid (MSAF). Meconium aspiration syndrome (MAS) is defined as respiratory distress in an infant born through meconium-stained amniotic fluid whose symptoms cannot be otherwise explained. When aspirated into fetal lungs, meconium particles mechanically obstruct the small airways. Meconium, or the chemical pneumonitis it causes, inhibits surfactant function, and inflammation of lung tissue contributes further to small airway obstruction. MAS is now rare in developed countries but still a significant cause of morbidity and mortality in developing countries.

Balchin et al[1] wished to estimate the rates of MSAF and adverse outcome in relation to gestational age and racial group, and to investigate the predictors of MSAF. They studied almost half a million infants born from 1988 to 2000 in London, England. The crude MSAF rates in preterm, term, and post-term births were 5%, 17%, and 27%, respectively; the rates in blacks, South Asians, and whites were 23%, 17%, and 16%, respectively. Independent predictors of MSAF included being black, vaginal breech, being South Asian, and being in an advancing week of gestation. Using white neonates born at 40 weeks as reference, the absolute risks of adverse outcome at 41 and 42 weeks were 2% and 5% in whites, 3% and 7% in South Asians, and 7% and 11% in blacks. Balchin et al[1] concluded that MSAF rates are different among races and across gestational age, and overall risk of adverse outcomes in MSAF is low.

Dargaville et al have documented that lung lavage with dilute surfactant does not reduce the duration of mechanical ventilation but may reduce mortality, especially in units where extracorporeal membrane oxygenation (ECMO) is not available. Ever since the first attempts at randomized controlled trials of lung lavage, the investigators have been hampered by slow to nonexistent rates of enrollment. In this multicenter trial, there are only 65 infants with 3 of 30 deaths or need for ECMO in the lavage group compared with 11 of 35 in the control group. The lack of blinding raises the possibility that choice of treatments after randomization, including inhaled nitric oxide and ECMO, was biased by knowledge of the allocation group. Also, the slow rate of recruitment meant that experience with lung lavage in each participating center was limited, which may have had an impact on the effectiveness of the therapy. Also, the long time to obtain consent resulted in an approximately 14-hour delay before therapy was initiated. This may account for the lack of efficacy regarding duration of mechanical ventilation. On the other hand, there is no evidence of harm. Lung lavage with dilute surfactant can therefore be available for selected patients with severe MAS and respiratory failure.

A. A. Fanaroff, MD, FRCPE, FRCP&CH

Reference

1. Balchin I, Whittaker JC, Lamont RF, Steer PJ. Maternal and fetal characteristics associated with meconium-stained amniotic fluid. *Obstet Gynecol.* 2011;117: 828-835.

Randomized Controlled Trial of Lung Lavage with Dilute Surfactant for Meconium Aspiration Syndrome

Dargaville PA, on behalf of the lessMAS Trial Study Group (Royal Hobart Hosp and Univ of Tasmania, Australia; et al)
J Pediatr 158:383-389, 2011

Objective.—To evaluate whether lung lavage with surfactant changes the duration of mechanical respiratory support or other outcomes in meconium aspiration syndrome (MAS).

Study Design.—We conducted a randomized controlled trial that enrolled ventilated infants with MAS. Infants randomized to lavage received two 15-mL/kg aliquots of dilute bovine surfactant instilled into, and recovered from, the lung. Control subjects received standard care, which in both groups included high frequency ventilation, nitric oxide, and, where available, extracorporeal membrane oxygenation (ECMO).

Results.—Sixty-six infants were randomized, with one ineligible infant excluded from analysis. Median duration of respiratory support was similar in infants who underwent lavage and control subjects (5.5 versus 6.0 days, $P = .77$). Requirement for high frequency ventilation and nitric oxide did not differ between the groups. Fewer infants who underwent lavage died or required ECMO: 10% (3/30) compared with 31% (11/35) in the control group (odds ratio, 0.24; 95% confidence interval, 0.060-0.97). Lavage transiently reduced oxygen saturation without substantial heart rate or blood pressure alterations. Mean airway pressure was more rapidly weaned in the lavage group after randomization.

Conclusion.—Lung lavage with dilute surfactant does not alter duration of respiratory support, but may reduce mortality, especially in units not offering ECMO.

▶ Despite significant efforts by our obstetrical colleagues to avoid prolonged pregnancies, meconium aspiration syndrome (MAS) still happens. Aspiration of meconium may result in surfactant inactivation or dysfunction as well as obstruction of airways and the development of chemical pneumonitis. Lavaging the lung with exogenous surfactant makes good sense. Surfactant has detergent-like properties that could help solubilize particulate meconium and restore the pool of functional surfactant. A smaller earlier trial by Wiswell et al demonstrated the proof of concept, but a larger trial was needed.[1]

This investigation of the lessMAS study group achieved similar results, with a reduction in the need for extracorporeal membrane oxygenation and improved survival, and there was also a faster reduction in mean airway pressure, which could potentially improve cardiac performance and reduce the incidence of air leaks in a larger sample. The lavage technique appeared to be reasonably well tolerated, especially considering that enrolled infants were quite ill, with an entry alveolar-arterial oxygen difference > 450 torr. I wonder if the results would have been even better if entry criteria were not as stringent.

S. M. Donn, MD

Reference

1. Wiswell TE, Knight GR, Finer NN, et al. A multicenter, randomized, controlled trial comparing Surfaxin (Lucinactant) lavage with standard care for treatment of meconium aspiration syndrome. *Pediatrics.* 2002;109:1081-1087.

Safety of Surfactant Administration before Transport of Premature Infants
Biniwale M, Kleinman M (Keck School of Medicine of the Univ of Southern California, Los Angeles, CA; Children's Hosp Boston, MA)
Air Med J 29:170-177, 2010

Objective.—To assess the safety of surfactant administration prior to transport of premature infants.

Design/Methods.—We performed a retrospective review of 24- to 34-weeks premature infants admitted to the Newborn Intensive Care Unit (NICU) between July 1, 1999 and September 30, 2004. Outcome measures were the presence of hyperventilation (PCO2 <40 mm Hg) and/or pneumothorax on admission to the NICU. Factors associated with the presence of hyperventilation and pneumothorax were identified.

Results.—955 infants born at 24 to 34 weeks' gestation were admitted to the NICU during the study period. 217 (22.7%) received surfactant prior to transport within 48 hours of birth. The incidence of hyperventilation was 18.9%. Hyperventilated infants had longer transport times, lower birth weights, and lower PCO2 on blood gases obtained prior to transport. Pneumothorax occurred in six subjects (2.9%). Neonates with pneumothorax had lower APGAR scores.

Conclusions.—We found the administration of surfactant prior to transport to be safe as evidenced by a low incidence of pneumothorax. Pneumothorax was more likely to occur in infants who needed significant resuscitation at birth. The incidence of hyperventilation appeared to be high and was inversely associated with birth weight.

▶ This retrospective review attempted to document the safety of administration of surfactant to preterm infants of 24 to 34 weeks' gestation prior to transport. The outcome measures chosen for safety were carbon dioxide tensions and presence or absence of pneumothorax. Additional analyses were performed based upon the demonstration of hyperventilation, which the authors defined as a $PaCO_2 < 40$ mm Hg on the first arterial, venous, or capillary blood gas obtained after admission to the neonatal intensive care unit.

Since this was a nonrandomized trial, there is little we can take from this study. There do not appear to be any major drawbacks to administering surfactant at referring hospitals. What the study does tell us is that we are not able to assess ventilation very well during neonatal transport. While most, if not all, infants are monitored by pulse oximetry during transport, $PaCO_2$ evaluation is a completely different matter. Point-of-care blood gas analyses are available, but their expense is high, and they add another level of equipment to the transport. End-tidal carbon dioxide monitoring is also not effective in this setting, as the authors indicated. Perhaps the newest generation of transcutaneous $PaCO_2$ monitoring will help to alleviate the situation.

Of note, the investigators did find a trend toward a longer duration of mechanical ventilation and length of stay in the hyperventilated infants, a conclusion similar to the observation of Kraybill et al in 1989.

This article also raises 2 other issues. The first is definitional. To me, hyperventilation is a term that suggests a deliberate attempt to lower carbon dioxide tension to a lower than physiologic level. Had this been a hyperventilation study, many of us would question whether a $PaCO_2$ of 39 mm Hg met that criteria. Second, we need to be more articulate in presenting statistics, which although statistically significant have little clinical relevance. The authors stated that "infants with hyperventilation received significantly lower peak inspiratory pressures (21.56 vs 22.93 cm H_2O, $P = .48$) at the beginning of the transport." Can our transport ventilators even detect differences that small?

S. M. Donn, MD

Type and Timing of Ventilation in the First Postnatal Week is Associated with Bronchopulmonary Dysplasia/Death

Dumpa V, Northrup V, Bhandari V (Yale Univ School of Medicine, New Haven, CT; Yale Ctr for Clinical Investigation, New Haven, CT)
Am J Perinatol 28:321-330, 2011

The type and timing of respiratory support in the first week affecting bronchopulmonary dysplasia (BPD)/death have not been evaluated. We compared outcomes of premature infants on nasal intermittent positive pressure ventilation (NIPPV) or nasal continuous positive airway pressure (NCPAP) to those on endotracheal tube (ETT). We retrospectively reviewed data (1/2004 to 6/2009) of infants ≤30 weeks' gestational age (GA) who received NIPPV in the first postnatal week. National Institutes of Health consensus definition was used for BPD. Infants were categorized into three groups based on their being on a particular respiratory support mode for majority of days in the first week. There was no difference in the mean GA and body weight in the three groups: ETT ($n = 65$; 26.7 weeks; 909 g), NIPPV ($n = 66$; 27.1 weeks; 948 g), and NCPAP ($n = 33$; 27.4 weeks; 976 g). Use of surfactant was significantly different. In multivariate analysis, compared with ETT, NIPPV ($p < 0.02$) and NCPAP ($p < 0.01$) groups were less likely to have BPD/death. Infants on ETT ($n = 97$) during 1 to 3 days were more likely to have BPD/death compared with those on NIPPV ($n = 38$): 67% versus 47% ($p = 0.035$). Infants on ETT ($n = 30$) during 4 to 7 days were more likely to have BPD/death compared with those extubated to NIPPV ($n = 36$): 87 versus 53%

($p = 0.003$). Extubation to NIPPV or NCPAP in the first postnatal week is associated with decreased probability of BPD/death.

▶ This report adds new data to the ongoing comparison of invasive and noninvasive strategies for assisted ventilation of the preterm infant. Based on a retrospective analysis, the authors conclude that "Extubation to [nasal intermittent positive pressure ventilation (NIPPV)] or [nasal continuous positive airway pressure (NCPAP)] in the first postnatal week decreases the probability of [bronchopulmonary dysplasia (BPD)]/death in premature infants." Because this is not a prospective, randomized trial, this conclusion must be met with some skepticism. It appears to be at odds with the report of no significant difference in BPD/death between infants extubated to NIPPV at 4 to 7 days and those who were on NIPPV at 1 to 3 days and remained so at 4 to 7 days in this cohort. In addition, infants treated with ventilation via an endotracheal tube were less likely to have mothers with pregnancy-induced hypertension, were more likely to have Apgar scores ≤3 or 5 at 1 and 5 minutes, were more likely to receive surfactant or more than 2 doses of surfactant, and had higher rates of intraventricular hemorrhage. Since these infants were clearly sicker than those in the NIPPV or NCPAP groups, it is not surprising that their outcomes were less favorable. Nonetheless, it remains possible that the initial choice of ventilation strategy had a causal role in the need for surfactant and rates of intraventricular hemorrhage. That hypothesis is not supported by the SUPPORT Study,[1] the largest randomized comparison of ventilation strategies in this population to date, which did not demonstrate a reduction in the combined outcome of death or BPD among infants initially treated with NCPAP.

W. E. Benitz, MD

Reference

1. Finer NN, Carlo WA, Walsh MC, et al. Early CPAP versus surfactant in extremely preterm infants. *N Engl J Med.* 2010;362:1970-1979.

Ventilation Practices in the Neonatal Intensive Care Unit: A Cross-Sectional Study

van Kaam AH, on behalf of the Neovent Study Group (Emma Children's Hosp, Amsterdam, the Netherlands; et al)
J Pediatr 157:767-771, 2010

Objective.—To assess current ventilation practices in newborn infants. *Study Design.*—We conducted a 2-point cross-sectional study in 173 European neonatal intensive care units, including 535 infants (mean gestational age 28 weeks and birth weight 1024 g). Patient characteristics, ventilator settings, and measurements were collected bedside from endotracheally ventilated infants.

Results.—A total of 457 (85%) patients were conventionally ventilated. Time cycled pressure–limited ventilation was used in 59% of these patients, most often combined with synchronized intermittent mandatory ventilation (51%). Newer conventional ventilation modes like volume targeted and pressure support ventilation were used in, respectively, 9% and 7% of the patients. The mean tidal volume, measured in 84% of the conventionally ventilated patients, was 5.7 ± 2.3 ml/kg. The mean positive end-expiratory pressure was 4.5 ± 1.1 cmH$_2$O and rarely exceeded 7 cmH$_2$O.

Conclusions.—Time cycled pressure–limited ventilation is the most commonly used mode in neonatal ventilation. Tidal volumes are usually targeted between 4 to 7 mL/kg and positive end-expiratory pressure between 4 to 6 cmH$_2$O. Newer ventilation modes are only used in a minority of patients.

▶ This article reported on the results of a survey conducted at 2 time points (April 2007 and May 2008) to ascertain the ventilation practices in 173 neonatal intensive care units in 21 European countries. The results can be characterized by "good news, bad news." The bad news: traditional (as in nearly 50 years old) time cycled pressure–limited (TCPL) ventilation was practiced in nearly 60% of units, with more than half using synchronized intermittent mandatory ventilation. Newer modes and modalities of ventilation, such as volume targeting and pressure support, were seldom used despite an increasing evidence base for both safety and efficacy. It is hard to determine where the reluctance originates. Change is difficult; it involves expanding one's knowledge base and experience. The new technology is also expensive, so there may be economic constraints (although the survey occurred before the most recent downturn in the economy). Perhaps the imposed limitation on duty hours of trainees has also had a role. Examination of the averaged ventilatory parameters is also troublesome. Not only are clinicians mired in TCPL but it also looks like the "Rate of 40, Pressures of 20/4, one size fits all" approach is still being practiced. So what's the good news? First, clinicians are finally paying attention to tidal volume delivery and seem to be getting this right. Second, there's lots of room for improvement and wonderful opportunities for further research.

Finally, there may be 1 other message emanating from this survey. We need to find a better way to infuse the technology into clinical practice. The proliferation of advanced forms of mechanical ventilation came at a rapid pace, not always adequately tested, and often times too intimidating for many to embrace. Yet we need to start approaching each baby as a unique patient, and we have the means available to individualize treatment strategies and objectively assess the baby's response. It's time we move the knee jerk to a higher cortical level.

S. M. Donn, MD

Ventilation Practices in the Neonatal Intensive Care Unit: A Cross-Sectional Study

van Kaam AH, on behalf of the Neovent Study Group (Emma Children's Hosp, Amsterdam, the Netherlands; et al)

J Pediatr 157:767-771, 2010

Objective.—To assess current ventilation practices in newborn infants. *Study Design.*—We conducted a 2-point cross-sectional study in 173 European neonatal intensive care units, including 535 infants (mean gestational age 28 weeks and birth weight 1024 g). Patient characteristics, ventilator settings, and measurements were collected bedside from endotracheally ventilated infants.

Results.—A total of 457 (85%) patients were conventionally ventilated. Time cycled pressure–limited ventilation was used in 59% of these patients, most often combined with synchronized intermittent mandatory ventilation (51%). Newer conventional ventilation modes like volume targeted and pressure support ventilation were used in, respectively, 9% and 7% of the patients. The mean tidal volume, measured in 84% of the conventionally ventilated patients, was 5.7 ± 2.3 ml/kg. The mean positive end-expiratory pressure was 4.5 ± 1.1 cmH$_2$O and rarely exceeded 7 cmH$_2$O.

Conclusions.—Time cycled pressure–limited ventilation is the most commonly used mode in neonatal ventilation. Tidal volumes are usually targeted between 4 to 7 mL/kg and positive end-expiratory pressure between 4 to 6 cmH$_2$O. Newer ventilation modes are only used in a minority of patients.

▶ Using a cross-sectional survey strategy, these authors characterized approaches to mechanical ventilation in 173 neonatal units across Europe. They describe an unexpected degree of consistency in the approach to assisted ventilation. Conventional ventilation is used much more commonly (85%) than high-frequency ventilation (15%). Use of synchronization is nearly universal (93%) among conventionally ventilated infants. Although automated volume-controlled or volume-targeted modes were not commonly used (11%), most patients (84%) had measurements of tidal volumes. Practitioners appear to have adopted low–tidal volume strategies; among infants with measured tidal volumes, 66% fell between 4 and 7 mL/kg, but larger tidal volumes were used in 18%. Similarly, there is an apparent consensus on use of positive end-expiratory pressure at 4 to 5 cm H$_2$O. Calling for future trials to better define optimal use of ventilation modes and strategies, the authors point out that the empirical evidence supporting this consistency is rather thin. Studies in human infants are needed to determine how to best use conventional ventilation modes and to compare those familiar approaches with newer methods, such as volume-targeted and pressure support ventilations.

W. E. Benitz, MD

Remifentanil for endotracheal intubation in neonates: a randomised controlled trial
Choong K, AlFaleh K, Doucette J, et al (McMaster Univ, Hamilton, Ontario, Canada; King Saud Univ, Riyadh, Saudi Arabia; McMaster Children's Hosp, Hamilton, Ontario, Canada; et al)
Arch Dis Child Fetal Neonatal Ed 95:F80-F84, 2010

Objective.—To evaluate the efficacy and safety of remifentanil as a premedication in neonates undergoing elective endotracheal intubation.

Design.—A double-blind randomised controlled trial.

Setting.—Tertiary care neonatal intensive care unit.

Patients.—Haemodynamically stable term and preterm neonates requiring elective endotracheal intubation.

Interventions.—Infants in the intervention arm received remifentanil (3 µg/kg) and normal saline placebo. The control group received fentanyl (2 µg/kg) and succinylcholine (2 mg/kg). Both groups also received atropine (20 µg/kg) as part of the premedication regime.

Main Outcome Measures.—The primary outcome was time to successful intubation. Secondary outcomes included time to return of spontaneous respirations, oxygen saturation, heart rate and blood pressure changes during the procedure, adverse events and a survey of intubation conditions.

Results.—A total of 15 infants were randomised to each group. Baseline characteristics were similar in both groups. The median time to successful intubation was not statistically different (247 s in the remifentanil group vs 156 s in the fentanyl group, p=0.88). The intubation conditions were rated more favourably with fentanyl by the intubators. Although not statistically significant, chest wall rigidity was observed more commonly with remifentanil.

Conclusions.—Although remifentanil is comparable to fentanyl and succinylcholine in attenuating adverse physiologic responses during neonatal intubation, muscle rigidity is a concern at doses of 3 µg/kg. Further trials are required to evaluate ideal dosing regimens and combinations of agents for use with remifentanil in neonates.

▶ Intubation is greatly facilitated by adequate muscle relaxation, usually obtained by using a neuromuscular blocker. Adequate sedation/anesthesia must also be provided to attenuate the stress response to intubation. Typically a rapid-onset neuromuscular blocker, such as succinylcholine, has been used in combination with an anesthetic reduction agent or, in neonates, a narcotic such as fentanyl or morphine. Neuromuscular blockers, especially succinylcholine, are associated with various side effects. Intubation can be accomplished with sedation/anesthesia alone if the depth of anesthesia is enough to provide relaxation and optimal intubation conditions.

Remifentanil is a potent, synthetic narcotic with rapid onset of action and equally rapid extinction of action due to cleavage of nonspecific plasma and tissue esterases. It is 200 times more potent than morphine and twice as potent as fentanyl. It also costs 4 times as much as fentanyl. Because of its rapid inactivation, larger doses can be given without concerns for clearance and recovery. This study investigated whether remifentanil alone, without muscle relaxant, would provide adequate intubation conditions compared with a typical regimen using fentanyl and succinylcholine. The remifentanil cocktail did indeed attenuate physiologic responses during intubation comparable with those of the control group who received succinylcholine with fentanyl, but there were problems. The dose of remifentanil given did not achieve adequate intubation conditions in 3 of the 15 infants, whereas 2 of the 5 developed stiff chest syndrome, which would have been obviated by the use of a neuromuscular blocker. Of course, stiff chest syndrome can also be seen with fentanyl in the absence of neuromuscular blockade. One could look at this another way: 11 of the 15 patients taking remifentanil were adequately sedated and did not require a muscle relaxant for trouble-free intubation. Having to administer a muscle relaxant if the first induction agent does not provide adequate relaxation for a procedure is an everyday occurrence in the pediatric operating room. Like the pediatric anesthesiologist, physicians who use these drugs need to understand how to assess the infant for adequate relaxation before proceeding with intubation and provide additional medication as necessary. Unless larger randomized trials prove otherwise, I plan to continue using fentanyl and a fast-acting nonpolarizing muscle relaxant.

Whether a vagolytic drug like atropine is necessary in most controlled intubations is not clear to me. We have atropine available during nonemergent intubation in the neonatal intensive care unit (NICU) at Rainbow Babies & Children's Hospital but seldom use it, as intubating a relaxed and well-sedated neonate rarely induces bradycardia. Has this issue been adequately studied? The answer is no! There is a recent clinical report published by the American Academy of Pediatrics on premedication for nonemergent endotracheal intubation in the neonate, which provides a thorough and very readable review of what few randomized trials have done in this area. The report by Praveen Kumar and the Fetus and Newborn Committee[1] outlines the efficacy of drugs in use currently but also details several glaring gaps in knowledge referable to our use of anesthetic drugs in the NICU. Hopefully, larger randomized trials will address these issues in the future. The bottom line is no induction protocol is going to work ideally in 100% of patients. Neonatologists therefore need to become very familiar with how these drugs work and for how long and know the side effects and the trade-offs for using multiple drugs as opposed to a single induction agent.

E. K. Stork, MD

Reference

1. Kumar P, Denson SE, Mancuso TJ, Committee on Fetus and Newborn, Section on Anesthesiology and Pain Medicine. Premedication for nonemergency endotracheal intubation in the neonate. *Pediatrics.* 2010;125:608-615.

16 The Fetus

A Randomized Trial of Prenatal versus Postnatal Repair of Myelomeningocele

Adzick NS, for the MOMS Investigators (Children's Hosp of Philadelphia and the Univ of Pennsylvania School of Medicine; et al)
N Engl J Med 364:993-1004, 2011

Background.—Prenatal repair of myelomeningocele, the most common form of spina bifida, may result in better neurologic function than repair deferred until after delivery. We compared outcomes of in utero repair with standard postnatal repair.

Methods.—We randomly assigned eligible women to undergo either prenatal surgery before 26 weeks of gestation or standard postnatal repair. One primary outcome was a composite of fetal or neonatal death or the need for placement of a cerebrospinal fluid shunt by the age of 12 months. Another primary outcome at 30 months was a composite of mental development and motor function.

Results.—The trial was stopped for efficacy of prenatal surgery after the recruitment of 183 of a planned 200 patients. This report is based on results in 158 patients whose children were evaluated at 12 months. The first primary outcome occurred in 68% of the infants in the prenatal-surgery group and in 98% of those in the postnatal-surgery group (relative risk, 0.70; 97.7% confidence interval [CI], 0.58 to 0.84; P < 0.001). Actual rates of shunt placement were 40% in the prenatal-surgery group and 82% in the postnatal-surgery group (relative risk, 0.48; 97.7% CI, 0.36 to 0.64; P < 0.001). Prenatal surgery also resulted in improvement in the composite score for mental development and motor function at 30 months (P = 0.007) and in improvement in several secondary outcomes, including hindbrain herniation by 12 months and ambulation by 30 months. However, prenatal surgery was associated with an increased risk of preterm delivery and uterine dehiscence at delivery.

Conclusions.—Prenatal surgery for myelomeningocele reduced the need for shunting and improved motor outcomes at 30 months but was associated with maternal and fetal risks. (Funded by the National Institutes of Health; ClinicalTrials.gov number, NCT00060606.)

▶ Despite folic acid fortification, the incidence of myelomeningocele has stabilized at 3.4 per 10 000 live births in the United States.[1] Live born infants with myelomeningocele have a death rate of approximately 10%. Long-term survivors have major disabilities, including paralysis and bowel and bladder dysfunction. Damage to the spinal cord and peripheral nerves is usually evident at birth and is irreversible despite early postnatal surgical repair. The severity of the neurologic disability in the lower limbs is correlated with the level of the injury to the spinal cord.

Human prenatal myelomeningocele repair by hysterotomy was first performed in 1997, and by 2003, more than 200 fetuses had undergone the procedure. Early data suggested a dramatic improvement in hindbrain herniation in comparison with historic controls but also showed an increased maternal risk, including preterm labor and uterine dehiscence and a substantially increased risk of fetal or neonatal death and preterm birth.[2,3] Despite encouraging results,[4] there was an urgent need for a randomized trial because fetuses with myelomeningocele were inundating those centers where prenatal surgery was available.

Many professional and lay people have eagerly awaited the results of this important study. After an unbearably long gestational period with apparently some recruitment issues, the results are finally available. The news is mixed. The good news that despite having more severe lesions and more preterm babies delivered before 30 weeks' gestation, the prenatal surgery groups had significantly better outcomes than those operated on following delivery. The authors suggest that the earlier timing of the repair permits more normal nervous system development later and the reduced hindbrain herniation improves the flow of cerebral spinal fluid and diminishes the need for shunting. This also translated into better ambulation and intellect. The benefits of the prenatal surgery must be weighed against the risks of uterine dehiscence, uterine scarring, intraoperative complications, and prematurity complications. It is encouraging to see better outcomes for the baby, and perhaps over time less invasive means of doing the corrective surgery in utero will be developed.

A. A. Fanaroff, MD, FRCPE, FRCP&CH

References

1. Boulet SL, Yang Q, Mai C, et al. Trends in the postfortification prevalence of spina bifida and anencephaly in the United States. *Birth Defects Res A Clin Mol Teratol.* 2008;82:527-532.
2. Tulipan N, Bruner JP, Hernanz-Schulman M, et al. Effect of intrauterine myelomeningocele repair on central nervous system structure and function. *Pediatr Neurosurg.* 1999;31:183-188.
3. Sutton LN, Adzick NS, Bilaniuk LT, Johnson MP, Crombleholme TM, Flake AW. Improvement in hindbrain herniation demonstrated by serial fetal magnetic resonance imaging following fetal surgery for myelomeningocele. *JAMA.* 1999;282:1826-1831.
4. Danzer E, Finkel RS, Rintoul NE, et al. Reversal of hindbrain herniation after maternal-fetal surgery for myelomeningocele subsequently reduces the incidence and severity of brainstem dysfunction and cranial nerve compression. *Neuropediatrics.* 2008;39:359-362.

A Randomized Trial of Prenatal versus Postnatal Repair of Myelomeningocele

Adzick NS, for the MOMS Investigators (Children's Hosp of Philadelphia and the Univ of Pennsylvania School of Medicine; et al)
N Engl J Med 364:993-1004, 2011

Background.—Prenatal repair of myelomeningocele, the most common form of spina bifida, may result in better neurologic function than repair deferred until after delivery. We compared outcomes of in utero repair with standard postnatal repair.

Methods.—We randomly assigned eligible women to undergo either prenatal surgery before 26 weeks of gestation or standard postnatal repair. One primary outcome was a composite of fetal or neonatal death or the need for placement of a cerebrospinal fluid shunt by the age of 12 months. Another primary outcome at 30 months was a composite of mental development and motor function.

Results.—The trial was stopped for efficacy of prenatal surgery after the recruitment of 183 of a planned 200 patients. This report is based on results in 158 patients whose children were evaluated at 12 months. The first primary outcome occurred in 68% of the infants in the prenatal-surgery group and in 98% of those in the postnatal-surgery group (relative risk, 0.70; 97.7% confidence interval [CI], 0.58 to 0.84; P < 0.001). Actual rates of shunt placement were 40% in the prenatal-surgery group and 82% in the postnatal-surgery group (relative risk, 0.48; 97.7% CI, 0.36 to 0.64; P < 0.001). Prenatal surgery also resulted in improvement in the composite score for mental development and motor function at 30 months (P = 0.007) and in improvement in several secondary outcomes, including hindbrain herniation by 12 months and ambulation by 30 months. However, prenatal surgery was associated with an increased risk of preterm delivery and uterine dehiscence at delivery.

Conclusions.—Prenatal surgery for myelomeningocele reduced the need for shunting and improved motor outcomes at 30 months but was associated with maternal and fetal risks. (Funded by the National Institutes of Health; ClinicalTrials.gov number, NCT00060606.)

▶ This landmark article is the first to report a substantial benefit for fetuses managed with prenatal surgery via hysterotomy. This trial was difficult to organize and conduct, and could not have been done without the support of other pediatric surgeons across the country, who agreed not to offer this procedure outside of trial until it could be completed. The investigators are to be commended for their diligence in bringing it to completion.

The trial enrolled 183 women from 1087 candidates. At 12 months of age, fetuses who underwent open prenatal surgical repair were less likely to die or require ventriculoperitoneal shunting (68% vs 98%), to require a shunt (40% vs 82%), or to have hindbrain herniation (64% vs 96%) or brainstem kinking (20% vs 48%). At 30 months, they were more likely to have motor functional levels better than the anatomical levels of their defects (43% vs 21%); to walk independently (42% vs 21%); and to have higher scores for psychomotor development, locomotion, object manipulation, and mobility. These results came at a price, however: higher rates of bradycardia during the repair (10% vs 0%) and of delivery before 34 (46% vs 5%) or 37 weeks of gestation (79% vs 15%), resulting in higher rates of apnea (36% vs 22%) and respiratory distress syndrome (21% vs 6%). Pregnancy complications were more frequent: chorioamniotic membrane separation (26% vs 0%), oligohydramnios (21% vs 4%), placental abruption (6% vs 0%), and spontaneous labor (38% vs 14%) or membrane rupture (46% vs 8%). Maternal effects included more pulmonary edema (6% vs 0%) and more frequent need for blood transfusion at delivery (9% vs 1%). At delivery, the hysterotomy site was very thin or dehiscent in 36% of the cases.

These results are not easily generalized. The subjects are a select subset of women carrying an affected fetus. The highly skilled teams that performed the procedures, following precise protocols, are not easily replicated. Their results should not be extrapolated to patients who do not meet stringent enrollment criteria or to future cases at less-experienced facilities. Long-term effects on bowel and bladder control, reproductive health, and cognitive development await further study. Implications for future pregnancies, which must be delivered by cesarean and may hold other hazards for both mother and fetus, also remain unaddressed. Progress in this field will require development of new ethical constructs for balancing fetal benefits and maternal harm and new strategies for noncoercive informed consent for these mothers, who most certainly are vulnerable subjects. There should be no rush to offer this intervention at other centers.

W. E. Benitz, MD

A Randomized Trial of Prenatal versus Postnatal Repair of Myelomeningocele
Adzick NS, for the MOMS Investigators (Children's Hosp of Philadelphia and the Univ of Pennsylvania School of Medicine; et al)
N Engl J Med 364:993-1004, 2011

Background.—Prenatal repair of myelomeningocele, the most common form of spina bifida, may result in better neurologic function than repair deferred until after delivery. We compared outcomes of in utero repair with standard postnatal repair.

Methods.—We randomly assigned eligible women to undergo either prenatal surgery before 26 weeks of gestation or standard postnatal repair. One primary outcome was a composite of fetal or neonatal death or the need for placement of a cerebrospinal fluid shunt by the age of 12 months. Another primary outcome at 30 months was a composite of mental development and motor function.

Results.—The trial was stopped for efficacy of prenatal surgery after the recruitment of 183 of a planned 200 patients. This report is based on results in 158 patients whose children were evaluated at 12 months. The first primary outcome occurred in 68% of the infants in the prenatal-surgery group and in 98% of those in the postnatalsurgery group (relative risk, 0.70; 97.7% confidence interval [CI], 0.58 to 0.84; P<0.001). Actual rates of shunt placement were 40% in the prenatal-surgery group and 82% in the postnatal-surgery group (relative risk, 0.48; 97.7% CI, 0.36 to 0.64; P<0.001). Prenatal surgery also resulted in improvement in the composite score for mental development and motor function at 30 months (P = 0.007) and in improvement in several secondary outcomes, including hindbrain herniation by 12 months and ambulation by 30 months. However, prenatal surgery was associated with an increased risk of preterm delivery and uterine dehiscence at delivery.

Conclusions.—Prenatal surgery for myelomeningocele reduced the need for shunting and improved motor outcomes at 30 months but was associated with maternal and fetal risks. (Funded by the National Institutes of Health; ClinicalTrials.gov number, NCT00060606.)

▶ Prenatal myelomeningocele repair by hysterotomy was first performed in 1997, and by 2003 more than 200 fetuses had undergone the procedure. Early reports from the centers offering the procedure suggested an improvement in hindbrain herniation in comparison with historical controls, but also showed serious maternal complications, including preterm labor and uterine dehiscence, and a substantially increased risk of fetal or neonatal death and preterm birth. As a consequence, the Management of Myelomeningocele Study (MOMS) was designed to assess the risks and benefits of prenatal surgery as compared with postnatal repair. The trial was conducted at 3 maternal-fetal surgery centers in the United States; all other fetal intervention centers in the United States agreed not to perform prenatal surgery for myelomeningocele while the trial was ongoing. The trial was stopped after the recruitment of 92% of projected enrollment, approximately 10 years after its initiation. More than 1087 women underwent preliminary screening and of the 299 referred to 1 of the 3 participating centers, 183 underwent randomization (15%). The article includes the short-term outcomes of 158 (86%) of the 183 subjects enrolled in the trial and the 30-month outcome for 134 (73%).

Prenatal surgery resulted in a significant reduction in the combined primary outcome of infant death or the need for placement of a cerebrospinal fluid shunt at 1 year of age, a finding entirely driven by a substantially lower frequency of shunt placement in the prenatal cohort. When objective criteria for shunt placement were applied, however, only 40% of the infants in the prenatal group who met criteria underwent shunt placement compared with 89% in the postnatal group, and 5% of the infants in the postnatal group had a shunt placed even though criteria were not met, suggesting that the decision to place a shunt was influenced by the infant's treatment allocation. There was also a significant reduction in the second co-primary outcome of a composite score based on the Bayley Scores of Infant Development Mental Developmental Index (MDI) and assessment of motor development at 30 months of age, but prenatal intervention had no significant effect on MDI alone. The rates of maternal complications were significantly higher in the fetal intervention group: spontaneous rupture of the membranes (46% vs 8%), oligohydramnios (21% vs 4%), chorioamniotic separation (26% vs 0%), and placental abruption (6% vs 0%), as was the rate of premature births (79% vs 15%). None of the infants in the late surgery group were born prior to 30 weeks of gestation compared with 13% in the early surgery group. The percentage of infants born at less than 34 weeks of gestational age was eightfold higher in the late group (43% vs 5%). As a consequence, the frequency of neonatal respiratory distress was significantly higher in the early surgery group (21% vs 6%).

Although the results of the MOMS were significant, they are modest, with only a 20% absolute improvement in ambulation. As other centers launch their own programs, fetal results may not be as good as those in the MOMS, and maternal complications most likely will increase as individuals hone their skills. Additionally, ascertaining the true risk/benefit of the procedure will need a longer period of follow-up of both the women who undergo the procedure and their infants to determine the impact on maternal reproductive health and the effect of prematurity on later outcome.

L. A. Papile, MD

Delivery outcome after maternal use of antidepressant drugs in pregnancy: an update using Swedish data
Reis M, Källén B (Natl Board of Forensic Medicine, Linköping, Sweden; Univ of Lund, Sweden)
Psychol Med 40:1723-1733, 2010

Background.—Concerns have been expressed about possible adverse effects of the use of antidepressant medication during pregnancy, including risk for neonatal pathology and the presence of congenital malformations.

Method.—Data from the Swedish Medical Birth Register (MBR) from 1 July 1995 up to 2007 were used to identify women who reported the use of antidepressants in early pregnancy or were prescribed antidepressants during pregnancy by antenatal care: a total of 14 821 women with 15 017 infants. Maternal characteristics, maternal delivery diagnoses, infant neonatal diagnoses and the presence of congenital malformations were compared with all other women who gave birth, using the Mantel—Haenszel technique and with adjustments for certain characteristics.

Results.—There was an association between antidepressant treatment and pre-existing diabetes and chronic hypertension but also with many pregnancy complications. Rates of induced delivery and caesarean section were increased. The preterm birth rate was increased but not that of intra-uterine growth retardation. Neonatal complications were common, notably after tricyclic antidepressant (TCA) use. An increased risk of persistent pulmonary hypertension of the newborn (PPHN) was verified. The congenital malformation rate was increased after TCAs. An association between use of paroxetine and congenital heart defects was verified and a similar effect on hypospadias was seen.

Conclusions.—Women using antidepressants during pregnancy and their newborns have increased pathology. It is not clear how much of this is due to drug use or underlying pathology. Use of TCAs was found to carry a higher risk than other antidepressants and paroxetine seems to be associated with a specific teratogenic property.

▶ This analysis of more than 15 000 infants born to Swedish women who reported treatment with antidepressant medication neatly demonstrates both the capabilities and limitations of studies on population-based health registries. Comparison of infants exposed to these medications with a reference group of more than 1 million unexposed infants provides strong evidence of an increase in adverse outcomes, including preeclampsia, premature rupture of membranes, and caesarean section. All 3 medication classes (tricyclic antidepressants, selective serotonin-reuptake inhibitors [SSRIs], and selective norepinephrine reuptake inhibitors) were associated with preterm birth, suggesting an association with the underlying condition rather than with drug exposure. In contrast, relatively severe malformations, cardiovascular defects, and ventricular septal defect/atrial septal defect were more common in infants exposed to tricyclic antidepressants but not to SSRI or serotonin-norepinephrine reuptake inhibitor agents. Paroxetine, but not other SSRIs, was associated with increased risks of cardiovascular defects and hypospadias. These more specific associations suggest a role for the drugs themselves. These are important observations. However, the reported association of persistent pulmonary hypertension of the newborn (PPHN) with SSRI exposure is a curious one. Analysis of that association was restricted to infants delivered after 34 completed weeks of gestation because of a previously reported marked increase in PPHN in less mature infants in this population.[1] This suggests that the diagnosis was not the sort of PPHN associated with precocious muscularization of pulmonary arterioles as described by Murphy and colleagues in the early 1980s,[2] which is more common in postterm and distinctly unusual in preterm infants. The magnitude of the risk for and exact nature of the association between SSRI exposure and postnatal respiratory problems therefore remains ill defined, and the intriguing implication of SSRI agents as potential causes of PPHN reported by Campbell et al[3] remains unconfirmed.

W. E. Benitz, MD

References

1. Källén B, Olausson PO. Maternal use of selective serotonin re-uptake inhibitors and persistent pulmonary hypertension of the newborn. *Pharmacoepidemiol Drug Saf.* 2008;17:801-806.
2. Murphy JD, Rabinovitch M, Goldstein JD, Reid LM. The structural basis of persistent pulmonary hypertension of the newborn infant. *J Pediatr.* 1981;98:962-967.
3. Chambers CD, Hernandez-Diaz A, Van Marter LJ, et al. Selective serotonin-reuptake inhibitors and risk of persistent pulmonary hypertension of the newborn. *N Engl J Med.* 2006;354:579-587.

Long-term developmental follow-up of infants who participated in a randomized clinical trial of amniocentesis vs laser photocoagulation for the treatment of twin-to-twin transfusion syndrome
Salomon LJ, Örtqvist L, Aegerter P, et al (Université Paris Descartes, France; Ambroise Paré Hosp, Boulogne, France)
Am J Obstet Gynecol 203:444.e1-444.e7, 2010

Objective.—We sought to assess long-term neurodevelopment of children who were treated prenatally as part of the Eurofoetus randomized controlled trial.

Study Design.—The study population was composed of 128 cases of twin-to-twin transfusion syndrome (TTTS) included and followed up in France. Survivors were evaluated by standardized neurological examination and by Ages and Stages Questionnaires (ASQ). Primary outcome was a composite of death and major neurological impairment.

Results.—A total of 120 children (47%) were alive at the age of 6 months and were followed up to the age of 6 years. At the time of diagnosis, only treatment and Quintero stage were predictors of a poor outcome (hazard ratio, 0.61; 95% confidence interval, 0.41−0.90; $P=.01$ and hazard ratio, 3.23; 95% confidence interval, 2.19−4.76; $P<.001$, respectively). Children treated by fetoscopic selective laser coagulation (FSLC) had higher ASQ scores at the end of follow-up ($P=.04$).

Conclusion.—FSLC was significantly associated with a reduction of the risk of death or long-term major neurological impairment at the time of diagnosis and treatment.

▶ In the Eurofoetus trial, a multinational randomized controlled trial comparing fetoscopic selective laser coagulation (FSLC) and amniodrainage (AD) as a first-line treatment for twin-to-twin transfusion syndrome (TTTS), FSLC treatment resulted in a significantly higher survival rate and fewer neurological sequelae in surviving infants at 6 months of age.[1] The article describes the outcome of a subset of the study cohort at 5 years of age.

Of the 142 women with monochorionic twins and TTTS enrolled in the original trial, the offspring of 128 (90%) are included. Overall mortality was high (51%) with most of the deaths occurring in utero (73%). Fetal deaths were comparable in the 2 groups; however, twice as many infants in the AD cohort died after birth, most within the neonatal period. No additional deaths occurred in either group after 6 months of age. The initial finding of fewer neurosensory problems in the FSLC cohort at 6 months of age was no longer evident at 5 years of age. Major impairment was noted in 12% and 13% of the FSLC and AD cohorts, respectively. From these results, it would appear that FSLC is a powerful intervention for reducing mortality after birth by 50%, but does not have any effect on neurosensory outcome. The latter is not surprising, given the hemodynamic perturbations that occur with TTTS, only some of which are mitigated by treatment.

L. A. Papile, MD

Reference

1. Senat MV, Deprest J, Boulvain M, Paupe A, Winer N, Ville Y. Endoscopic laser surgery versus serial amnioreduction for severe twin-to-twin transfusion syndrome. *N Engl J Med.* 2004;351:136-144.

Prenatal intraabdominal bowel dilation is associated with postnatal gastrointestinal complications in fetuses with gastroschisis
Huh NG, Hirose S, Goldstein RB (Univ of California at San Francisco School of Medicine)
Am J Obstet Gynecol 202:396.e1-396.e6, 2010

Objective.—The purpose of this study was to determine whether prenatal intraabdominal bowel dilation (IBD) is associated with increased postnatal complications in fetuses with gastroschisis.

Study Design.—A retrospective review was performed on all maternal-fetus pairs with prenatally diagnosed gastroschisis that was treated at the University of California San Francisco from 2002-2008. Postnatal outcomes were compared between fetuses with and without IBD.

Results.—Forty-three of 61 maternal-fetal pairs met the criteria for inclusion. Sixteen fetuses (37%) had evidence of IBD. Fetuses with IBD were significantly more likely to have postnatal bowel complications (38% vs 7%; *P* =.037). The presence of multiple loops of IBD (*n* = 6) as opposed to a single loop (*n* = 10) was associated highly with bowel complications and increased time to full enteral feeding and length of hospital stay (100% vs 0% [*P* =.001]; 44 vs 23 days [*P* =.034]; 69 vs 27 days [*P* =.001], respectively).

Conclusion.—IBD is associated with increased postnatal complications in infants with prenatally diagnosed gastroschisis; however, this association seems to be limited to those with multiple loops of dilated intraabdominal bowel.

▶ The decreased mortality of gastroschisis in the past 4 decades has been a triumph of neonatology, pediatric surgery, and obstetrics, with current survival greater than 90%. The use of prenatal ultrasound has enabled detection of this condition and allowed for the preparation of the parents and the medical caretakers once the baby is born. Prediction of severity of the disease has been a challenge. This article evaluates the predictive value of intra-abdominal bowel dilation (IBD) seen on fetal ultrasound to subsequent outcome. In this study of 61 maternal-fetal pairs with gastroschisis, 37% had evidence of IBD. Interestingly, these babies were delivered an average 2 weeks earlier than those who did not demonstrate IBD. The reasons for the earlier delivery were not clearly provided. Nevertheless, those babies with IBD, but not those with dilatation of the externalized bowel, were significantly more likely to have bowel-related complications than those fetuses without IBD (38% vs 7%). The presence of multiple loop dilatations also appeared to increase the risk of subsequent complications and the associated length of hospitalization, which was an average 42 days longer in those babies with multiple loops affected. Several of the babies with multiple loops of dilatation had obstructions, but only 1 developed necrotizing enterocolitis. This provides interesting and potentially helpful predictive information. Perhaps the immediate care after birth may not be different, but the more realistic expectations of more complications and longer hospitalization if the fetus exhibits dilatation, especially of multiple loops of intestine, may be helpful.

J. Neu, MD

Article Index

Chapter 1: Behavior and Pain

Chapter 2: Cardiovascular System

Chapter 3: Central Nervous System and Special Senses

Chapter 4: Epidemiology and Pregnancy Complications

Chapter 5: Ethics

Chapter 6: Gastrointestinal Health and Nutrition

Chapter 7: Genetics and Teratology

Chapter 8: Hematology and Bilirubin

Chapter 9: Infectious Disease and Immunology

Chapter 10: Labor and Delivery

Chapter 11: Miscellaneous

Chapter 12: Pharmacology

Chapter 13: Postnatal Growth and Development/Follow-up

Chapter 14: Renal, Metabolism, and Endocrine Disorders

Chapter 15: Respiratory Disorders

Chapter 16: The Fetus

Author Index

321

Printed and bound by CPI Group (UK) Ltd, Croydon, CR0 4YY

08/05/2025

01864677-0010